ECOLOGICAL PUBLIC HEALTH

What is public health? To some, it is about drains, water, food and housing, all requiring engineering and expert management. To others, it is the State using medicine or health education and tackling unhealthy lifestyles. This book argues that public health thinking needs an overhaul, a return to and modernisation around ecological principles. Ecological Public Health thinking, outlined here, fits the twenty-first century's challenges. It integrates what the authors call the four dimensions of existence: the material, biological, social and cultural aspects of life. Public health becomes the task of transforming the relationship between people, their circumstances and the biological world of nature and bodies. For Rayner and Lang, this is about facing a number of long-term transitions, some well recognised, others not. These transitions are Demographic, Epidemiological, Urban, Energy, Economic, Nutrition, Biological, Cultural and Democracy itself. The authors argue that identifying large-scale transitions such as these refocuses public health actions onto the conditions on which human and eco-systems health interact. Making their case, Rayner and Lang map past confusions in public health images, definitions and models. This is an optimistic book, arguing public health can be rescued from its current dilemmas and frustrations. This century's agenda is unavoidably complex, however, and requires stronger and more daring combinations of interdisciplinary work, movements and professions locally, nationally and globally. Outlining these in the concluding section, the book charts a positive and reinvigorated institutional purpose.

Both authors have long been active in the international public health movement as practitioners, advocates, researchers and thinkers. **Geof Rayner** is an independent social scientist working in public health, and is currently a Research Fellow at the Centre for Food Policy, City University London and Professor Associate at Brunel University. **Tim Lang** is a social scientist specialising in food, public health, the environment and social justice, and is Professor of Food Policy at City University London.

ECOLOGICAL PUBLIC HEALTH

Reshaping the conditions for good health

Geof Rayner and Tim Lang

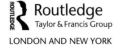

Routledge
Taylor & Francis Group

LONDON AND NEW YORK

First published 2012
by Routledge
2 Park Square, Milton Park, Abingdon, Oxon OX14 4RN

Simultaneously published in the USA and Canada
by Routledge
711 Third Avenue, New York, NY 10017

British Library Cataloguing in Publication Data
A catalogue record for this book is available from the British Library

Library of Congress Cataloging in Publication Data
Rayner, Geof.
  Ecological public health: reshaping the conditions for good health /
  Geof Rayner and Tim Lang.
    p. ; cm.
  Includes bibliographical references and index.
  I. Lang, Tim. II. Title.
  [DNLM: 1. Environmental Health.
  2. Ecological and Environmental Phenomena.
  3. Health Promotion. 4. Public Health. WA 30.5]
  362.1—dc23
  2011045337

ISBN 978–1–84407–831–8 (hbk)
ISBN 978–1–84407–832–5 (pbk)
ISBN 978–0–203–13480–1 (ebk)

Typeset in Bembo
by Swales & Willis Ltd, Exeter, Devon

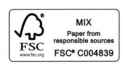

Printed and bound in Great Britain by the MPG Books Group

This book is dedicated to our families, friends and colleagues in the public health movement.

CONTENTS

FIGURES

TABLES

PREFACE: FROM THE HISTORY TO THE FUTURE OF PUBLIC HEALTH

Our motive for this book was dissatisfaction with some contemporary thinking and conventional approaches to public health. Centrally, the book grapples with the immensity of the changes facing public health in the twenty-first century. It attempts to clarify some distinctions in thinking about the world of public health which we felt warranted scrutiny and which were not being adequately integrated into a useful working perspective. This book champions what we and others call Ecological Public Health, a perspective which has deep roots and offers rich insights for the future but needed clarification.

The book starts by acknowledging the enormous impact of past public health measures on the well-being of humanity. Despite this success story, public health remains strangely marginal in public discourse, as well as patchy in execution, a state of affairs we want to address. The book is in three parts. Part I sets out the problem of defining and articulating what is meant by public health. Part II explores nine transitions which we suggest now define the terrain on which public health operates. These transitions are what modern public health has to address. Part III draws out the implications of those transitions for a reinvigorated public health framework appropriate for the twenty-first century.

The book outlines some conventional everyday notions of health – not just public health – because, in the public mind, 'public health' is a somewhat vague entity or rather old-fashioned concern. It is often seen as mainly applicable to developing countries today but not surely to the rich Western world. We profoundly disagree with this assessment, so our account of the various images of health (Chapter 1) leads directly into the difficulty of defining public health (Chapter 2) and a range of intellectual models about what public health is (Chapter 3). We there outline five main models of public health emerging over the last two centuries or more. All these models have features to recommend them, and pass the test of time. We argue that the conventional dichotomy of medical versus social models, or other such conventions, is not helpful. Such models narrow and fragment the complexity of the public health challenge. That said, we give particular attention to the Cinderella among public health models which sees public health through the ecological lens. We believe that Ecological Public Health thinking offers richer understandings than have previously been acknowledged. Indeed, we assert more strongly that the crises facing humanity in the twenty-first century are unlikely to be successfully addressed unless there is a strong Ecological Public Health perspective.

We then, in a series of chapters in Part II (Chapters 4–12), outline in some detail a series of fundamental dynamics, here called transitions. These alter what public health interventions can do and have effects on human health, both directly and indirectly. Some of these transitions are familiar to people in the public health world, such as the Demographic and Epidemiological Transitions. Others are less familiar, such as the Energy, Nutrition, Cultural and Democratic Transitions. We make the case for why these transitions collectively shape the population's health and how people live their lives.

In Part III we ask what difference it makes to look at public health in this way. We propose a number of implications which might help guide the actions of proponents of public health. Our case is that looking at health through the Ecological Public Health lens sharpens focus, explains connections otherwise buried, brings together people and professions too easily separated, and provokes an integrated understanding of the collective task.

This book is in some respects a panorama of public health. It goes back in history, looking at events, people and ideas, as well as looking at the present and hazarding thoughts about the future. It draws extensively on thinking and debates which some practitioners might find arcane. We are unapologetic. We argue that the huge challenges facing the population's health in coming decades cannot be properly understood without drawing on the work of people who are long gone. The process of public health requires to be constantly updated, of course, but perspective is improved if there is some clarity about whence problems arise and how they have been argued over. The book in this respect is our plea that contemporary public health thinking should better acknowledge its own rich history, much of which has not necessarily happened under the banner of public health.

Our case is that public health is an interdisciplinary project, and not merely the preserve of particular professionals or titles. Indeed, one of the themes of the book is that public health is often improved by movements and by people prepared to challenge conventional assumptions and the status quo. This view has never been popular, although ironically the benefits of public health action have often been claimed by subsequent establishments. In these cynical academic times, when thinking is too often set within narrow economistic terms – What can we afford? What is the cost–benefit of health action? – and when the notion of the 'public' is often replaced by the 'individual' or the 'private', this book offers an analysis of public health which is unashamedly *pro bono publico*, for the public good. We try to articulate what is meant by social progress, and what role health thinking and practice have in a civilised society.

Geof Rayner and Tim Lang
London, February 2012

ACKNOWLEDGEMENTS

Many people have helped us formulate the thinking reflected in these pages and have provided settings and support for our deliberations. This book, like all books, is not just the work of its nominal authors but also reflects countless hours discussing, reading, listening and analysing what is meant by public health with many other people around the world in the rich networks of public health. They are too numerous to list. We only hope that they recognise points of argument for which we are in their debt.

We have been hugely influenced by participation in various bodies, and we thank our friends and colleagues in them, particularly the UK Public Health Association, the Faculty of Public Health, the Chartered Institute of Environmental Health, the Department of Health Expert Advisory Group on Obesity, the Chief Scientist's Foresight process, Sustain, the UK's Sustainable Development Commission, the World Public Health Nutrition Association, and colleagues at the Centre for Food Policy at City University London. We owe debts, too, to the many research projects and editorial and advisory boards with which we have worked; we do not underestimate how many questions have been raised or avenues of thought suggested by our engagement in the practical world of public health.

We owe special thanks to those who have helped us in this task by encouraging us and debating ideas over meals, meetings and the internet. Some have read sections of the book, but responsibility for what is here is, of course, ours not theirs. They include: Fiona Adshead, Thomas Alam, Pascale Allotey, Miriam Armstrong, Terry Bilharz, Anita Borch, Malcolm Bruce, William Buckland, Geoffrey Cannon, Charlie Clutterbuck, Maggie Davies, Jay Glasser, Nigel Goldie, Jo Goossens, Sian Griffiths, Corinna Hawkes, Liselotte Hedegaard, Lois Jones, Fred Kavalier, Geoffrey Lawrence, Phil Mackie, David Pencheon, Daniel Reidpath, Harry Rutter, Fiona Sim, Andrew Simms, Esther Trenchard-Mabere and Philippe Vandenbroeck.

We discussed our ideas at a variety of fora including the Academy of Social Sciences of Australia and a symposium at Deakin University, a special session at the American Public Health Association convention in San Diego, financially supported by the journal *Public Health* and Elsevier publishers, the Annual Public Health Forum of the UK Public Health Association, the Faculty of Public Health annual conference, the Royal Society for Public Health, the Royal Society of Edinburgh, the Royal College of Defence Studies, the Food and Agriculture Organisation, the Institut Scientifique de Recherche Agronomique, the British Sociological Association Food Studies Group, the European Public Health and Agriculture Consortium, the European Society for Rural Sociology, National Heart Forum-UK, the Chinese University of Hong Kong, and, prior to publication, a conference on the book organised by Aalborg University, Denmark and the Danish Cancer Society. We thank everyone involved in arranging these events.

We would also thank the editors and reviewers of various journals which have published early thinking now incorporated into this book. They include: *British Medical Journal, Eurohealth, Globalization and Health, Health Promotion International, Journal of Epidemiology and Community Health, Journal of Hunger and Environmental Nutrition, Public Health, Public Health Nutrition, Obesity Reviews, Journal of European Social Policy, Social Policy & Administration*, and *The Lancet*.

Of the many colleagues who have inspired the authors, we make special mention of Peter Draper and David Player who for years have championed the Public Health Imagination.

The book would not have been written without Tim Hardwick's patience in waiting for us to complete, and Jonathan Sinclair-Wilson for encouraging us to do it in the first place. Jonathan Appleyard of City University was a tremendous help in devising our graphics. We thank all those in the production team at Earthscan, Routledge and Taylor & Francis, and the copy-editor Helen Moss. Finally, we give huge thanks to Gina Glover, not least for the cover photograph, and Liz Castledine for their endless patience and unstinting support.

While every effort has been made to trace and acknowledge ownership of copyright material used in this volume, the Publishers will be glad to make suitable arrangements with any copyright holders whom it has not been possible to contact.

Figure sources and credits

Figure 1.1a http://sphtc.org/timeline/19th8.jpg. Public domain.

Figure 1.1b US Department of Health and Human Services, CDC, *Principles of Epidemiology in Public Health Practice*, 3rd edn (Atlanta, GA: Centers for Disease Control and Prevention, 2006).

Figure 1.2 http://www.nobelprize.org/nobel_prizes/physics/laureates/1903/curie_lab_photo.jpg. Public domain.

Figure 1.3 http://en.wikipedia.org/wiki/File:SirEdwinChadwick.jpg. Public domain.

Figure 1.4 Original data source: J.-N. Biraben, *Les hommes et la peste en France et dans les pays européens et méditerranéens* (Paris: Mouton, 1975). Graphed data source: N. Voigtländer and H.-J. Voth, *The Three Horsemen of Growth: Plague, War and Urbanization in Early Modern Europe* (London: Centre for Economic Policy Research, 2009). Permission granted by the authors.

Figure 1.5 Engraving by Paul Fürst, http://tinyurl.com/6wcjqyz. Public domain.

Figure 1.6 Oxfordshire Health Archives. Permission granted.

Figure 1.7 Arena/MGM TV/The Kobal Collection. Permission granted.

Figure 1.8 Fox TV/The Kobal Collection. Permission granted.

Figure 1.9 G. Dahlgren and M. Whitehead, Tackling Inequalities in Health: What Can We Learn from What Has Been Tried? Working paper prepared for the King's Fund International Seminar on Tackling Inequalities in Health, September 1993, Ditchley Park, Oxfordshire. Accessible in G. Dahlgren and M. Whitehead, *European Strategies for Tackling Social Inequities in Health: Levelling up Part 2* (Copenhagen: WHO Regional Office for Europe, 2007). Permission granted.

Figure 1.10 Derived from U. Bronfenbrenner, *The Ecology of Human Development* (Cambridge, MA: Harvard University Press, 1979).

Figure 1.11 O. Solar and A. Irwin, *A Conceptual Framework for Action on the Social Determinants of Health*, Social Determinants of Health Discussion Paper 2 (Policy and Practice) (Geneva: World Health Organization, 2010), p. 6. Permission granted by World Health Organization.

Figure 1.12 A.H. Dolan, M. Taylor, B. Neis, R. Ommer, J. Eyles, D. Schneider *et al.*, Restructuring and Health in Canadian Coastal Communities (*EcoHealth* 2005, 2, 3: 195–208). Permission granted.

Figure 1.13 P. Martens and J. Rotmans, Transitions in a Globalising World (*Futures* 2005, 37: 1133–1144). Permission granted.

Figure 1.14 P. Martens, M. Huynen, S. Akin, H. Hilderink and C.L. Soskolne, Globalisation and Human Health: Complexity, Links and Research Gaps (*IHDP Update* 2011, 1 (January): 2–6). Permission granted.

Figure 1.15 Photo by Robin Meldrum/MSF. Permission granted.

Figure 1.16 International Baby Milk Action. Permission granted.

Figure 1.17a Columbia/The Kobal Collection. Permission granted.

Figure 1.17b Public domain.

Figure 2.1 US Library of Congress. Open source.

Figure 3.1 *Illustrated Evening News*. Open source.

Figure 3.2a http://upload.wikimedia.org/wikipedia/commons/e/e4/Ignaz_Semmelweis_1863_last_image.jpg. Open source.

Figure 3.2b Bildarchiv Preussischer Kulturbesitz (BPK), Berlin. Open source.

Figure 4.1 Keith Montgomery, University of Wisconsin – Marathon County, http://www.marathon.uwc.edu/geography/demotrans/demtran.htm. Permission granted by the author.

Figure 4.2 UN Population Division, *World Population Prospects: The 2010 Revision* (New York: UN Population Division, Department of Economic and Social Affairs, 2011). Open source.

Figure 5.1 E. Grundy, Commentary: The McKeown Debate: Time for Burial (*International Journal of Epidemiology* 2005, 34(3): 529–533). Permission granted by Oxford University Press.

Figure 6.1 M.P. Walsh, *Motor Vehicle Pollution Control*, Paper to China Fuel Economy Workshop, Hong Kong, 13 December 2004, http://tinyurl.com/6oq84zs (Arlington, VA: Carlines, 2004). Permission granted.

Figure 7.1 US Energy Information Administration, *International Energy Outlook 2010* (Washington, DC: US Energy Information Administration, 2010). Open source.

Figure 8.1 Herman E. Daly, Uneconomic Growth: Empty-World Versus Full-World Economics, in *Sustainable Development: The Challenge of Transition*, ed. Jurgen Schmandt and C.H. Ward (Cambridge: Cambridge University Press, 2000), ch. 3, pp. 63–78. Permission granted by Cambridge University Press.

Figure 8.2 Facundo Alvaredo, Anthony B. Atkinson, Thomas Piketty and Emmanuel Saez, *The World Top Incomes Database*, Paris School of Economics, http://g-mond.parisschoolofeconomics.eu/topincomes/, 19 January 2012. Permission granted.

Figure 8.3 OECD, *Divided We Stand: Why Inequality Keeps Rising* (Paris: OECD Publishing, 2011). Permission granted by the OECD.

Figure 9.1 B.M. Popkin, An Overview on the Nutrition Transition and Its Health Implications: The Bellagio Meeting (*Public Health Nutrition* 2002, 5, 1A: 93–103). Permission granted by the author.

Figure 9.2 USDA Economic Research Service, Major Trends in U.S. Food Supply, 1909–99 (*Food Review* 2000, 23, 1: 8–15). Permission granted by USDA and the authors.

Figure 9.3 USDA Economic Research Service, Food Expenditures by Families and Individuals as a Share of Disposable Personal Income 1929–2008, http://www.ers.usda.gov/briefing/CPIFoodAndExpenditures/Data/, in *Food CPI and Expenditures: Food Expenditure Tables* (Washington, DC: US Department of Agriculture Economic Research Service, 2008). Permission granted.

Figure 9.4 N. Alexandratos, The Mediterranean Diet in a World Context (*Public Health Nutrition* 2006, 9, 1A: 111–117). Permission granted by the author.

Figure 10.1 C. Darwin, *On the Origin of Species by Means of Natural Selection, or the Preservation of Favoured Races in the Struggle for Life* (London: John Murray, 1859). Public domain.

Figure 10.2 National Library of Medicine, http://cohaforum.org/2011/10/11/ scientific-progress-at-an-inhuman-cost/. Public domain.

Figure 10.3 American Academy of Microbiology, *Clinical Microbiology in the 21st Century: Keeping Up the Pace* (Washington, DC: American Academy of Microbiology, 2008), p. 13. Permission granted by the American Academy of Microbiology.

Figure 10.4 E. Haeckel, *Generelle Morphologie der Organismen* (Berlin: Georg Reimer, 1866). Open source.

Figure 10.5 N. Stern, *The Stern Review of the Economics of Climate Change: Final Report* (London: HM Treasury, 2006). Open source.

Figure 10.6 Millennium Ecosystem Assessment, *Ecosystems and Human Well-Being: Synthesis* (Washington, DC: Island Press, 2005). Permission granted.

Figure 11.1 R. Inglehart and W.E. Baker, Looking Forward Looking Back: Continuity and Change at the Turn of the Millennium (*American Sociological Review* 2000, 65, 1: 19–51). Permission granted.

Figure 13.1 Foresight, *Tackling Obesities: Future Choices* (London: Government Office of Science, 2007), fig. 8.1.

Table sources and credits

Table 2.1 http://www.cdc.gov/about/history/tengpha.htm

Table 5.1 A.R. Omran, Epidemiological Aspects of Health and Population Dynamics: Proceedings of a Faculty Seminar in India (*Bulletin of the Gandhigram Institute of Rural Health and Family Planning* 1969, 4, 1), quoted in G. Weisz and J. Olszynko-Gryn, The Theory of Epidemiologic Transition: The Origins of a Citation Classic (*Journal of the History of Medicine and Allied Sciences* 2010, 65, 3: 287–326).

Table 6.1 UN Habitat, *Global Report on Human Settlement 2011: Cities and Climate Change* (Nairobi: UN Habitat, 2011), table 1.1.

Table 6.2 C. Kennedy, J. Steinberger, B. Gasson, Y. Hansen, T. Hillman, M. Havránek *et al.*, Greenhouse Gas Emissions from Global Cities (*Environmental Science and Technology* 2009, 43, 19: 7297–7302).

Table 7.1 BP, *BP Statistical Review of World Energy, June 2010* (London: BP, 2010).

Table 7.2 R. Fouquet, *The Slow Search for Solutions: Lessons from Historical Energy Transitions by Sector and Service*, BC3 Working Paper Series 2010-05 (Bilbao: Basque Centre for Climate Change, 2010), plus present authors' additions.

Table 9.1 Alexandratos (2006, 2009), quoted in Foresight, *The Future of Food and Farming: Challenges and Choices for Global Sustainability*, Final report (London: Government Office for Science, 2011), table C1.1.

Table 10.1 B. Spellberg, R. Guidos, D. Gilbert, J. Bradley, H.W. Boucher, W.M. Scheld *et al.*, The Epidemic of Antibiotic-Resistant Infections: A Call to Action for the Medical Community from the Infectious Diseases Society of America (*Clinical Infectious Diseases* 2008, 46, 2: 155–164).

Table 12.1 T. Lang and M. Caraher, Influencing International Policy, in *Oxford Handbook of Public Health*, 3rd edn, ed. C. Guest, I. Kawachi, I. Lang and W. Ricciardi (Oxford: Oxford University Press, 2012).

ABBREVIATIONS

AMR	antimicrobial resistance
APHA	American Public Health Association
ASEAN	Association of Southeast Asian Nations
BINGO	business interest non-governmental organisation
BMI	body mass index
BMJ	*British Medical Journal*
BSE	bovine spongiform encephalopathy
bn	billion
CO_2	carbon dioxide
CDC	US Centers for Disease Control and Prevention
CFCs	chlorofluorocarbons
CSR	corporate social responsibility
EC	European Commission
EU	European Union
EBM	evidence-based medicine
FAO	Food and Agriculture Organization (of the UN)
GATT	General Agreement on Tariffs and Trade
GDP	gross domestic product
GRID	gay-related immune deficiency
HIV/AIDS	human immunodeficiency virus, the cause of acquired immune deficiency syndrome
HTLV-III	human T-cell lymphotropic virus type III
ILO	International Labour Organization (of the UN)
IPR	intellectual property rights
MNC	multinational corporation
NCD	non-communicable diseases
MMR	measles, mumps and rubella (vaccine)
NAFTA	North American Free Trade Agreement

NHS	National Health Service (UK)
NGO	non-governmental organisation
NO$_x$	mono-nitrogen oxide
OECD	Organisation for Economic Co-operation and Development
ppm	parts per million
PPP	public–private partnership
PR	public relations
q-Btu	quadrillion British thermal units (a measure of energy)
RCT	randomised controlled trial
SO$_2$	sulphur dioxide
TB	tuberculosis
UK	United Kingdom (of Great Britain and Northern Ireland)
UN	United Nations
UNCED	UN Conference on Environment and Development
UNCTAD	UN Conference on Trade and Development
UNDP	UN Development Programme
UNESCO	United Nations Educational, Scientific and Cultural Organization
Unicef	UN Children's Fund
USA	United States of America
USSR	Union of Soviet Socialist Republics
WHO	World Health Organization (of the UN)
WTO	World Trade Organization

PART I

Images and models of public health

1

INTRODUCING THE NOTION OF ECOLOGICAL PUBLIC HEALTH

This chapter introduces conventional understandings of public health. It explores some images of what is meant. It concludes by laying out some characteristics of what a twenty-first-century public health entails. Public health is literally the health of the public, but to protect and promote it requires recognition of the complexity of the task. It is rare for there to be any simple 'silver bullets' for public health. Improving public health today requires: recognition of the scale of change dynamics and societal transitions; political involvement and leadership; interdisciplinary collaboration; commitment to democracy and progress; and an ecological framework of thinking.

Making the invisible visible

This book is about what is meant by public health. It explores various traditions and ways of thinking about health. It argues that public health is sometimes completely marginal to mainstream thinking and lives, yet they depend entirely upon the population having a modicum of good health. The key notion of public health is that good health flows from the population level to the individual rather than the other way round. No one, however rich, however well-endowed with 'good genes', living in any circumstances, can outweigh the impact of the collective experience or poor conditions threatening their individual health. Public health literally means 'the health of the public'. Calling it a field, a profession, a task, a set of interventions or a set of laws or technologies comes after that founding perspective that health is a public and not just personal phenomenon. Public health is ultimately about all of humanity – how we live together, our shared circumstances and infrastructure (air, water, soil, food, housing, work, etc.), the causes of our illnesses, the quality of our lives and the causes and quality of our deaths. For us, public health is a synecdoche, an indicator of progress both for and of human society.

We set out a critical assessment of public health, arguing that the notion of health-as-public or public health suffers from cultural invisibility. It lacks a good story for modern politics, and therefore suffers too much from a deficit of high-level championship. While it has successes, which are discussed in this book, these are seen as episodic, the resolution of crises, or occasional moments of action. Public health is associated with the drama of threat. Few politicians will ignore a crisis, not least since they do not want their names associated with failure to respond. Equally, they are content to marginalise public health when concentrating on conventional political aspirations such as job creation, growing the economy, or getting re-elected. Then, public health is too often painted as a drag on lively economies, what 'we can or cannot afford'.

A different interpretation of public health and its invisibility points to a paradox. Successful societies are those which embrace public health principles but often, in the act of applying these principles and investing in their implementation, lose sight of the rationale for why the actions have been pursued. Success in preventing ill health quickly breeds collective amnesia. Sight is lost of causation and what went into its resolution. Political memories fade. The result may leave changed daily behaviour but lacks rationale. The rules of driving cars on the road, for example, came about because the number of people killed on roads by motor traffic was considerable. Traffic lights, rules of how to drive, and collective awareness of other drivers transformed the 'freedom' of the individual early driver. Civility, law and good sense worked together to discipline what otherwise was initially a free-for-all, symbolised by Mr Toad's driving behaviour in Kenneth Grahame's Edwardian novel *Wind in the Willows* – a mad individualist who hogs the road, threatening others and endangering himself.[1]

Mr Toad, apart from his clammy green skin, eccentric language and dress sense, represents the twenty-first-century not just early-twentieth-century individualist, everything reduced to his needs, no one else's. His counterparts today might be the presenters of television series celebrating the interests of the motorist, such as the BBC's successful *Top Gear* programme, whose motoring stunts and light humour draw 350 million viewers worldwide. In contrast, public health seems killjoy, imposing rules, stopping individual motorists putting their foot down in pursuit of motoring freedom.

Public health thus easily represents a rather sober case for investing in and accepting the need for measures which are designed to improve the lot of the public. If so, who does it? Whose interests triumph? Hence the accusations that public health is the killjoy. Yet public health provides the rationale for creating healthy, sustainable transport systems and, for that matter, also decent water supplies, or setting minimum wages or cleaning up food adulteration or preventing children dying prematurely from preventable diseases. This positive image of public health is easily swamped by the individualist perspective which too often tacitly encourages young people to see road rules as against their interests. In fact, the more people survive road carnage, the better road safety has become. In 1926 Britain, there were 2.9 fatalities per 1,000 vehicles on the roads. By the end of the century, the ratio had fallen to 0.1.[2]

Behind this public health success story lies huge investment in road safety, car design, driver regulation, skills and policing, all of which generated a culture of civility, based on thinking and negotiating with one another. Rules on alcohol use and seat belts, for example, were successfully injected into motor car use, transforming social norms of accepted behaviour. On the other hand, the less pleasant news is that, over this period, cycle use has plunged and parents have become increasingly wary of their children using bicycles. Children are car-driven to school, to parks and to parties, insulating them from knowledge of where they live and from necessary but stunningly ordinary means of gaining physical exercise such as walking and cycling. Improving safety in one mode of transport has thus compromised another. From a public health perspective, critics of motorised transport also rightly point to its contribution to obesity, disconnected social life, changes in the physical environment, and wasteful use of finite energy resources.[3] It needs to be said that the positive trends in Britain and other developed economies may not be the case elsewhere. Approximately 1.3 million people die each year on the world's roads, and 20–50 million sustain non-fatal injuries. Roughly half of the victims are pedestrians.[4]

Part of the invisibility of public health, such examples suggest, is that societies come to rely on the investments championed in the name of public health. Those improvements are then taken for granted and even attacked as unnecessary or 'nannying'. Part of the challenge for twenty-first-century public health is to articulate the principles by which this century's health can be improved. In this book, we explore the principles and institutions of public health, and how they are or are not providing the necessary new clarity. Making a healthy society requires institutionalisation of investment, commitments, and rules of civil engagement and everyday life. If movies of car-driver mayhem divert people away from poor driving on the road, so to the good, but the effects have to be understood and acknowledged. Mangled bodies or frightened pedestrians are not ultimately topics of entertainment.

We are not alone in seeing this paradox – success leading to silence leading to underemphasis on the centrality of public health – as the denial of a civilising force. The philosopher John Searle has highlighted the way humans think they are acting in freedom and spontaneity but how in reality behaviours are contextualised by a hidden framework of prior decisions, laws, institutions, habits and tacit everyday rules which guide our behaviour and mental reflexes:

> I go into a café in Paris and sit in a chair at a table. The waiter comes and I utter a fragment of a French sentence. I say, 'un Demi, Munich, à pression, s'il vous plaît.' The waiter brings the beer and I drink it. I leave some money on the table and leave.

Searle points out that this simple everyday episode – ordering and drinking a beer in a café – is more complex than it appears to be at first:

> [T]he waiter did not actually own the beer he gave me, but he is employed by the restaurant which owned it. The restaurant is required to post a list of

the prices of all the boissons, and even if I never see such a list, I am required to pay only the listed price. The owner of the restaurant is licensed by the French government to operate it. As such, he is subject to a thousand rules and regulations I know nothing about. I am entitled to be there in the first place only because I am a citizen of the United States, the bearer of a valid passport, and I have entered France legally.[5]

Everyday exchanges, he argues, have behind them a vast number of hidden institutional rules and conventions, built up over time, and negotiated between and within cultures, which guide our behaviour and actions. In similar manner, public health is more than individual genes or the size of bank accounts. Public health is part of the fabric of how society operates. Who could be against public health, the right to live in a state of health? Most people desire health for themselves, their families and their fellows. But for this to come about requires collective action.

Some argue that public health merely needs better public relations. We think its problems are more profound than can be resolved by spending on publicity. Certainly, public health, when compared to other aspects of health provision, is often low in the list. David Hemenway, a US public health specialist working in the field of violence and firearms, has asked why this is so, and he suggests that its lack of profile is systemic, not least because it sits alongside medicine, which has a far higher profile and funding.[6] Unlike medicine, where the linkage to patients is immediate and direct, the benefits of public health programmes often lie in the future, and whereas the beneficiaries of medicine are easily identified – and at some time it will be us – the beneficiaries and even benefactors of public health may be unknown. When lives are saved and when the population's health improves, it is unclear whose lives they are, and people may not even recognise that they have been helped. They become anonymised in mass statistics, the health profile of a nation or group. To complicate further, some lines of public health effort encounter not just disinterest but out-and-out opposition. For Hemenway, firearms – less of a feature in Europe than in some parts of the world – are a case in point.

The invisibility of public health is not recent, but has dogged its history. In 1937 Richard Shryock (1917–72), a US historian of public health, observed that, 'by the simple process of forgetting' its past efforts, the public health movement had become irrelevant. He expressed a worry that 'indifference to the past' might promote 'complacency in the present'.[7]

There are also powerful intellectual reasons why public health is such a thorny issue. The process of identifying problems and solutions is often furiously difficult, whether the problem is death due to famine or infectious disease, or death due to firearms or tobacco. The case for public health always has to be built, argued and won. And, once won, it continues to need to be argued for. Thus public health requires a movement which champions it. The more people are engaged in thinking about public health, the more their health is likely to be improved and/or maintained. That is why this book and the model of public health that we elaborate here – Ecological Public Health – see social engagement about health as so important. The health of the public is actually a measure of societal progress. Indeed, public health *is* the health of societies and is the ultimate yardstick by which most people value existence for themselves and their loved ones.

So why is there such opposition to public health, and why is it frequently presented as unwarranted intervention or busybodying? Arguments offered against public health include that public health measures:

- come at too high a price for the taxpayer;
- interfere with private decision-making;
- act as a restraint on trade and economic growth;
- impose an unnecessary burden on business;
- disrupt moral or religious norms (e.g. between the sexes, parents and children);
- are expressions of self-interest by State-funded interest groups;
- represent an overextension of legitimate public health action into unnecessary terrain;
- are not evidence-based or are based on insufficient evidence for benefit;
- infantilise the general public by assuming our need for paternalism and oversight;
- result from the manipulation of moral panics;
- are a smokescreen for social engineering; and
- are ultimately self-defeating.

Again, these arguments are not new. A similar list of potential objections to his plans for the promotion of public health in Boston, USA was compiled by Lemuel Shattuck (1793–1859) in the late 1840s. Objections frequently voiced against measures to promote the public health, said Shattuck, were that they were:[8]

- too complicated;
- 'not applicable to us';
- too statistical;
- interfering with private matters;
- interfering with private rights;
- creating an unnecessary expense;
- promoting quackery;
- alarming the people;
- interfering with Providence; and
- a diversion of time.

These arguments are essentially that public health is overweening and self-aggrandising. But they also expose how health interventions are moral and societal dilemmas. They are sometimes the result of the collision between social conservatism and progressivism, the precedence of the short term over the long term, or powers held by the few over the many. While we speak of public health being aligned with social progress, it would hardly be of surprise if these and other dimensions of philosophical disagreement were not also reflected within public health. While we argue that the discussion and promotion of public health by its nature represents social progress, acknowledgement also needs to be made of the fact that public health interventions can be received as oppressive, retrospectively irrelevant, or interest-laden. A serious critique of public health is that its manifestation may result from or ignore long-standing injustices. Too often the history of public health is written as a continual line of progress. For example, *A History of Public Health*, published in 1958 and written by the eminent historian George Rosen (1910–77), gives an otherwise luminous account of US public health history and humankind's struggle to improve its lot. The book does not give attention, however, to critical failures in the US public health system, in particular its long accommodation to racial oppression, a point now addressed in a posthumous introduction to his book by contemporary historian Elizabeth Fee.[9]

The failure to set public health within the maelstrom of everyday life leads it to being painted as either wholly good or wholly bad. Nowhere is this moral dichotomy more illustrated than in the issue of sexual health, an enduring concern worldwide. In 1864 the United Kingdom Parliament passed the first of several Contagious Diseases Acts which allowed the police to arrest prostitutes – in more modern language, sex workers – in ports and army towns and to enforce compulsory checks for 'venereal disease' – a term which itself reflected the presumed source of the infection. The motivating cause was the very high rate of infections among servicemen, which was serious enough, but the measures enacted provided easier but also repressive routes of remedy. If the women were deemed to be suffering from sexually transmitted diseases, they were placed in locked hospital wards until 'cured'. Many of the women arrested were not prostitutes but were forced to go to the police station to undergo humiliating medical examinations. Some modern scholarship has employed the analysis of Michel Foucault (1926–84), the French historian of ideas, to interpret these events as illustrations of medicine and public health being vehicles for 'biopower' and social control.[10]

By the late nineteenth century, far more was known about gonorrhoea and syphilis. The evidence base had improved, and the focus on effective prevention and treatment began to collide overtly with middle-class moral codes.[11] Gradually, sexually transmitted infections began to be seen as just another category of transmissible disease by public health authorities. In the US, this new approach was defined by Prince Morrow (1846–1913), a European-trained physician, who established the new 'social hygiene' movement, insisting that such infections were not moral but public health problems. Even so, he averred they were not 'a purely sanitary problem' since they were not just 'diseases of the human body but diseases of the social organism', caused by ignorance, shame, an ineffective medical response and widespread irresponsibility in which the male was 'the chief malefactor'.[12] But if some leaders made the connection between public health science and the ridding from society of repressive social rules, others shamed the public health field by traditions of unequal and racist technical practice. The Tuskegee syphilis experiment by the US Public Health Service was set up to assess the progress of untreated syphilis in poor, black populations in Alabama. The experiment ran from 1932 to 1972 on 399 black men in the late stages of syphilis; they were mostly illiterate sharecroppers who were not told what they had. The disease was studied but not tackled, despite effective drugs becoming available during the course of the 'experiment'. In all, 28 died of syphilis, 100 died of related complications, 40 wives were infected and 19 children were born with congenital syphilis.[13] This is hardly a proud episode in public health history. President Clinton apologised to the remaining survivors in 1997.

What should we make of these brief vignettes? That in public health, as in any other field, intentions are mixed and judgements often reflect the conditions and thinking of wider society. The movement for improved sexual health, illustrated above, expressed the best and the worst: the best was represented by outspoken, maverick but always imperfect people defying convention; the worst was what the British refer to as the 'jobsworth' tendency, people willing to adopt practices and moral codes in the name of health which they think are morally right or pragmatic, or as purely technical measures. Tuskegee, in particular, was a glaring example of how measures ostensibly to promote health can be repressive and morally flawed, both at the State and the individual level of responsibility. Another example in the literature is the solitary treatment of a woman known as Typhoid Mary. She was a well but highly infectious typhoid carrier incarcerated by New York City public health authorities early in the twentieth century.[14] Our point here, in this first chapter, is that public health is inevitably complex, raising questions of judgement, truth and evidence, social as well as individual rights.

What's the point of public health?

The orthodox answer to this question was originally voiced by utilitarianism, the British philosophical movement which provided some of the core concepts to modern economics (think of the concept 'utility'). This philosophical system was named by one of its most prominent members, John Stuart Mill.[15] For Mill, utilitarianism had to be 'grounded on the permanent interests of man as a progressive being'.[16] The specific promoter of the cause of utilitarianism in public health was Edwin Chadwick (1800–80), a name we will return to time and again, who was a lawyer–civil servant and follower (indeed secretary) of Jeremy Bentham (1748–1832), the founder of this school of thought. In his report on an inquiry into the sanitary conditions of the English working class in 1842, Chadwick posited the argument that the purpose of public health was to secure the economic advance of society by reducing mortality among economically active heads of households.[17] Improving public health thus reduces the potential dependency of the ill on others but particularly on the State. It was not based upon the provision of some basic set of human rights. Chadwick, note, worked for the British government for much of his life, but had been a journalist who had learnt from Paris's formative experience of the science and statistics of health.[18] As his fame spread, Chadwick was not only knighted but elected a corresponding member of the Institutes of France and Belgium and of the Societies of Medicine and Hygiene of France, Belgium and Italy. His views were adopted into international thinking.

The same essentially utilitarian approach to health, with variations, was offered 160 years later by the World Health Organization's Commission on Macroeconomics and Health, which reported in 2002. Chaired by Jeffrey Sachs, the US economist, the Commission argued that investment in public health aids social development. Disease, being a determinant of poverty, acts as a brake on development. Vice versa, investment in health thus unleashes development: 'We believe that the additional investments in health – requiring of donors roughly one-tenth of one percent of their national income – would be repaid many times over in millions of lives saved each year, enhanced economic development, and strengthened global security.'[19] The new dimension since Chadwick is that, whereas in his day the financial transfer was intra-state, by the twenty-first century the main dynamic being posited was interstate.

Critics of this utilitarian position include those who argue that public health is a 'fundamental human value, worthy of investment for its own sake'.[20] The origins of this position lie within a different philosophical tradition, associated with the German philosopher Immanuel Kant (1724–1804), which proposes that values are fundamental. We judge the rightness or wrongness of actions in and of themselves and not subject to circumstance, contingencies or collective trade-offs. Values are essential truths. Like utilitarianism, this argument runs throughout this book. We don't necessarily see values in complete opposition to the utilitarian position, but the argument does raise questions about the variation in rationales for public health. We suggest that public health is at the heart of what societies want from their economies and political systems. It defines what is meant by progress. It is both economic and value-driven. But there are other dimensions too. It is also 'fear-driven'.

Friedrich Engels (1820–95), in his 1892 introduction to the English edition of his *Condition of the Working Class in England*, originally published in 1845 in German only, noted that the bourgeois under threats from 'cholera, typhus, smallpox and other epidemics . . . had shown the urgent necessity of sanitation in his towns and cities if he wishes to save himself and family from falling victims to such diseases'.[21] This was self-interest rather than altruism. It is and was a structural-functionalist argument. The function of the State, said Engels, was to protect the position of the elite by mitigating the poor circumstances of the masses. A similar logic, we see later, can be constructed for a range of matters, from the extension of democratic participation in Britain to the development of social security in Prussia. Such actions and thinking bound the British and the Prussian elites in the nineteenth century into a form of elite corporatism, but other national elites have not necessarily followed this self-interested argument.

So far we have considered only three positions on what public health is: a utilitarian position, one which is values-led and another which is structural-functional. We have assumed that public health is about the public in the larger, more collective sense, to use another, closely akin term, 'population health', which some have suggested substitutes for public health in some countries' discourse.[22] But it also seems unlikely that we can speak of populations without actually addressing real people in their real environments; that's where public health started after all. Whereas it may seem desirable to speak about public health in the general sense, it may be impossible to avoid addressing the personal too. A person is always a member of the public, and the public would mean very little without individual people within it. In sum, there may be many arguments about the purpose of public health, but most, not to dismiss the others, centre on either utilitarianism or value-based arguments. The case of Typhoid Mary, cited earlier, can be interpreted through either with different consequences. From the utilitarian perspective, to confine her was right, to protect the wider public. From a values perspective, her incarceration was an affront to decency and civilisation. A fuller list of rationales offered for public health action includes the following:

- self-interest and protection of immediate family and household;
- democratisation and improvements in everyday quality of life;
- equalisation of health status of men and women and across other social divides;
- the reduction of population growth that follows from the emancipation of women;
- economic efficiency and modernisation of the economy;
- international development and social justice;
- global trade and international exchange, not just of goods, but of people and ideas.

All of these arguments are being altered by the new discourse around humans and the environment, a huge challenge for the twenty-first century. In the past, there were three lines of thinking found within public health thinking about the environment. The first was sanitarian: to address the environment, and it was usually the urban environment, resulting in measures to combat filth, overcrowding and other insults to the eye, nose and moral sensitivities. These basic issues of sanitation still afflict many parts of the world and shape public health priorities.

The second line of thought within environmental approaches to health in the past was to appreciate how urban environments depended for their literal sustenance on the rural environment. Like others, Chadwick for example championed the return of organic detritus (faeces, etc.) from the city to the land to improve it, an idea current again today as an answer to improving both plant yield and sanitation.[23]

A third line of thinking focused on a broader conception of the environment, a recognition that human activity was altering nature, and that humans depend on that environment, not least through food. This argument has returned in modern times with the realisation of the impact of climate change, biodiversity loss, global interconnectedness through the oil-based economy, and multinationals' systems of governance. A new ecological sense of public health is emerging based on the recognition of the limits on nature, that nature no longer offers an endless cornucopia of its resources for human use or that the biological world can be ceaselessly altered to human advantage. As many have argued, the Western debt-fuelled consumerist approach to happiness and health – the later rendition of the original utilitarian model – is now facing major difficulties about sustainability.

The challenge now is to work out the meaning and purpose of public health in an era of ecological threat. Over two centuries and more, there appears to have been a persistent capacity for public health and economic development not to match with the environment. Now, the scale of twenty-first-century ecological change casts all the hesitant past relationships of human to environmental health in a new and stark light. To help 'read' this mismatch, in much of this book we apply a template for thinking which we propose to clarify problems and solutions. This is to juxtapose what we term four 'dimensions of existence', namely firstly the material nature of things, secondly the biological processes of life, thirdly societal and human relations, and fourthly cultural or cognitive experience. These four dimensions of existence – material, biological, social, cultural – clarify the complexity of life and health and the conditions which shape public health. They are integral to the approach we refer to as Ecological Public Health.

Conventional understandings of public health

A common-sense view is that public health is just what the juxtaposition of the two words says it is, centrally about health and the public dimension of health rather than the individual or personal aspects. In the world's first legislation on public health per se, the Public Health Act of 1848, which applied to England and Wales, the words 'public health' had a flat meaning, shaped by utilitarianism and pragmatism. Yet, as we have already intimated above, what it means is fiercely argued over. The very notion of public health is intellectually and politically problematic, because it comes replete with societal meanings and associations.

Public health is also claimed by some societal institutions and sectional interests. There are professions with the term 'public health' in their job titles or descriptions. There is a branch of medicine termed 'public health'. There are public health nurses, working in the community. Some of these professions are old, such as the UK's and Ireland's environmental health officers, formerly sanitary officers, whose *raison d'être* was to protect the public health as enshrined in the Victorian-era public health laws. 'Sanitary' meant health. There are also academics whose work centres on public health. Epidemiologists study the development of diseases and what makes them, at population level. Health educators set out, as their title implies, to educate the public about how to prevent ill-health. Community nurses and 'frontline' practitioners visit people in their homes and engage directly with the public, often centred on the vulnerability of children, and helping parents, mostly mothers. Public health clearly engages with people's daily lives at certain points and life stages. But what does the public think about public health?

Public opinion

If public health, as we have argued, is an invisible concept, can the general public be expected to have views about it? Of course, people do have views, and they are formed in complex ways – family, friends, childhood, media input, life experiences, and more. Mostly, when people are asked about health the topic is not about health at all. They are usually asked about healthcare, not health. Health services are not the same thing as public health, yet polling on that dwarfs every other type of focus. People are asked, too, about components of public health, notably their views on their experience of and attitudes to diseases and risks. It is therefore hard to generate a rounded view of public opinion on public health. Many opinion polls, as we will see, are misleading, not because they are designed to mislead (although this may also be the case, depending on the poll's funder) but because the questions they ask tap ephemeral issues, something around which a media narrative has been constructed. Modern politics is heavily influenced by the ebbs and flows of such 'public opinion', often translated by and filtered through powerful media interests.

Public opinion is an elastic concept with many influences. This is not surprising; most people have vagueness and ambivalences in their own thinking and attitudes, let alone behaviour. People change their opinions. They hold contrary opinions according to where they are, who they are with or last talked to, and probably the time of day and whether the sun is shining. Opinions may shape behaviour, and they may not, although an entire psychological edifice – constructed around the 'health belief model' and the idea that people's attitudes and beliefs are under their personal control[24] – has been constructed on the proposal that they are related. Understanding what opinions are and how they were shaped is often investigated by specialist organisations, many of which are marketing companies themselves in the business of shaping opinions, or guiding the emotional responses (for example towards brands) underneath those opinions. Should the world of public health therefore be wary of these claims? We think yes.

One typical example of polling on healthcare shows the difficulty of trying to establish a consistent and reliable picture of opinions. In June 2004 the International Research Institute, a body composed of marketing companies all over the world, conducted a study through members across 23 countries asking the public questions about the state of their national healthcare arrangements.[25] About half (52 per cent) of a sample of the British public thought their healthcare was 'in crisis'; this was also true of majorities in 19 other countries. These included France, where 58 per cent of people felt their nation's healthcare system was 'in crisis', the USA (65 per cent), Germany (78 per cent) and Poland (the highest at 93 per cent). Five years later, another set of polls, again by a reputable organisation (in this case Ipsos-Mori), asked questions around public 'concern' (not 'crisis') about healthcare. This time the level of concern was around 20 per cent in France and in the UK around 15 per cent. Poland was still the highest at above 50 per cent. Poles either think their healthcare system is in crisis or at least consistently worry about it, but people in France and the UK apparently are less concerned. Perhaps the question was posed differently, prompting a significantly different response. In US studies, people's responses over time appear more consistent.[26] But this may also be due to consistent narratives over time helping to form people's opinions, crowding out other options. In the US, for example, the healthcare industry, formed of insurance and drug companies, lobby groups and others, has spread a consistent message since the 1930s that government should stay out of healthcare, which should be left to the private market, and that poor insurance coverage was less important than the maintenance of market freedom. This may help explain the wide divergence in views between the USA and the UK.[27]

Similarly, and away from healthcare, it appears that many people, at least in the US, do consider health to be their top priority in life. In one opinion survey in 2009, over 1,000 people told US pollsters that their health (not public health) was deeply important to them. Among the survey respondents, 91 per cent said they would rather be talked about as someone who is 'healthy' than as someone who is 'wealthy', and 71 per cent said they would prefer to be described as someone who 'looks really healthy' than as someone who looks 'well put together or well dressed'. The pollsters also found that 58 per cent of respondents 'prefer not to socialise with people who lead unhealthy lifestyles'. The conclusion of that report overtly linked the polling with the company's 'insight-driven approach to help our clients understand the new consumer psyche for both consumer and prescription products'.[28] In this example, like many others, pollsters might be accused of aping the Delphic Oracles of ancient Greece, whose unintelligible utterances were interpreted by a priesthood and passed on to the unwary inquirer as truth. In the modern era, the new priesthood of predictions might well be the marketing companies.

Not all inquiries into public belief have this commercial orientation or are in thrall to narrative feedback. More than a decade ago, the US Centers for Disease Control and Prevention (CDC), a government body, recognised how public health invisibility limited their effectiveness in making a case for public health efforts.[29] They may have been surprised though by the degree of invisibility that emerged from their inquiry. Respondents were asked by CDC: 'When you hear the term "public health", what do you think of?' and then given a choice of four descriptions. Approximately half (57 per cent) of the respondents could not define public health as either protecting the population from disease or policies and efforts that promoted healthy living conditions. Interviewers then defined public health and asked respondents to rate (excellent/good/fair/poor) the current system for protecting public health. Most (57 per cent) respondents offered negative evaluations of the public health system. Respondents also were asked whether sufficient resources were being dedicated to public health. In all, 65 per cent said that the United States should do more. When asked to compare public health as a spending priority, most said public health was more deserving of additional funds than building roads (80 per cent), missile defence (73 per cent) and cutting taxes (63 per cent). Only education was viewed as a greater priority for additional resources (24 per cent). When asked about environmental factors such as pollution and their relation to public health, 85 per cent said they believed that environmental factors were important determinants of disease and health problems. Of these, 38 per cent considered environmental factors very important.

With all the reservations about prompted answers, we could conclude that public health is both invisible *and* visible. People cannot define it easily, but prompted by interviewers they appear to like the idea. Perhaps they might offer the same verdict if the rationale for roads or missiles was explained. While it is true that, in the US, there is general support for public health, with people appearing to recognise the simple adage that spending money to prevent disease and illness saves money later, support starts to wane when particular items of public health intervention are mentioned. Sexual health is one prominent area where fissures quickly emerge.[30]

In the UK and in other Anglophone countries these divisions are less apparent. In the UK, polls suggest that, while public health is highly valued, its positive reception is tempered by the fear that it may also represent government interference in everyday life.[31] This is often invoked in the UK as 'the nanny state' problem, when individual liberties are constrained by an overweening, interfering busybody. Public opinion should therefore not be assumed to be constant. It is a contested area, shaped by many forces which are not evenly matched. Some health-related industries have very large funds at their disposal. On the other hand, even poorly funded public health causes – we look at some of them later – can be remarkably effective in waging what in power terms are asymmetric campaigns.[32]

Images of public health

Part of the difficulty public health has in the early twenty-first century is that there are competing images of what is involved. National histories, literature, television and radio shows, books, family histories, stories in newspapers, and song lyrics all convey narratives about public health. These provide a living, changing cultural library on what is meant by health, public health and the role of those who work in and on those issues and realities. These narrative storylines convey appeals for collective imagination about what public health means, who is involved and the processes underlying it. They construct emotional as well as scientific fictions about health. We do not demean fictions. They are important. They drive and populate events. They fix identities. They provide enduring metaphors which frame not only intellectual but emotional understanding. In each of the images of health which we now explore below – not intended as a definitive list – we ask: What is the picture of health being given? Who is involved? What roles and characters are played? How is the landscape portrayed? Who has the power and how is authority assigned in the situation? Who is watching? How are outcomes measured? What lessons are learnt? We repeat: these are *images* of public health. They are not offered as discrete or entirely separate images but to show that public understanding has a rich store of culturally resonant existing notions of what public health entails and what it draws upon. There is a blurring of lines between health and public health, official and popular understandings, and scientific and everyday meanings.

Image 1: People constructing knowledge-based interventions

One of the most pervasive images of public health is the notion that there is someone who applies systematically derived knowledge in the interests of health. In Western science, this person is white-coated and expert in modern science. In other cultures, the person may be shamanic, and culturally different. Whether the person is white-coated or a witch doctor, the notion is that knowledge is powerful and that health requires knowledge-based interventions.

In Western health, the power of the image of great men and women working on our collective 'public' behalf to make things safe is considerable. Wilson Smillie's 1955 chronology of public health in the USA required, he said, 'the study of great men'. Smillie (1886–1971) ought to have added women too. Freeing people

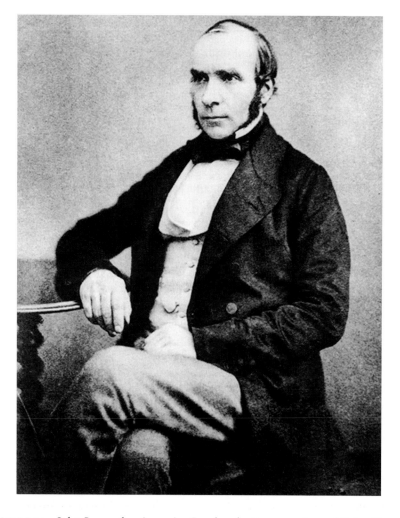

FIGURE 1.1a John Snow, the pioneering London doctor protecting public health

from fear is a core aim of civilisation. Advances in public health are 'an accurate index of our advancing civilization in all its aspects and connotations'.[33] The UK and world public health movement lionises Edward Jenner (1749–1823) for pioneering vaccination, John Snow (1813–58) for his action in removing the pump handle in Broad Street, London to tackle cholera (see Figure 1.1b), and William Farr (1807–83) for medical statistics. In Germany, there was the hygienist Johann Peter Frank (1745–1821) and more famously Rudolf Virchow (1821–1902), who pioneered cellular pathology and chaired the Sanitary Committee of Berlin, where a statue sits today in his honour. He combined social reform with liberal politics and a prodigious appetite for scientific investigation. In the USA, key figures in the public health movement were often anti-slavers such as Henry Ingersoll Bowditch (1808–92), the Blackwell sisters, Elizabeth (1821–1910) and Emily (1826–1910), trained in medicine, and freethinkers like Lemuel Shattuck, who saw the cause of health improvement based in research, health statistics and public administration.

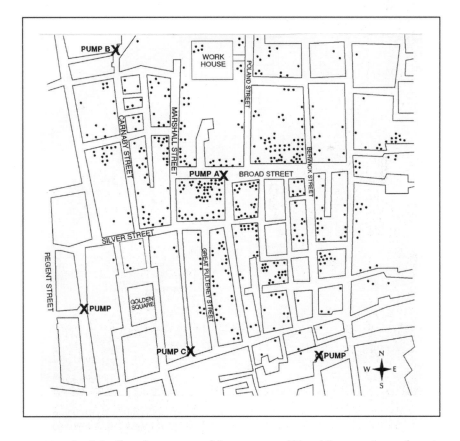

FIGURE 1.1b John Snow's spot map of the area around Broad Street, redrawn for epidemiology courses run by the US CDC

In France, figures like Louis-René Villermé (1782–1863) pioneered social epidemiology, showing the links between poverty and death rates.[34] Indeed it has been argued that France was the original source of the public health movement, which only later ceded leadership to the British.[35] The French pioneered hygiene and scientific medicine, with Marie Curie (1867–1934) possibly pre-eminent as inheritor and heroine of this tradition a century later (see Figure 1.2).

For the USA, Smillie catalogued and ranked those he called 'public health pioneers', setting a start date of 1610.[36] He could have set the time clock much further back in the past, beginning with the ancient Greeks. A strong strand of thinking

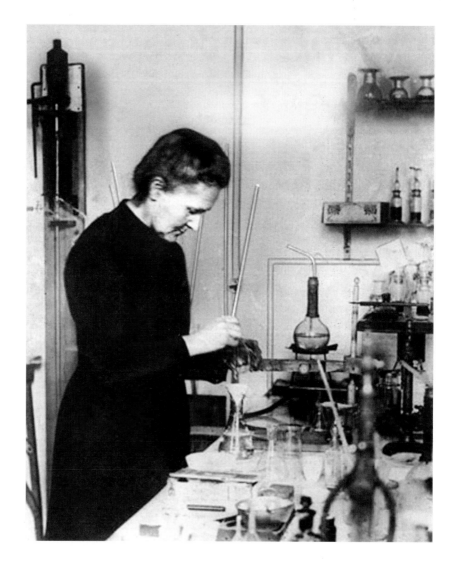

FIGURE 1.2   Marie Curie, Polish-French laboratory scientist

about health, the environment, and the mitigation and prevention of disease does indeed flow back to the Greeks for Westerners. But it might also be observed that the modern public health movements, particularly from the nineteenth century on, also benefited from an international trade in ideas, methods, interventions, policies and strategies. Increasingly public health has operated within a common language.

Core to this image is the promise that public health horrors can be mitigated, if not rolled back, by the actions of pioneers and reformers. The archetype location is perhaps a cataclysm such as the Crimean War, which saw the coincidence of Florence Nightingale (1820–1910) pioneering nursing and preventing unnecessary collateral damage in wounded troops with Alexis Soyer (1810–58), French chef fresh from the London Ritz, who pioneered mass catering for the troops, preventing death by feeding troops better and more efficiently. While Curie was laboratory-based, Soyer invented his field kitchens to make good hospital feeding possible to aid recovery as well for fighting men.[37]

Public health here is posed as a series of battles for hearts and minds, and for control over the body politic. It is presented as made by heroes and heroines, actors in a ripping yarn of Good mostly triumphing over Evil and Dread. This image captures some essential ingredients in the history of public health. It is about hard work and dogged attention to detail; leadership, vision, and preparedness to restructure; occasional breakthroughs; and opportunism and political nous. The rewards in earlier times were a posthumous statue and a footnote in history books. The rewards today are Nobel Prizes, although, as the British historian Dorothy Porter has noted, in recent years too there's been a countertrend which scoffs at any 'heroisation' of public health as a great achievement of Enlightenment rationalism.[38] Behind the narrative is the search for a presumed key fact or intervention point which will improve public health. Technology, science and research are crucial, whether statistics, the microscope and lens, or the means of organising human scientific effort. Observation and development of systematised knowledge are the key.

Image 2: Public health as State intervention: people in uniforms

In the USA, the Public Health Service is a uniformed branch of government. In the 1950 Hollywood film *Panic in the Streets* (directed by Elia Kazan), a disease outbreak at the port of New Orleans is managed by a uniformed medical officer who, with unerringly steady judgement, steers a course through local scepticism and objections to save the city from a pandemic. The plot is not entirely what it seems. Thickly accented foreigners and Cold-War fears are filtered through an otherwise simple story of science and detective work defeating mysterious bacteria.[39] In 2011, half a century on, another Hollywood film, *Contagion* (directed by Steven Soderbergh), explored the theme of unseen biological threats to health and civilisation. Again, experts and laboratory-based science are required to explain and address the crisis.

This image is one of public health as due to the actions and/or influences of the State, guided by experts who have the public's best interests at heart. The core function is to protect hygiene and to prevent or contain contagion, often by engaging with worrying outside influences. The State thus has to reform itself to be in the position to act as a positive force for good. There are benign and authoritarian versions of this image. These can both be represented in the husband–and–wife team of Sidney (1859–1947) and Beatrice (1858–1943) Webb, architects and archetypes of Fabian (UK reformist) approaches to health and welfare at the turn of the nineteenth and twentieth centuries. On the one hand, the Webbs were modernisers who saw the State as the delivery mechanism of the public good. Their narrative changed over time. Sidney began with promoting the role of municipal enterprise and intervention as the mechanisms for delivering health improvement. But later in their lives the couple saw the advantage of more authoritarian mechanisms for controlling individual behaviours of the lower classes. The narrative of the State as health provider becomes on the one hand welfare support and on the other hand eugenicism, the imposition of controls over the fertility of particular social groups. The State can easily become draconian once national efficiency is defined in population terms.

The epitome of the State health official is probably Edwin Chadwick (Figure 1.3), albeit uniformed not in a white coat but in a frock coat. He invented the methodologies of State management, cost–benefit analysis and arguments on the need for officials to act for the public health. In England, his case led directly to the creation of the sanitary inspector. His articulation of the tough role for the State created many enemies. Despite being rigorous, energetic and determined he was also described as tactless, humourless, impatient and dogmatic. George Rosen notes that, when in 1854 the government decided to release Chadwick from its employment, *The Times* responded to this event with a jubilant leader article which announced that, '[i]f there is such a thing as a political certainty among us, it is that nothing autocratic can exist in this country. . . . Mr Chadwick and Dr Southwood Smith have been deposed, and we prefer to take our chance of cholera and the rest than be bullied into health.'[40] Southwood Smith (1788–1861) will be considered later. Economic considerations lay behind the dismissal of Chadwick's efforts. His modus operandi threatened private property with new responsibilities and costs, confronting ratepayers and landlords directly with the bill for urban improvement. Local opposition to public health measures, it has been suggested, 'was grounded in self-interest, not ignorance'.[41]

Institutionally, this image of public health is deeply embedded in State functions, although private entities deliver public health services. Whole government bodies have the term 'public health' as their title, as we have seen. Entire divisions of State at local, sub-national, national and international levels now all espouse the promotion and protection of public health. The English Department of Health, for instance, listed in 2010 under 'Public health' on its website that it 'is responsible for health protection, health improvement and health inequalities issues in England, including pandemic influenza, seasonal flu, patient safety, tobacco, obesity, drugs,

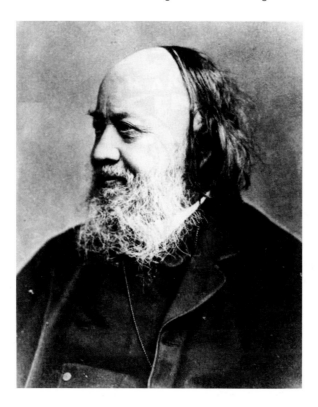

FIGURE 1.3   Edwin Chadwick, the British public health reformer

sexual health, and international health'.[42] At the international level, the World Health Organization (WHO) stresses how public health is about disease prevention. The State and its agents are promoted as acting for the public interest. The formation of these national, international and global institutions is discussed in Chapter 12.

Image 3: Public health as responding to pandemic disease

For a time, at least until the early 1980s, it appeared that infectious diseases were in long-term retreat, with infectious disease judged by the West as a problem for far-away places and chronic diseases barely acknowledged in population terms. In the USA infectious disease mortality declined during the first eight decades of the twentieth century from 797 deaths per 100,000 in 1900 to 36 deaths per 100,000 in 1980.[43] A similar picture emerges elsewhere in the developed world: until HIV/AIDS, that is. This new disease, first diagnosed in the early 1980s, revived once-dormant fears about the plague. In the language of the time it was the 'gay plague' and given unknown disease aetiology, ineffectiveness of treatment and apparently rapid spread. The public narrative was constructed around the fear that HIV might spread 'to the rest of us'. This soon faded into another story, that HIV was a feature of particular ways of life, drug use, risky sex and chance contact. This became yet another story, that of the affliction of HIV/AIDS on Africa and elsewhere, with the infection taking root in the social interstices between poverty, poor health literacy and sexual mores.

It has been suggested that epidemics should be seen as physical events which can lead to a destabilising social crisis which leads to a narrative that knits its other aspects together.[44] That was always true. The plague occurred in three huge pandemics starting from the sixth century, with millions of deaths and numerous smaller epidemics and sporadic cases (see Figure 1.4).[45] The plague has a powerful role in imagination (see Figure 1.5). In the fourteenth century alone it is estimated to have killed 200 million people. The great pandemics revealed disease to be arbitrary and capricious, placing humankind in a fluctuating state of fear and uncertainty. In the face of this metaphysical reality, what were the common human responses?

The social character of disease panics is available in a variety of on-the-spot accounts. In the early eighteenth century bubonic plague was causing havoc in Marseilles, France. Predictions were rife that it would soon reach England. The authorities issued new regulations, including *cordons sanitaires* and restrictions on shipping from countries known to be infected. These and other practical measures were documented in the journal of Daniel Defoe (1659–1731), the prolific author of *Robinson Crusoe*, whose account also gave attention to

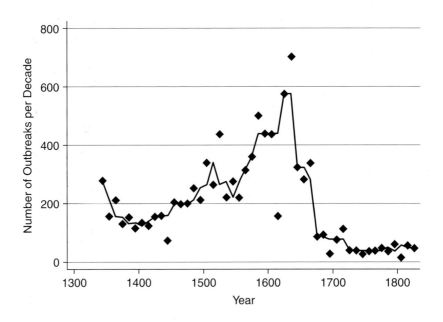

FIGURE 1.4   Plague outbreaks in Europe 1300s–1800s

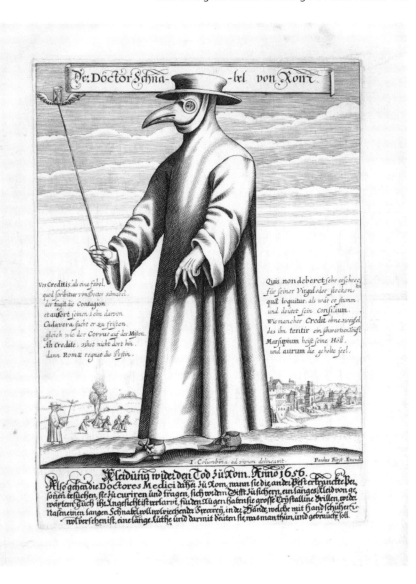

FIGURE 1.5   Doctor Schnabel von Rom, plague doctor, in 1656

complaints from the pulpit that disease represented God's wrath for sins of avarice and religious slovenliness.[46] By the nineteenth century, efforts to counter infectious disease had taken a more practical bent. The town of Wakefield, like many others across England, experienced cholera epidemics in the 1830s and 1840s, the first of which led to 62 deaths. The town responded with a variety of efforts, from actions against vagrants to improvements in the diet of the town's prison population (see Figure 1.6).

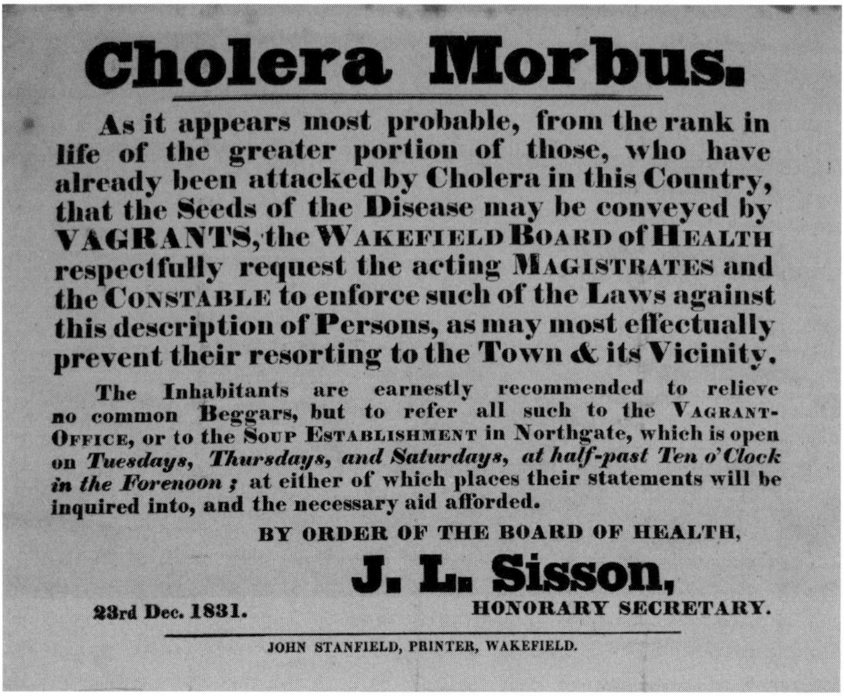

Cholera Morbus.

As it appears most probable, from the rank in life of the greater portion of those, who have already been attacked by Cholera in this Country, that the Seeds of the Disease may be conveyed by VAGRANTS, the WAKEFIELD BOARD of HEALTH respectfully request the acting MAGISTRATES and the CONSTABLE to enforce such of the Laws against this description of Persons, as may most effectually prevent their resorting to the Town & its Vicinity.

The Inhabitants are earnestly recommended to relieve no common Beggars, but to refer all such to the VAGRANT-OFFICE, or to the SOUP ESTABLISHMENT in Northgate, which is open on *Tuesdays, Thursdays, and Saturdays, at half-past Ten o'Clock in the Forenoon*; at either of which places their statements will be inquired into, and the necessary aid afforded.

BY ORDER OF THE BOARD OF HEALTH,

J. L. Sisson,

23rd Dec. 1831. HONORARY SECRETARY.

JOHN STANFIELD, PRINTER, WAKEFIELD.

FIGURE 1.6 Cholera poster, Wakefield, Yorkshire, England, 1832

By their nature pandemic diseases, when they occur rapidly, result in a high level of social disintegration and breaches in the normal rules of civility. Albert Camus's novel *La Peste* (The Plague), first published in 1947 and for which he won the Nobel Prize for literature, is set in Algeria in the mid-nineteenth century. Camus (1913–60) reveals all possible forms of reactions to the approaching threat, from the cowardly to the brave and decisive. People shift their focus as they confront their fears. The plague reveals the worst of human qualities but also the best. Camus's analysis is subtle. We should be cautious in making assumptions based on sensational reports. Panic too is infectious. The spread of severe acute respiratory syndrome (SARS) and swine flu in the early 2000s saw the widespread wearing of surgical masks in public, most obviously in Japan. The sight of so many people wearing surgical masks, with no intrinsic preventive benefit, might itself have led to the spread of fear. Another panic reaction is the search for the cause of the spread of disease among particular groups, be these migrants, 'foreigners in our midst', or racial, ethnic or sexual minorities. We considered earlier how prostitutes have been identified as health threats, but the demonisation of particular groups of people, usually minorities, varies from one society to another.

Many millions of people die prematurely with little accompanying sense of public panic. In some cases the death is accepted because the path of causation is normalised, even commercialised, as in the case of tobacco. If panic speaks to over-reaction, at times the sense of enhanced threat can help engineer a shift in culture and social policy towards dealing with the causes of the harm rather than ignoring it. The fight over the acceptability of tobacco across the twentieth century to today is a case in point.

Image 4: Public health as rescue, saving individual lives

The image of public health as an act of rescue is highly dramatic, and for that reason features much in TV drama. But it is questionable whether this is *public* health at all, merely an image of health workers, particularly doctors, acting heroically to save individual lives. The image is pervasive, however, and frames public understanding. The importance of this image has grown as technological possibilities have expanded. The USA spent comparatively little on healthcare in 1950, only 4.4 per cent of gross domestic product (GDP). The reason, says William Schwartz of the Brookings Institution in Washington, was that, for a large percentage of patients, 'doctors really couldn't do much'.[47] Since then the USA has pursued a highly technological form of medicine, spending heavily on devices such as the iron lung, the dialysis machine and the respirator.[48] By 2009 the USA was spending the equivalent of 17.4 per cent of its GDP on healthcare, almost double the 'rich country' average.[49] By 2040 the proportion is expected to rise to 29 per cent.[50] Nevertheless this level of spending did not improve its health performance. The USA was placed 37th out of 191 countries in health performance rankings in 2000 by the Organisation for Economic Co-operation and Development (OECD). By contrast, the United Kingdom spent just 6 per cent of GDP but ranked 18th.[51] By 2009, UK healthcare spending had risen to 9.8 per cent.[52]

From the 1950s the USA entered a new age of technological, heroic medicine, with doctors becoming celebrities for their apparently lifesaving surgical breakthroughs. As the sociologist Marcia Millman pointed out, the real heroes in fact were the patients who bore the risks.[53] Three celebrated and popular TV series in the UK and the USA illustrate her point and the nature and power of this image, and its changing form.

Dr. Finlay's Casebook was a television series based on a book written by A.J. Cronin (1896–1981) featuring a general medical practice in Scotland during the late 1920s. This is a form of medicine quite unlike that found in the USA today. Dr Finlay, the young doctor, is placed in a dynamic with his older fellow general practitioner Dr Cameron and their doughty and well-informed housekeeper, Janet. The depiction represents the country doctor socially above yet in touch with his patients, often through local knowledge provided by non-medic Janet. It represents the doctor as professional person in a community dispensing wisdom with remedies sometimes based on science and sometimes on pragmatism and common sense. For public health, Dr Finlay represents the voice of reason and judgement, based on a canny understanding of people's everyday lives. Public health requires human not just medical knowledge. Dr Finlay is learning at the feet of Dr Cameron and Janet.

Dr Kildare was a US film, TV and radio series from the late 1930s to the 1970s, created by a wonderfully named writer called Frederick Faust. This represented the doctor as glamorous persona, inhabiting the American system where the doctor straddles community and hospital (as 'attending physician'). Dr Kildare – the young medic – again is learning from the older and wiser Dr Gillespie, the hospital senior doctor. Dr Gillespie tells Dr Kildare at one point: 'Our job is to keep people alive not to tell them how to live.' This represents the new hospital-based medicine, wearing a formal white coat, with stethoscope around the neck, but relaxed, hands in pockets. Here, public health is represented as scientific, the application of modern methods which require technologies and specialism.

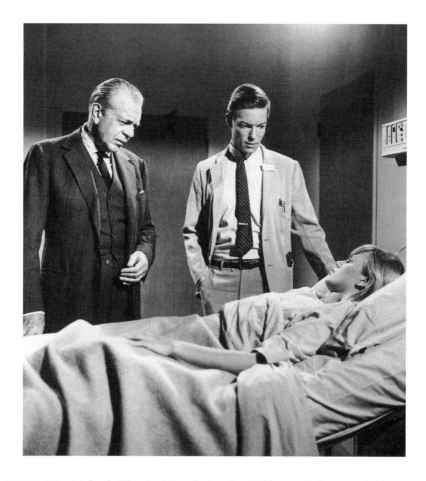

FIGURE 1.7 Richard Chamberlain playing Dr Kildare and Raymond Massey as Dr Gillespie

A third variant of this image is the fictional Dr Gregory House in the US block-buster TV series *House* in the 2000s. It was the most widely watched TV pro-gramme in the world in 2008. Gregory House is presented as a flawed human being, more Sherlock Holmes than a man with a good bedside manner. Indeed, House *is* – as the name itself implies – Holmes. Conan Doyle, a practising physi-cian himself until the Sherlock Holmes stories made him rich enough to give up his practice, may have patterned the character of Sherlock Holmes after his professor, Dr Joseph Bell of the Royal Infirmary of Edinburgh. House cares about his patients but, like Holmes, he fails to empathise with them. His role is to apply deductive science to health problems. He is an irritant, always on the point of being sacked from the hospital, but grudgingly accepted by the powers-that-be as the brightest and best. He's up against bureaucracy. His role centres on diagnosis: finding out what is the real problem in the patient's world. He asks: what is it that has caused the disruption to health, manifest in the patient's symptoms? It may be genetics or a pollutant in the home. Dr House is part public health sleuth, part semiotician:

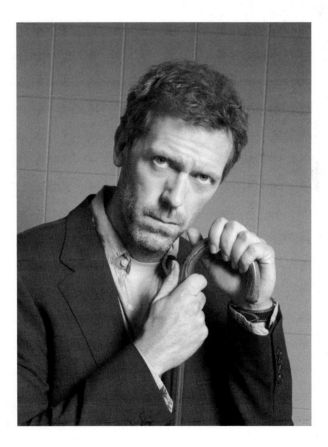

FIGURE 1.8   House MD, the Sherlock Holmes of US TV medical dramas in the 2000s, played by Hugh Laurie

an investigator of signs. He casts a radical image as outsider, only interested in the disease and completely disinterested in the patient's financial capacity to pay for health services. This is indeed a heroic stance for a medical doctor in the USA. His casual clothes and unshaven appearance are antithetical to the business-besuited professional ideal-type. Dr House differs in one substantial respect from Dr Finlay and Dr Kildare. He is the epidemiologist of the solitary body, aided by a precocious understanding of the human body and an expensive investigative medical technology far beyond either of his predecessors.

Of course, there are many more images of rescue than these, such as the popular US series *ER* and the local equivalents around the world. Viewers are confronted by a blizzard of big drama storylines. One would not be pleased to be the patient. Fortunately, the television set affords safe distance.

Image 5: Focusing on individuals shaped by wider determinants

The key narrative in this image is that individuals are surrounded by forces which shape their health. The image has various versions. In all, the individual or family or household or group is located in a web of influences, usually arranged concentrically around the human. The problem for public health is how to marry the attention on the individual or group with the weight of the surrounding forces. There are multiple external forces which are named but not specified. Actors are hidden and rarely identified. How this arrangement came into being is not explained. It just is. In early models, the relative weight of one factor against the others is not assessed; the influences are not calibrated. Do forces combine, overlap or amplify? It is not clear. Pictorially, however, we are given the immediate impression of a rainbow of influences, bearing down on the individual and household. This is a domestic-oriented pressure image. Later versions refine the relationship of the influences.

The most cited and used version of this image is that by Goren Dahlgren and Margaret Whitehead (Figure 1.9). Here individuals are presented in central focus, and all other forces are displayed on a proximal–distal dimension, some close, some distant. The image portrays health as running from individual to family to community to living and working social status to external forces of society, economy, culture and environment.

This rainbow image, although heralded as new in the 1990s, in fact draws on older cultural roots. In *City of God*, written in 426 AD, the Christian thinker St Augustine articulated a conception of the world which put humans at the centre, in the *domus* or household; above is the *civitas* or public space; and beyond that is the *orbis terrae*, the whole earth and all human society which inhabits it. Beyond that is the *mundus* or universe.[54] This doctrine also reflected the ideas of Claudius Ptolemy (*ca.* 100–170), who placed the earth at the centre of the universe of celestial objects orbiting around it and also incorporated Greek views on the nature of matter, being constructed of each of the four elements: earth,

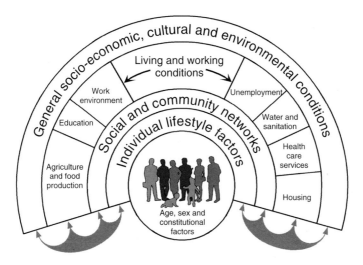

FIGURE 1.9 Dahlgren and Whitehead's much-cited graphic: The main determinants of health, revised version, from 1983

water, fire and air.[55] The Ptolemaic, or heliocentric, notion of the universe placed the universe as a series of concentric circles, radiating outwards, much as Dahlgren and Whitehead pitch public health forces surrounding the individual and household. This was the 'truth' which Copernicus and Galileo confronted, and before them a host of Islamic scholars.[56] The significance of these astronomical discoveries, according to the Oxford philosopher R.G. Collingwood (1889–1943), consisted not so much in displacing the world's centre from the earth to the sun as in 'implicitly denying that the world has a centre at all'.[57] Nevertheless, heliocentricity has been maintained as a convenient metaphor. The Russian-American child development theorist Urie Bronfenbrenner (1917–2005) also developed a not dissimilar model of radiating influences in the 1970s.[58] He posited these as three levels of proximity, wrapped around the individual, and later as four (see Figure 1.10, which shows only three levels). Bronfenbrenner's studies and advocacy of support for family-centred social policy form the basis of much socio-ecological thinking in health.

Such depictions are deceptively attractive. While they usefully present a picture of the world as having influences on the individual, they subtly sell a story that politics, economics and 'the environment' are distant and 'out there', when in fact they closely infuse intimate reality. They are both proximal and distal, in us and far away. At the same time the rules or organisational principles governing systems at one level may be different for another level. They are both material and mental, hard and soft, and are also intimately biological, which we discuss in Chapter 10. This is what the philosopher John Searle was trying to capture in

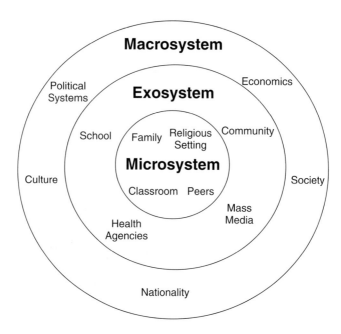

FIGURE 1.10   Urie Bronfenbrenner's ecology of child health

the quotation cited earlier. All apparently immediate actions and events have an infrastructure which may be hidden. Behind what we experience in immediate reality lies a complex web of supporting presences. It has been argued that, in nature as well as biology, scientists – including, by implication, social scientists – need to see things differently and to attune their metaphors to different properties of scale.

Image 6: Health as the operation of systems

The narrative of this image is of a complex interplay of interconnected forces. The image is of systemic linkages. They may be presented almost as hydraulic relationships and influences or, in modern computer-influenced metaphors, as cybernetics. This may be a truncated version of cybernetics, almost schematic rather than the total complex systems such as those espoused by Gregory Bateson (1904–80).[59] This image too comes in different versions. Some depict health *as* a system. Others depict it as influenced *by* systems. Still others paint it as the *outcome* of systems. The question raised implicitly is: what is the health *of* the system? The picture being painted is that health is complex but orderly. The task of public health improvement is to capture the relationships, and unpick the complexity, in order to be able to control it all. Systems, once understood, can be mastered and redirected. The image proposes that possibility.

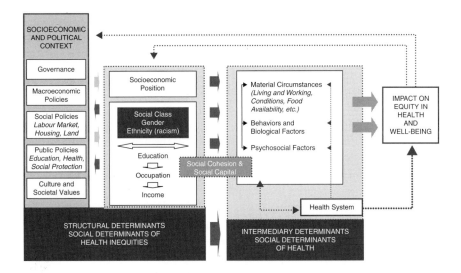

FIGURE 1.11   WHO Commission on Social Determinants of Health's model of health and health inequalities

The WHO Commission on Social Determinants of Health was an ambitious overview of public health and how to address the twenty-first-century challenges. It was chaired by Professor Sir Michael Marmot, a British epidemiologist. The Commission took the systems image and gave more emphasis to the shaping forces and the potential for change, but also the vulnerabilities. It needed an image which was appropriate for hugely different countries – rich and poor, developed and underdeveloped, small and large. It needed to suggest potential points of entry for modern public health. It injected the importance of social position as determining health. It hinted at the importance of health governance, how decisions are made and by whom, as a factor shaping health systems (see Figure 1.11). Its version of this image, like Dahlgren and Whitehead's, suggests gradations of influence. The image is of a filtration process with an output. The Commission was set up to explore societal pressures and thus downplays the environmental or planetary factors in public health (the Commissioners were acutely aware of that).

Image 7: Public health as interactions and transitions

This image goes beyond systems thinking yet is also systemic. The image presents health as located in a web of relationships, all of which are undergoing change. Everything is in motion. The narrative is that everything is connected and has an impact on health. It addresses the health of the system, not just health as an outcome of the system. The message is that human health depends on maintaining eco-systems and the wider context.

Holly Dolan and her colleagues in Canada have proposed a model of health which still draws on the concentric circles of the previous image but gives a stronger emphasis to the environment (see Figure 1.12). Health is depicted as framed by four great 'restructurings': environmental, industrial, political and social.[60] The entire system is in transition, a reflection of the health and economic circumstances of a marginalised coastal community fallen into crisis owing to the diminution of the environment resources and over-harvesting of marine resources.

A variant of this image has been provided by the Dutch systems and sustainability thinkers Pim Martens and Jan Rotmans (Figure 1.13).[61] They draw attention to systems in transition. For them a transition is a social transformation process which is structural to society, long-term and large-scale, and interacts at different scale levels. Everything works at the same time, suggesting difficulties in disaggregating influences. The larger context is presented as three forms of capital: ecological (natural), socio-cultural and economic. Health is presented as just one, but a key, factor in sustainable development dynamics. Health is one 'cog' in the interplay of economics, society and the environment. The presence of unlabelled cogs suggests other multiple forces of transition. Forces or cogs are both modifying and modified because the entire process is integrated. Change is universal but can be brought to a standstill if any one cog seizes up. Health is located in wider dynamics.

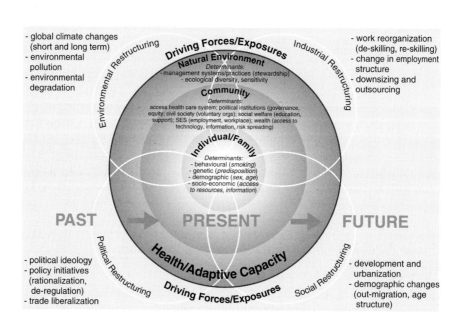

FIGURE 1.12 A socio-ecological framework of restructuring and health, based on research among Canadian coastal communities in the early 2000s

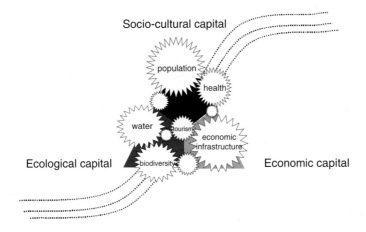

FIGURE 1.13   Health as part of a developmental 'machine' of multiple, interacting transitions

The same authors helped provide another version of this image (Figure 1.14). Here, population not individual or family health is placed at the centre, with globalisation forces at the extremity. Again, the image suggests a dimension of immediacy, ranging from proximal to distal to contextual. What is interesting in this version is that we are asked to think of public health in macro terms. It could be criticised for losing the personal.

Image 8: Public health as social movements and causes

This image is more collective, the appeal made for public health by social causes and movements. These, by definition, tend to be at the societal level. They include broad-based developmental campaigns such as anti-poverty, or appeals to resolve particular public health problems, from leprosy to blindness caused by infection, by Oxfam or WaterAid.

Today this kind of public health work often draws upon old images. Médecins Sans Frontières (Doctors Without Borders), for instance, presents an image where the expert-led (doctor-fronted) NGO takes the place of the solitary backroom scientist. This is medicine in blue jeans (but still wearing a white coat or gilet) on the front line (see Figure 1.15). It couples public health intervention with welfare. The World Bank typology divides such bodies into operational types delivering services and advocacy-based work.[62] Many do both, of course. The online edition of the *Yearbook of International Organizations* contains profiles of 63,056 active and inactive international NGOs in 2011. This was up from 6,000 in 1990.[63]

Some campaigns and movements in public health are and have been enormous. The originating model of such movements is arguably the anti-slavery movement

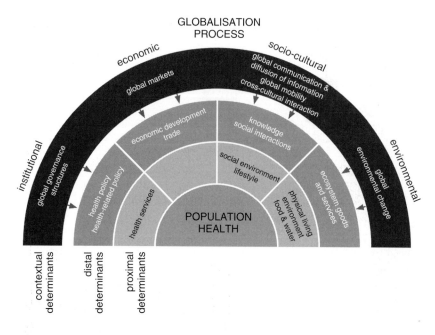

FIGURE 1.14   A conceptual framework for globalisation and population health

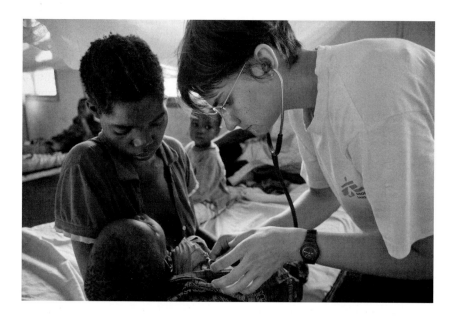

FIGURE 1.15   Dr Luisa Carnino doing the ward round in the paediatric department of Niangara hospital, Democratic Republic of Congo, June 2011

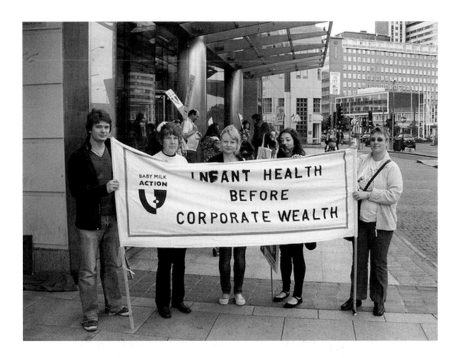

FIGURE 1.16   Demonstration against the corporate marketing of breastmilk substitutes in London in the early 2000s

of the early nineteenth century. Another was the mid-nineteenth-century campaign against child labour in the UK. Some such social movements are well organised and effective beyond their actual resources. An example of a late-twentieth-century public health movement which has been persistent, noisy and effective is the International Baby Food Action Network (IBFAN). For nigh on four decades, this global coalition of committed people has championed tighter controls on sales of breastfeeding substitutes, a particular concern in developing countries, where contaminated water being used in baby foods can and does kill. The image here is of campaigners fearlessly tackling giant interests; in IBFAN's case, this is often Nestlé, the world's largest food company (see Figure 1.16). Here, protecting public health means entering boardrooms, confronting boards and holding public bodies to account, to ensure that they are not seduced into accepting poor health standards. IBFAN campaigns with the WHO and Unicef, and also lobbies them, to ensure public hospitals support new mothers to breastfeed rather than accept 'soft' sold breastfeeding substitutes, when and if mothers are experiencing difficulties learning to breastfeed.[64]

Image 9: Public health as nanny or Big Brother

Our final image is one offered by vociferous critics of the existence of public health interventions. This too has a long pedigree across a wide range of politics but has been loudly voiced by, and to some extent is now owned by, New Right philosophers and neoliberal-supporting media.[65] It is of public health as nanny – interfering and bossy – or worse as Big Brother, as in George Orwell's novel *1984*.[66] Big Brother is all-controlling, fearsome and to be resisted.

At its most extreme, this image covers those who deny there is such a thing as the public health in the first place, arguing that people are all individuals. Most who subscribe to this image, however, accept a baseline of public health, but question strongly how far this should be extended in daily life. They resist unnecessary growth of power over the individual's right to determine his or her state. This is an economic libertarian position. It resists nannies. The nanny is presented as someone who knows better than you do, who protects you from yourself. It is an image which can be benign or malign.

Richard Epstein, a lawyer at Chicago University, argues that there is a baseline of activity which should be reserved as public health. This is the realm of infectious disease and contamination which no individual can see or control. Such threats to health warrant collective action by someone and some organisations beyond the individual's remit. This is the realm of what economists call public goods, as opposed to the realm of individual choice where the State should not enter.[67] In public health this means a distinction can be made between threats to health and who provides the healthcare. In this image, the heroes are ultimate individualists, and individuals are the heroes. Robert Nozick (1938–2002), a Harvard philosopher, argued that the State has no right to be in policy zones such as education or healthcare. There should be only a 'minimal state', having the characteristics of a nightwatchman, someone employed directly to warn citizens of threats, not necessarily to act on them.[68] In the lexicon of its more simplified exponents, this translates all social reality into ownership relations, 'where the government acts only as a policeman that protects man's rights'.[69]

Michel Foucault, the French historian of ideas, generally seen as of the political Left, saw fields like public health as an expression of disciplinary power – what he termed 'biopower' – by the State, companies, professions and others.[70] Public health is the imposition of an external order over individuals' bodies which becomes a form of internal order. This takes the nanny criticism towards social libertarianism not just economic libertarianism. The common themes are freedom, individual rights, and the exertion of moral power. This latter point also troubled, much earlier than Foucault, the Anglo-Irish writer George Bernard Shaw (1856–1950), who fought a long battle against vaccination, arguing that it constituted a form of professional tyranny, that its effectiveness was unproven and that it distracted social reformers' attention from where they ought to put their political attention, namely transforming society. Shaw saw vaccination as accepting an unnecessary level of dirt, squalor and poverty. In modern terms, he was

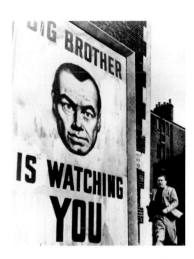
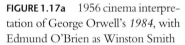

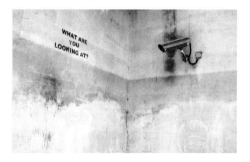

FIGURE 1.17a 1956 cinema interpretation of George Orwell's *1984*, with Edmund O'Brien as Winston Smith

FIGURE 1.17b The new reality is presented by satirical street artist Banksy highlighting now-ubiquitous CCTV

arguing that vaccination was a technical fix.[71] Many people promoting vaccination would not have seen it this way. Sanitarians stood on both sides of this argument, as we see in Chapter 10.

Utilitarianism, the calculus of pleasure and pain in which John Stuart Mill's (1806–83) thinking was originally embedded, has been the common basis of justification for public health interventions even today. But this image of an overweening State or the illegitimate exercise of power also traces its lineage back to Mill and other liberal, and sometimes socialist, thinkers of the Enlightenment. Mill's arguments have been deployed by those who regard the advocacy of public health to defeat the tobacco industry as a 'tyranny'.[72] We question later whether Mill's ideas can be used in this way. Mill, after all, believed in the nationalisation of land and co-operative ownership of the means of production.

Today a new strand of intellectualisation of these issues is the field of 'public health ethics'. One writer in this field claims that 'the principal issue of public health is that of paternalism'.[73] This focuses on discussion and application of Mill's 'harm principle', drawn from his book *On Liberty*, written in 1869.[74] The principal focus of public health ethics appears to be the interventions themselves rather than the state of public health, the social lines of inequality or how health is influenced by the wider determinants of public health. The tone of US public health advocates especially is often defensive.[75] Questions of the ethical or legitimate basis of action – the language of paternalism is only its more superficial representation – cannot be lightly dismissed. It surely needs to be understood in terms of the world confronting citizens, how they are informed and their opportunities for deliberating on such questions. It also needs to recognise that not everyone will agree and that not all measures are designed for everyone. Some measures may be centrally concerned with social justice, for example, but not all.[76] And what some call paternalism, be it the improvement of school meals or the banning of tobacco advertising, may accord with the informed collective will. It is there to enhance the conditions of life confronting the individual. The framing or shaping metaphors of such disputes are never neutral.

This list of images is not intended to be comprehensive. We could have spoken of many more. There is the image of public health as social care. This is composed of nurses, social workers and others in long-term relationships with people to help manage lives, distress, disabilities, families or poverty. Of course, most public health in this image occurs within families. Public health exists in retail settings too, as with community pharmacies, often with low-key advice but ubiquitous and often helpful in their presence. Public health is ever-present, often hidden in the background, in law, in risk environments, such as factories, kitchens, even dwellings; think of noisy neighbours. In workplaces many staff voluntarily take on duties such as first aid or health and safety monitoring. There are many more images, differing in form and function and varying from place to place and with different names and under guises in different societies. Many, as we argued, often have a limited presence in public consciousness, except of course when they are needed. We encounter these services and hidden functions as patients, users, customers, householders, pedestrians and drivers, and in many other ways.

These images, however, shape our understanding of health and help define it. Their cultural currency means people are being appealed to for support and recognition. The images may both extend and limit collective understanding of health. They are images, however, and thus are reduced versions of the real world, metaphors and metonyms with which to explore the thickets of knowledge and experience. We have explored these images to underline how the subject of this book is not abstract. Our consciousness of public health is already primed. There isn't a blank sheet of paper. The images exist. They are shared, often whether we recognise the process or not. The reality if not the image of public health is deeply embedded in the structure of society.

2

DEFINING PUBLIC HEALTH

The difference between the images we presented in the previous chapter and the formal definitions of public health, to which we now turn, further exposes the complexity of our task of trying to pin down what is meant by public health. We can look at health in terms of the simple origin of words and dictionary definitions. Here we find that the word 'health' is of Germanic origin, related to 'whole'; the simplest dictionary definition indicates that it means being free from illness or injury. English also used words like 'sanitary', from Latin, or 'hygiene', from Greek, which have a strong contemporary resonance in other European languages.

Our point is that in culture there are many images and meanings of what health is, some which persist over long periods, vying for attention. Others go through transformation over time. Health, sanitary, hygiene: all are related; all provoke varying inflections of meaning over time. Formal definitions, however, are generally encountered upon entering a field of thought and activity. Academics and scientists like definitions, which set the terms of intellectual engagement. We therefore now explore different definitions of health and public health, and how they emerged and whence they stem. This sketches the evolution of the words and meanings of health, disease and public health. Whereas the previous chapter suggested that the terrain of public health and policy is cut across by existing images and appeals, this chapter explores how the notion of public health has been fiercely and tightly nailed down in the past, with definitions being offered and countered. While there have been many attempts to define disease or health, there have been fewer attempts to define public health from outside the public health field. An example was a review of the terms 'health' and 'disease' by Swedish philosopher Lennart Nordenfelt, who barely mentions public health.[1] People working within public health have tended to coin their own definitions without the assistance of philosophers. That does not mean they have not drawn upon philosophical reasoning.

Before looking at some definitions it is pertinent to ask why anyone should bother with them at all. The simple answer is that definitions matter because people think they matter. Definitions bring into existence a special sort of social knowledge, a shared understanding among people about the objects of their world and how they ought to use language; this knowledge typically takes the form of an explicit, often authoritative articulation of the meaning of words and concepts and how they should be used to refer to reality. Although definitions provide a kind of security, what they offer can be deceptive. Definitions therefore might be better understood as a signpost to knowledge rather than the knowledge itself. The Swiss developmental psychologist and epistemologist Jean Piaget (1896–1980) once pointed to this issue: if representation of the world were in some sense a copy of the world, then we would have to already know the world in order to construct our copy of it![2] Definitions are a helpful route-stop on the way to knowledge, not the end of the journey.

This answer poses another question. What is the end of the journey? The classical answer, originating from within Platonic philosophy, and especially from Aristotle, is that a definition should lead to knowledge of the true essence of a thing. The more objective the understanding, the more free of subjective viewpoints and observer error, the more valid the knowledge. The Aristotelian approach thus leads to more objective knowledge and is therefore in accord with the physical sciences. The Enlightenment was launched on very different scientific premises. It was to be open-ended, experimental, expecting of the unexpected and driven by reason, not by metaphysics. Newton's theories on the motions of celestial bodies in the last decade of the seventeenth century, *Philosophiae naturalis principia mathematica* (Mathematical principles of natural philosophy) (1687), thought truly revolutionary at the time, provided Enlightenment thinkers, in particular the French *philosophes* (Voltaire attended Newton's funeral), with the scientific premises for a new age of rationalism. In one modern account, 'Newton paved the way by showing how reason enabled people to discover the natural laws to which all institutions should conform.'[3] However, the image of Newton as disinterested scientist or icon for a rational, secular age is essentially a mirage. Newton himself saw his discoveries merely as an investigation of God's plan.[4] To the question 'What is the end of the journey?' Newton's answer was simple: the discovery of God's intentions, not engagement with reason. Nevertheless, on this false attribution of intentions the Age of Enlightenment was launched.

Modern physics sees the role of humankind in rather different terms, although, in common background interpretations of science, Newtonian principles still rule. Although often castigated as unscientific, social science operates with the more humble but also more realistic principle that investigations into human behaviour operate with more muted principles of objectivity. Reflexivity is bound into its understanding; observer and observed are always linked. Only in the twentieth century was this same principle extended into natural science. One cannot now examine nature without altering it. This is the new principle. According to the physicist Werner Heisenberg (1901–75), the formulator of quantum mechanics:

Science no longer confronts nature as an objective observer, but sees itself as an actor in this interplay between man and nature. The scientific method of analysing, explaining and classifying has become conscious of its limitations, which arise out of the fact that by its intervention science alters and refashions the object of investigation.[5]

What do we draw from all of this? With definitions as with science, both natural and social, there is no possible end to the journey of ideas and meanings. This implies a more constructivist or pragmatic approach to the creation and use of definitions and a more historical understanding of the persistence of definitions. Definitions can be helpful, but if understood too rigidly might also be a hindrance.

In the section on images in Chapter 1, we skipped between health and public health, suggesting that images in mass consciousness use them almost interchangeably. We suggest now that definitions of health, like thinking about the role of definitions, began with Greek philosophy.

Greek thought has often been seen as the starting point for thinking about health. Rosen's *History of Public Health*, a book described as a 'grand narrative of progress',[6] provides an account of public health ideas from ancient times to the near-present (the mid-1950s).

There are several themes present in Greek thought. The first, their consideration of the human impact on the environment, has perhaps been the least mentioned. The chorus in Sophocles' *Antigone* sings of human dominion over the earth and its creatures, how humans subjugated the earth to their needs. There was certainly awareness among some Greeks that the biosphere was an organic whole, of which human existence was merely one part, and of environmental degradation. Plato noted that the hills of Attica were stripped of their forest cover and that the soil had disappeared. His is probably the earliest documentation of human environmental destruction.[7] One should be cautious in interpreting too much. No Greeks, as far as can be told, were environmentalists. The Greeks, Collingwood has argued, did not operate with the sense of nature that modern Europeans do, where it relates to the sum total or aggregate of natural things. Their response to the question 'What is nature?' was converted to the question 'What are things made of?'[8]

By the fifth century BC, the Greeks had come to recognise that evil spirits did not invade the body and cause disease and that magical incantations or potions were not curative. Nevertheless there were different viewpoints. Plato, following Socrates' commitment to the application of reason to build a comprehensive philosophy embracing both natural and social worlds, proposed that Truth resided in the realm of ideas or Forms. These were universal, unchanging and absolute. Aristotle thought that this approach ignored the material world. While the search for ultimate knowledge remained his final quest, he recognised that the human senses – sight, hearing, touch – were the means of investigation for phenomena and of real things.[9] The modern biological sciences are traceable back to Aristotle's investigations of nature.

Another group of thinkers, the Asclepiad medical community on the island of Kos associated with Hippocrates (460–370 BC), provides the fundamental

reference point for thinking about human health and its relation to the environment. It is not certain whether Hippocrates actually existed or his thoughts were
the product of multiple authors over time.[10] Whatever the truth, the Hippocratic
treatise *Airs, Waters, and Places* contains a mass of observations on how health is
influenced by prevalent winds, sunlight, water, soil, seasonal changes and local
vegetation and through the constitutional aspects of various populations in Europe
and Asia, which, when once formed by those influences, were carried forward by
heredity.[11] The treatise is a remarkable distillation of early wisdom. There are two
positive conceptions underlying the Hippocratic perspective, the synergy or co-
operation of the functions, and the action of the environment on the organism.
In the Hippocratic view a disease could not be treated without knowledge of 'the
whole', albeit this was an ambiguous term indicating either the body in general or
the patient's environment.[12]

These ideas might seem irrelevant or too loose for today. Health understanding
is more detailed. To return to the wisdom of the past, as some New Age philoso-
phies might design, would be to succumb to a world of painful teeth and possibly
early death from infected wounds. On the other hand, to say that health is now
managed on an industrial scale would be to think too small. In many countries the
healthcare industry is the largest employer, and as the population ages the sector
expands. What Greek thinking in contrast provides is a means of returning to some
first principles. It allows the modern world to examine its assumptions afresh and to
examine its modern disputes from an ancient, more holistic perspective.

This is precisely what occurred in the US public health world in recent decades.
The discussion of what the Greeks thought formed part of a long-running discussion about the fraying links between public health and medicine. So serious was
the issue of division between public health medicine and private personal medicine
thought to be in the 1990s that it led to a major research effort by numerous medical and public health bodies. Their study resulted in a report by the New York
Academy of Medicine in 1997. The authors of the report gave notable credit to
the medical philosophy of the Greeks. A return to the Greeks' outlook, they stated,
would help bond public health and medicine 'as a whole'. Indeed in the past the
combined effort by both sides of medicine 'served as a common ground for leaders
in medicine and public health from the mid-19th to the early 20th centuries'.[13] So
why deny that linkage? To some degree the august bodies involved in this enterprise were engaged in wishful thinking. Those with a sense of history would have
known it too, as we now see.

The contribution of Lemuel Shattuck

> What were the ideals with which the Fathers of Sanitation in New and
> in Old England began their work? They cannot be better expressed than
> in their own words . . . in the 1850 Report of the Massachusetts Sanitary
> Commission.
>
> *Sir Arthur Newsholme, 1920*[14]

The collision between public health and medicine in the USA has been long-standing, although the originators of the American Public Health Association (APHA) stood for a combined vision.[15] By the turn of the century, physicians constituted up to 80 per cent of the association's membership, and medicine and public health were often allies in nineteenth-century social and moral reform.[16] A major division, a harbinger of future strains, nonetheless appeared in the first serious attempt to establish a new infrastructure for public health in Massachusetts in the mid-nineteenth century. The lonely leader of this effort was one Lemuel Shattuck, later referred to as the 'founder' of public health in America[17] and by the APHA as its 'prophet'.[18] Shattuck's report has been referred to as one of the three main documents of US public health, the other two being *Medical Care for the American People*, the proposal for reform of medical care in the 1930s, and the 1964 Surgeon General's report *Smoking and Health*.[19]

Shattuck's efforts centred on the development of a health survey, following the example of Sir Edwin Chadwick's Sanitary Conditions Commission and report in England. Shattuck was not the first to conduct such an inquiry, but the first to do so systematically. Dr John Griscom's *Sanitary Condition of the Laboring Population of New York*, the title also reflecting the influence of Chadwick, had been published five years earlier. It had been compiled from requests for information among the concerned knowledgeable citizens of New York. Griscom was a Quaker.[20] Much of his account was an indictment of the social conditions afflicting the poor, especially immigrants, who Griscom argued were most afflicted by disease as they were

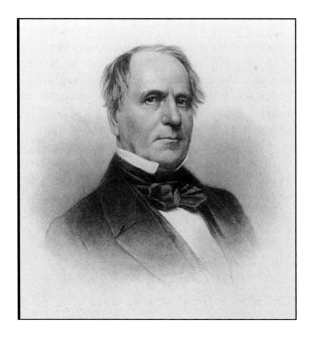

FIGURE 2.1 Lemuel Shattuck, public health reformer, in 1850s Boston, MA, USA

'required to live in dirt'.[21] By trade a bookseller and teacher, Shattuck was unusually skilful in social statistics, which he put to full use. Shattuck openly referenced his ideas to the ancient Greeks, summarised their ideas about health and how sanitary engineering had advanced in the Roman period, and then, jumping to his own times, commended the new field of hygiene as developed in France. The finale to his argument was the recently enacted English sanitary laws, which he presented as a role model for Massachusetts.

Shattuck's 300-page report was written for wide distribution, and 2,000 copies were printed. It was especially designed to appeal to the Bostonian culture and 'all the elements that are fundamental to Puritan doctrines'.[22] He knew his audience. He articulated a philosophical conception of health, a utilitarian justification for public investment, the authority of statistically endorsed facts, a values-based appeal, recommendations on health behaviours and the entreaty to different social groups for their involvement. His was a broad vision and appeal. His principal demand was that new institutions were needed, a general board of health on English lines, with promise of real improvement in health to follow. Today this would be called an 'evidence-based approach' based on its appeal to the 'abundant evidence in the history of sanitary experience'.[23] It was a highly imaginative construction.

Boston was not fertile ground for such ideas. The historian Wilson Smillie noted that in both city and state there was an absence of official health bodies, little or no understanding of disease, non-existent scientific research, and poorly trained local physicians with little interest in public health and indeed opposed to Shattuck. Nor was there any sense of a community unified and ready to mobilise behind public health reform. Following the publication of his study, Shattuck prepared a bill for legislature, which was rejected. He died nine years later, on the eve of the American Civil War. Without that war, others might have championed his plan; with it, the potential for support collapsed.

Shattuck's plan arguably lacked two essential ingredients for success: a public health movement to support him and a general public which recognised the problems he identified, both conditions which gave Chadwick room for political manoeuvre in England. The general board of health that Shattuck envisaged was not established until decades later, but Shattuck's conception of public health echoes down to today. Like Chadwick, he defined public health not as modes of intervention or an approach but as a state of society. He distinguished 'public health' from 'personal health', but also juxtaposed them. Both matter. Griscom had already made the distinction between 'public health' and 'individual health', noting their 'intimate connection' before Shattuck, with whom he was in active correspondence.[24] Shattuck placed disease in juxtaposition to broader social harms and made the case that prevention produces better results than curative medicine. Another feature of his ideas was the importance of making public health thinking understandable, relevant and popular. 'We would divest our subject of all mystery and professional technicalities; and as it concerns everybody, we would adapt it to universal comprehension, and universal application.'[25] The following passage, drawn from Shuttuck's report but quoted back to the members of Massachusetts

Board of Health in 1919 by the visiting Sir Arthur Newsholme (1890–1943), an English chief medical officer, is worth citing in full:

> WE BELIEVE that the conditions of perfect health, either public or personal, are seldom or never attained, though attainable; that the average length of human life may be very much extended, and its physical power greatly augmented; that in every year, within this Commonwealth, thousands of lives are lost which might have been saved; that tens of thousands of cases of sickness occur, which might have been prevented; that a vast amount of unnecessarily impaired health, and physical debility exists among those not actually confined by sickness; that these preventable evils require an enormous expenditure and loss of money, and impose upon the people unnumbered and immeasurable calamities, pecuniary, social, physical, mental, and moral, which might be avoided, that means exist, within our reach, for their mitigation or removal; and that measures for prevention will effect infinitely more, than remedies for the cure of disease.[26]

In this statement Shattuck contrasts a potential state of health and 'the conditions of perfect public health', and he also defines other terms such as 'sanitary' and 'hygiene', noting that they are just synonyms for health. He contrasts these with actual circumstances of disease, sickness and disability. Public health, in this account, is not itself an intervention but is obtained through intervention. Public health is aspiration to be measured against reality, and vice versa. This notion of a perfect or ideal state of health, outside the framework of disease, is today promoted by the World Health Organization, a century later. With Shattuck they were opposites held in tension, not entirely separate. In his time the principal threat to public health was infectious disease, but his notion of health was as both a population and an individual state – 'public health and personal health'. Public health is on the one hand something to be researched and acted upon and, on the other hand, a future state of 'perfect health' to be striven for. Shattuck's conceptualisation thus returns us to the discussion introduced earlier, that public health should be perceived as *both* a state, or potential state, and a set of methods, activities, professions, laws and more.

Since Shattuck, public health has come to be defined as an approach, a set of problems and a set of priorities. Seventy years after Shattuck's report, Charles-Edward Winslow (1877–1957), a bacteriologist at Yale University, defined public health in terms still resonant today:

> Public health is the science and the art of preventing disease, prolonging life, and promoting physical health and efficiency through organized community efforts for the sanitation of the environment, the control of community infections, the education of the individual in principles of personal hygiene, the organization of medical and nursing service for the early diagnosis and preventive treatment of disease, and the development of the social machinery which will ensure to every individual in the community a standard of living adequate for the maintenance of health.[27]

Winslow's definition, centring on the words 'the science and the art', is both abstract and substantive. In contrast to Shattuck, Winslow saw public health as a field of action. It was not just a state or condition of society but essentially concerned with the priorities and values. It was about what people working in public health *do*. In fact, the use of the term 'public health' in this particular sense was relatively new. The 1911 Index of the *American Journal of Public Health* contained no rubric for public health. Papers in the first volume appeared under State Medicine, or one of its sub-headings such as Public Hygiene, Hygiene of Occupations, Inspection of Food and Drugs, Sewerage, Water Supply, and a variety of disease headings categorised under Practice of Medicine such as Cholera Asiatica, Hydrophobia and Typhoid Fever. The *Index Medicus* only adopted the general term 'public health' in 1927.[28] Public health was now seen as a field, a set of professions and a set of aspirations and values to guide them.

Winslow's definition has defied time and obsolescence. The first two lines of the definition, with slight modification, feature as the official definition of public health across many English-speaking countries today. In this revised form it was adopted in England in 1988 at the behest of its then chief medical officer, Sir Donald Acheson (1926–2010). This was more than half a century after its original creation.[29] In this revision public health was defined as '[t]he science and art of preventing disease, prolonging life and promoting, protecting and improving health through the organised efforts of society'. Shorn of substantive details it stands almost as a mission statement. The fact that it started life as a US definition and was deployed by the English is deeply ironic. Winslow thought that British conceptualisations of public health influenced the early US public health movement and field. Here was a conceptualisation and definition making a round trip. Sadly, however, the discussion of the original definition and its purposes and context is often absent in current reviews of public health definitions.[30]

Modern definitions of public health are often criticised for being either too broad or too imprecise.[31] The field of public health has vastly expanded, and the practical sense in Shattuck's original definition has become obscured. Beginning with Winslow, public health has increasingly come to denote efforts or actions rather than public health as a state of society, although worries about threats to 'public health' remain an often-cited media narrative. In 1988 the US Institute of Medicine cut the definition and released a new, abbreviated definition. 'Public health is what we, as a society, do collectively to assure the conditions in which people can be healthy.'[32] This is now widely quoted. In speaking of the 'conditions' it does partially recall older concepts. Alongside the definition, the Institute added a more businesslike division of the definition into mission, substance and organisational framework. Thus the mission of public health is 'the fulfilment of society's interest in assuring the conditions in which people can be healthy'. The substance of public health is 'organized community efforts aimed at the prevention of disease and the promotion of health'. The organisational framework of public health 'encompasses both activities undertaken within the formal structure of government and the associated efforts of private and voluntary organizations and individuals'.[33] Another example of an everyday definition is one offered in an undergraduate course for public health trainees thus: '[t]he totality of all evidence-based public and private efforts that preserve and promote health and prevent disease, disability and death'.[34] This training definition, while having the advantage of brevity, presents public health with an impossible task: to base all public health on that which is 'evidence-based'.

Compared to these modern attempts to define public health, Winslow's 1920s definition appears the more satisfying. It has content. It draws upon his own working situation and knowledge. Winslow was a public health scientist, not a doctor, fully involved in, and cognisant of, the historical nature of the broad public health enterprise and the priorities of the day. Winslow understood too that conventional concepts of health and disease were always filtered through social constructs, even of an ancient kind. In a later book on the historical origins of disease, for example, he observed how even expressions like 'God bless you' or 'Gesundheit' to ward off TB and the use of curtains around a bed to combat smallpox were hangovers from the past which set the cultural framework of the present.[35] His understanding of priorities was drawn upon his experience, not simply academic theory of which there was very little. His mentor, Hermann Biggs (1859–1923), the Commissioner of Health for New York City, famous for the establishment of public health laboratories there, saw disease as the product of social and economic living conditions, urging action to improve these 'rather than a fight against germs'.[36] Winslow thought the field of public health was founded on sanitary engineering and laboratory science, but what he also understood was that it required medical support, an organised public health service, community health centres and universal health insurance.[37] One of the greatest difficulties for Winslow, as an academic teacher, was in persuading medical students to opt for a career in public health.[38] This is why, despite Winslow seeing the field of public health as a multidisciplinary enterprise, he was so keen to engender medical involvement. As we saw earlier in this chapter, the professional tension between public health medicine and medicine remains.

In contrast to the term 'public health', that of 'disease' might seem far easier to define. Disease appears as an objective state. It is an impairment of the body, something therefore definable in medical categories. The human body comprises many organ systems that have natural functions from which the systems can depart in many ways. Some of these departures from normal functioning are harmless or beneficial, but others are not. The latter are termed 'diseases'.[39] A disease is much like a weed being a plant in the wrong place, we might add. The language of disease does not stop with the body, however. It is also used to refer to things outside the body to which the body might or might not be susceptible. This adds confusion. Another common image, linked to some of the images discussed in the previous chapter, resonates with the Newtonian conception of nature. The diseased body is like a defective machine operating in a risky environment. However, the body is not a machine and, while every body is unique, it is also interconnected, not only with other bodies but with the environment. Some diseases, in fact, might not even be definable in organic terms at all, although there is always a temptation to look for organic causes. The battle over chronic fatigue syndrome might be viewed in these terms. Mental health problems may have an organic aspect, but which came first, the organic malfunctioning or the environmental stress?

The more disease is considered more fully, the less such apparently objective criteria seem to apply and the more it is necessary to call upon other disciplinary or philosophical standpoints. Understanding of disease then becomes a matter of perspective. The bio-medical approach looks for factors which explain individual differences.[40] Evolutionary biology might ask why members of species, or the species itself, are susceptible.[41] Sociologists might ask how a disease becomes defined and how and why we give meaning to it.[42] Each of these viewpoints is legitimate and reveals new knowledge. This is why we later examine different models of public health. No one definition, or model, will do. Nor is it helpful to term some definitions as 'scientific' and others as 'normative' or 'relational'. To group non-bio-medical understanding as non-scientific is itself interpretive. All conceptualisations, even bio-medical ones, are based upon created criteria which are subject to change. While there is often a desire to formulate value-free definitions, it may be impossible fully to extricate values from inquiry.[43] No single definition of disease can serve all the functions demanded of it. Professionally limited definitions have a practical form. They are functional. In the larger picture of the understanding of disease, however, definitions require some degree of interdisciplinary input.

So far we have discussed definitions of public health and disease. What of the definition of health itself? Our understanding of health, we saw, emerges from language. To say 'health' is to say 'wholeness', a concept familiar and understandable to Europeans and European-derived cultures, including, as we saw, the ancient Greeks. Wholeness implies some deep aspiration. It is not found in the practicality of the day-to-day. To be healthy, according to some, as we saw in Chapter 1, is to be one of the winners in the game of life. In everyday life too, we saw, the image of health so often becomes that of medicine or disease. The constitution of the World Health Organization, adopted in 1948, abandoned this dichotomisation of health and disease entirely. Drafted in 1946 by Dr Szeming Sze (1908–1998), a member of the Chinese delegation (trained at Cambridge University and St Thomas' Hospital, London) and later medical director for the UN and Dr Brock Chisholm (1896–1971), a Canadian psychiatrist who would become the WHO's first Director-General, it made the sharp distinction between disease and a more desirable state of health, to include both physical and mental health aspects. 'Health is a state of complete physical, mental and social well-being and not merely the absence of disease or infirmity.'[44] It is a statement of ideals, reminiscent of Shattuck's language of 'perfect health'. This new definition was coined after a devastating world war. New organisations of the UN were being formed to pool knowledge and action on economies, society and health. It is in the aftermath of war, said Richard Titmuss (1907–73), the British writer on social welfare, that people desire change, that social norms are disrupted, and when policy changes occur.[45] Such dreams of perfect health or complete health become possible.

The notion that perfect health and happiness were ever within humankind's possibilities, said the microbiologist René Dubos (1901–82), is a complete illusion which 'has flourished in many different forms throughout history'.[46] The reason he gave is the inevitable evolutionary mismatch between societal change and biological change. One mismatch he cited, which is considered later in this book, is the mismatch between the body's nutritional needs and the state of nutrition in society. Dubos, ever an insightful thinker, was perhaps being too categorical here. Societal aspirations have a real function, even if perfection will always be out of reach. Images of future possibility, which the WHO definition captures, were set against the realities of disease and death. Its drafters understood that. They also knew that at times of adversity, when the need for change is critical, aspirations may be a social necessity to ward off the fatalism which is so often the blockage to progressive social change.

The popular Irish playwright Oscar Wilde (1854–1900) saw such idealistic projections not as something for reproach but as a necessary element to any discussion of social progress. In *The Soul of Man under Socialism* he observed:

> A map of the world that does not include Utopia is not worth even glancing at, for it leaves out the one country at which Humanity is always landing. And when Humanity lands there, it looks out, and, seeing a better country, sets sail. Progress is the realisation of Utopias.[47]

Social progress is another persistent theme of this book. We saw already in examining varying images of health that concepts of social progress are contested. The ruling or dominant idiom of progress is enormously important for shaping social responses to new ideas.

The underlying assumptions of progress found in the WHO definition of health are now interpreted in the cooler light of market-led economics (discussed in Chapter 8). Certainly it falls outside the conventional bio-medical model. In other words it does not, according to one criticism, appear 'reasonable'.[48] The WHO definition was extensively debated on the occasion of its sixtieth anniversary in the *British Medical Journal* (*BMJ*), where many views were logged and blogged. A common theme was its impracticality. What was the function of speaking of ideals when 40 per cent of the world's population lacked clean water? Because the definition included the element of well-being, argued one epidemiologist, it corresponded more closely to happiness than to health and, since happiness was 'essentially boundless', it was promoting the unobtainable.[49] The *BMJ* debate's initiators, seeing the potential for almost endless discussion, proposed that:

> any attempt to define health is futile; that health, like beauty, is in the eye of the beholder; and that a definition cannot capture its complexity. We might need to accept that all we can do is to frame the concept of health through the services that society can afford, and modulate our hopes and expectations with the limited resources available, and common sense.[50]

The *BMJ* debate reveals how expectations have shifted. The provision of health, note, not the desirability of health, becomes principally a question of affordability. It is a product, 'a service'. Such thinking is a form of bio-medical utilitarianism, turning a discussion of health into a discourse on the rationing of medical products. But again, in utilitarian terms, what society could afford *not* to have its citizens have access to clean water? What society could not afford to ensure that all citizens had access to better medical care? The answer is, we later see, that for these questions even to be posed is to be located in history, in a certain democratic discourse of entitlements, progress and values.

Besides the main much-cited central phrase of the 1946 WHO definition, there were eight additional clauses, although these were barely mentioned in the *BMJ* debate. These clauses included the notion that the highest attainable standard of health is a fundamental right of everyone, that the health of all is fundamental to the attainment of peace, that the promotion and protection of health are of value to everyone, that unequal development is a danger, that the health of children is of basic importance, that the benefits of medical, psychological and related knowledge are essential, that promoting health requires the informed and active co-operation of the public, and that governments have a responsibility for the health of their peoples 'which can only be fulfilled by the provision of adequate health and social measures'.

No definition of health, for the reasons set out above, can be fully satisfactory. There have been offers of alternatives. It has been suggested that, given the difficulty of forming a unified definition of health, it may be better to speak of medical health, biological health or social health.[51] Others suggest that a redraft of the WHO definition is required which includes the loss of body functions, that poor health restricts lives and that the loss of health restricts relationships.[52] While worthy, such proposals may be beside the point. The notion of completeness in the WHO definition – for that matter the sense of 'wholeness' in the single word 'health' – already addresses everything. Turning it into a constantly updating list may be helpful, but only in restricted contexts. The WHO definition, despite criticisms, may be 'fit for purpose', to use a common epithet of public health organisational terminology. In fact, it probably does not really function as a definition at all. It is however a statement of universal aspiration. The central criticism is that the WHO definition of health is essentially impractical utopianism. The same objection might also befall the Universal Declaration of Human Rights or the numerous charters or declarations, often issued via the UN, which we list in Chapter 12 (see Table 12.1).

The broad ambitions of the WHO definition are periodically reconfirmed. Three decades after its original formulation, the Declaration of Alma-Ata added the line 'whose realization requires the action of many other social and economic sectors in addition to the health sector'.[53] In 1986 the Ottawa Charter for Health Promotion, adopted at the First International Conference on Health Promotion in Ottawa, Canada, stressing the importance of action outside the medical domain, extended the notion of health to that of 'a resource for everyday life'. According to the distinguished US epidemiologist Lester Breslow, this newer concept reflects the growing perception that people 'nowadays want health in order to live: to do the things important to them' and to build their capacities for health and life enjoyment.[54] All such additions speak to the continuing and perhaps necessary contestation of meaning and interpretation.

A summary of this discussion now seems in order. We suggested at the beginning of this chapter that definitions are best seen as signposts to knowledge, something which should promote rather than close discussion. We examined, all too briefly, some definitions of public health, disease and health. No definition, we suggested, offers crystal clarity, although the distinction between public health as a 'state of existence' and the interventions and policies to obtain that state does seem fundamental. In moving from the priority and task-driven definition offered by C.-E. Winslow to its attenuated form in recent official definitions of public health, we thought that historical anchors to practice had been lost. We also suggested that, while definitions of disease may appear to have an objective character, this occurred only in disciplinary-defined terms. A fuller concept of disease requires interdisciplinary formulation. In looking at the WHO definition of health, we saw that the idealism of the past is now subject to the financial and other pressures of the present. In these circumstances, practicality, said critics, should rule. In any case, from an evolutionary perspective, appeals to perfect health are illusory. For us, there is a role for both aspirational and functional definitions, which must therefore coexist.

Perhaps so, but what we have stressed has been the need for integration. And the return to a sense of integration alerts us to a question that has so far been inadequately formed in all these attempts to define health: the tension between the environment and human health. The Greeks thought health and disease were linked to the environment. It would be false to describe them as environmentalists in the modern sense, although they also understood that the human presence altered the environment. What all these definitions leave out is the human population's impact on the 'health' of nature, not just, we see later (see Chapter 10), the impact on flora and fauna but across the biological world as such. Thinking about the health of humans seems difficult enough, but introducing the health of the environment opens up a potentially vast terrain of inquiry and action.

Environmental feedback on health is growing, although it has been present since humankind first began to tame animals, establish agriculture and live a settled way of life. The ecological economist Robert Costanza has introduced the concept 'eco-system health' to link the health of populations and the health of the environment. This perspective resonates with our image of public health as a social-ecological set of relationships over time. For Costanza, a fuller and more systematic definition of health needs to be built from ecological and human health 'systems' operating together in order to achieve a desirable sustainable end point. It offers the prospect of a project no less ambiguous or difficult than the defining of human health. Assessing eco-system health, for Costanza, is more like assembling pieces of a puzzle, and no one part of the puzzle can ever be comprehensive enough or exact enough by itself.[55] Costanza refers to the eco-system, we refer here to 'eco-systems'. We prefer to see eco-systems as differentiated by many properties, histories and dynamics, which in combining together may be more or less vital to their sustainability. Of course, in terms of living circumstances humankind confronts many different types of climatic, biotic and abiotic environments. In our view it is possible to depict the relationship between human and

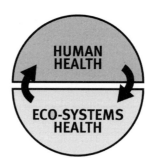

FIGURE 2.2 The dynamics of Ecological Public Health: a simple model

eco-systems health in simple terms pictorially. This is shown in Figure 2.2. Here human health is above, and depends upon, eco-systems health. They interrelate, interact and are in tension, but they are also inseparable. For us, this is the core dynamic tension at the heart of what we call Ecological Public Health.

While a new environmental conception of health, what we in this book call Ecological Public Health, might seem a difficult and complex task, that is now the twenty-first century's unavoidable task.

Twenty-first-century public health: the need for new ambitions

Some of our discussion of public health in Part I – its images, definitions and traditions – shows that public health does have some common themes and perspectives. Public health is obviously many things, but it starts off with a root point, simply given in the juxtaposition of the two words 'public' and 'health'. We now try to outline the characteristics public health has or might have in this century. We begin to ask: is public health now something new in the age of globalisation and climate change? Or is it merely changing focus but with the survival of early traditions, because the early problems remain albeit in new form? Or is public health no longer a coherent entity at all, and might it be good to abandon the notion of a coherent and integrated project? In short, we now begin to face a big question throughout this book: what is good public health?

Ambition 1: Recognise the challenge of complexity

The first challenge to be faced is complexity. We just saw one illustration of complexity, the puzzle-like character of eco-system health. The term 'complexity' is frequently encountered, but what does it mean? One frequent source of confusion is the word itself. 'Complex' is often a synonym for 'complicated'. Complexity does not mean complicated or else impossible to understand, although certainly the roots of complexity thinking are complicated and scattered. In its modern conceptualisation complexity occurs when the elements of a system interact in a non-linear fashion, that is to say where there is no necessary proportionality between causes and effects and when it is impossible to predict system behaviour from only knowledge of the elements themselves.[56] In a complex system there may be sensitivity to initial conditions, as well as numerous feedback loops and multiple chains of interaction.

This term is increasingly used across the natural and social sciences, although there are differences in emphasis. The theoretical physicist Murray Gell-Mann, winner of the Nobel Prize in physics in 1966 for the discovery of the quark, the simplest component of matter, is one of a group of scientific thinkers at the Santa Fe Institute in New Mexico, USA who think that the attributes of complexity extend across all features of life.[57] Although this group of scholars have achieved much in understanding complexity, applying it from biology to molecular evolution, they admit that they have been far less successful in providing answers to the problems the investigation of complexity has raised.

Complexity thinking has also been applied to the consideration of culture. According to cultural analyst Mark Taylor, 'We are living in a moment of unprecedented complexity, when things are changing faster than our ability to comprehend them.'[58] The idea is that the speed of change is upsetting humankind's sense of stability. We now live in conditions of modernity where everything once accepted is overturned. That is not a new thought. The German sociologist Jürgen Habermas has noted that the 'modern' displacing the traditional was first used in the fifth century, when it was used to discriminate between pre-Christian and Christian Rome.[59] It is, however, a serious proposition. Our discussion of the Cultural Transition in Chapter 11 takes up how far it is true and how it might influence health.

Complexity thinking has, by degrees, entered public health thinking. In fact, complexity was already there before the term became formed as an independent concept. Complexity arrived in biology through the discovery of natural selection by Darwin and Wallace. Complexity in the biological sense is what evolution is all about. What once used to be thought of in only simple terms, the existence and spread of bacteria, for example, is now conceived of in terms of biological complexity. As humankind has created new antibiotics, bacteria have developed an evolutionary response. That biological feedback exists was recognised in the 1940s, almost at the very moment of the discovery of antibiotics. Bacteria evolve, often through human influence, such as in reaction to antibiotics. This critically important issue is examined in Chapter 10. Another property of complexity thinking, non-linearity, is demonstrated through the notion that chronic diseases develop within a 'web of causality'.[60] Causal factors are not equal or direct. In the past the task of epidemiology was to isolate the causes that unidirectionally influence disease states. Today this perspective is being replaced by one based on layered, multilevel patterns of cause and dynamic feedbacks.[61]

Any new theoretical trend is likely to generate its faddish elements. On this basis complexity might seem like a new, muddying feature for contemporary public health, one which the originators of public health thinking fought against. Our counter is that, while past public health challenges may appear simple in retrospect, this belies their historical reality. Complexity occurred in the past as it does today. Today it is just that much easier to recognise it.

Cultural complexity often provides the overlay to other forms of complexity. In the section on images in Chapter 1, for example, it was argued that multiple factors combine to define and give context to public health. The implication is that all human understandings, not just of culture but of all science, are situated within a historical and social context. While there appear to be disease processes of illness having the characteristic of straightforward simplicity (a broken leg but not a common cold!), there is an equally long list of contemporary health problems which defy either simple characterisation or simple remedy. Most obviously this applies to the vaguely named non-communicable diseases (NCDs) – obesity, drug and alcohol misuse, coronary heart disease, strokes, etc. – but it also applies to infectious and communicable diseases. As an example of the latter HIV/AIDS has a theoretically simple means of spread – body fluids, blood, etc. – but the adaptability of the virus and complex cultural contexts mean that preventing and treating HIV/AIDS are anything but simple. HIV/AIDS is a classic example of a complex problem occurring on both the biological and the cultural plane.

Complexity, like the acceptance that some problems require subtle understandings or a long-term outlook, is not attractive for the media or politicians. Media narratives attempt to present health matters in simple, understandable, dramatic terms. A gene is found which 'explains' a disease or characteristic, like a crime. A politician plays a moral trump card – such as personal responsibility – which locates health within the hands of the unwell, but also forecloses discussion of its social determinants. To tackle public health in such a world requires complexity to be acknowledged and to be a key characteristic of the intellectual framework.

Twenty-first-century health challenges therefore are characterised by scale, scope and unevenness. These can be grasped only by complex rather than single-dimensional thinking. Although hygiene continues to be a major public health problem, particularly in the developing world, to see health as 'cleansing' is no longer adequate to the challenges known to exist. A list of twenty-first-century challenges includes:

- exploitation of finite resources previously thought to be infinite;
- mega-trends such as climate change or mass urbanisation;
- destruction of the natural environment 'commons' in the name of progress;
- economic policies accelerating inequalities;
- the rise of non-communicable diseases;
- the globalisation of culture around Western consumption models and lifestyles;
- the delocalisation of the economy and culture;
- political failure to grapple with the dynamics of health.

These need to be addressed in the name of public health. Like many, we accept the evidence of a powerful list of structural drivers and challenges ahead. They include:

- demographics and the rapid rise of anticipated populations;
- pressures on the food system;
- energy use and availability;
- water stress and threats to habitats;
- climate change and its knock-on effects such as spread of disease;

- social inequalities within and between societies;
- the fragility of paid employment and the relocation of work by powerful companies and economic forces;
- pressures on housing from, on the one hand, de-ruralised populations and, on the other hand, demographic change;
- the consequences of democratic deficits on the health conditions of the economically weak.

The scale and range of these problems require big thinking if proponents of public health are to reconnect and relocate their roles to help people and societal processes live within biological and natural processes and to fuse human and planetary health.

Ambition 2: Construct a narrative with contemporary appeal and bite

Public health is about dealing with current realities but facing future trends which might threaten ill-health. The history of public health already sketched suggests that it is made by a combination of threat and opportunities, if not opportunism. Contemporary literature currently lacks a good narrative to 'sell' to the public let alone politicians. The political leverage of public health is weak. It is associated with crisis rather than a good news story. Yet the classic appeal of public health has been through three features: crises (things need to be done); cost (pay now to save later); and consequences (if the leaders refuse to act, then they are culpable).

Part of the problem for public health today is that when systems are working it is a non-story. Yet the pages of public health journals are full of problems lacking political and public leadership. Time and again, public health proponents complain of failure by politicians to dare to confront powerful forces whose interests are threatened by any ameliorative action. Tobacco is an example. Half a century after the evidence of its ill-health functions emerged, tobacco is still legal, growing in world use and celebrated on stock exchanges as a reliable investment, even during economic downturns. Part of the challenge for twenty-first-century public health is to create narratives and to nurture leaders who will address complexity at all levels of politics, from global to local.

Ambition 3: Recast public health as interdisciplinary collaboration

By the mid-twentieth century, public health work had become a mainly medically dominated field. By the end of the century, medical public health practitioners accepted that, such was the breadth of public health challenges, a multidisciplinary response was called for. The problem with the multidisciplinary perspective is not just that some disciplines are accorded more power than others but that the conceptualisation of the field assumes that the Bio-Medical model (which we explore in the next chapter) is the main framework for addressing it. Medicine becomes the filter through which non-medical professions are included.

We see a tension between the reality of *multidisciplinary* public health (actually shaped by a 'pecking order' of value and skills) and the ideal of an *interdisciplinary*, more equal collaboration. A multidisciplinary model is about the arrangements of skills and conceptualisations. An interdisciplinary model is based on the assumption that the boundaries are neither fixed nor impermeable and may be a hindrance to the re-conceptualisation of the problem and the means of addressing it. Critical skills and perspectives may even be entirely absent. The interdisciplinary ideal is, however, threatening. It recalls an age before academic and professional divisions were enshrined and self-reinforcing.

We are not arguing for a collapse of disciplinary knowledge and skills. On the contrary. But we are arguing that public health improvement in the twenty-first century requires far better mutual understanding of different disciplines' training, publications and experience. A phenomenon of twentieth-century life was the growth of boundaries, specialisms and professions. The twenty-first century requires fluidity of boundaries and therefore, while retaining knowledge within disciplines, the development of interdisciplinary knowledge.

Table 2.1 gives the US government's Centers for Disease Control's list of ten great public health achievements in the USA in the twentieth century. This was produced to greet the new millennium. One can argue about the list. Why is there nothing on housing? Can we really celebrate tobacco when its use and export remain legal and when US tobacco firms, alongside British, dominate world markets? Why is inequality not included when the evidence of its impact on health is so strong? Yet the importance of this and such lists is that around a third of the achievements are securely within a bio-medical framework. Two-thirds are not.

We see public health as a debate between different traditions and support the notion that public health cannot rule professions in or out, if only because the shaping factors of health may be professional, non-professional or completely unrelated to any public-health-inspired actions at all. James Riley, a US professor of history, in his review of the factors underlying the Epidemiological and

TABLE 2.1   The US Centers for Disease Control's ten great public health achievements in the twentieth century

1	Immunisations
2	Motor-vehicle safety
3	Workplace safety
4	Control of infectious diseases
5	Declines in deaths from heart disease and stroke
6	Safer and healthier foods
7	Healthier mothers and babies
8	Family planning
9	Fluoridation of drinking water
10	Tobacco as a health hazard

Health Transition (see Chapter 5) has discerned six 'tactical areas' through which society-wide health improvement has occurred. These include public health, medicine, wealth and income, nutrition, behaviour and education.[62] The word 'tactical' implies directed actions and sources of change that may be unrecognised or uncoordinated. The list may be longer, for example he leaves out the environment. Nevertheless Riley points to a range of possibilities far beyond the narrow bio-medical that tends to dominate what is meant by public health. The central domain of public health for the twenty-first century may not be bio-medical but social. With evidence about social inequalities and determinants (such as from the WHO Commission cited earlier), the impact of fiscal or other measures to reduce inequalities may be among the most potent public health actions. As the Edinburgh University microbiologist Dorothy Crawford has observed: 'It is glaringly obvious . . . that poverty is the major cause of microbe-related deaths.'[63] And, with climate and water stress, environmental actions may well be the key to health improvement. This is a warning about the differentiation of categories through which health improvement occurs. The biological or bio-medical perspective cannot be lost but strengthened, requiring a realignment of biological practice to biological knowledge, particularly in the light of growing antibiotic resistance and the resurgence of infectious diseases.[64]

Our perspective on public health is shaped by our own training as social scientists, of course. And in part this book explores the contribution of social science to public health. We see two traditions feeding into our broad view of Ecological Public Health (which is outlined in greater depth in Chapter 10). One is broadly from the natural sciences and the other from social science. One is broadly about biological relations, the other about consciousness. This is an awkward intellectual stance. Academic and professional careers tend to be based on specialism, yet society needs interdisciplinary collaboration. This requires policy and political reprioritisation. There is little or no pressure for this to happen. Money tends to flow through and to disciplines in their 'silos'.

Ambition 4: Espouse public health as societal progress not just professional toolbox

Adam Smith, one of the founding fathers of political economy and hence of modern economics, saw an index of social progress as the pace of population expansion. Looking across to the (then) American colonies, he saw that their population was rising rapidly and deduced that people were socially and physically better off than in the mother country, the UK. He was right. The colonialists were taller than the British and even taller than the European aristocracy.[65] America had plenty of food; dispersed populations didn't suffer urban infectious disease as severely, although severely enough.[66] There was a more democratic and in today's parlance inclusive social milieu. But, by the early nineteenth century, these US anthropometric data had begun to show a steady decline. The failure to maintain material progress and the rise of the diseases of urbanisation were confounding health and social progress.

Karl Marx (1818–88) criticised but learnt from political economists like Smith. In his essay 'The Holy Family', Marx praised the French thinker Charles Fourier (1772–1837) for declaring progress to be an 'inadequate abstract phrase', not only because 'even the most favourable brilliant deeds seemed to remain without brilliant results, [and] to end in trivialities', but also because 'all progress of the spirit has so far been progress against the mass of mankind'.[67] But he was speaking here of progress 'of the spirit', in the realm of ideas alone, and lack of progress for the majority of the population. He was quite ready to admit to progress in the material development of productive forces, in technology and in what he referred to as the 'movement of the great mass', found in their craving for knowledge and cultural development. Progress, this implied, came with two faces, the ideal and the material. Real progress required the realignment of both, said Marx and the nineteenth-century progressives such as J.S. Mill.

What's at stake here is how to measure public health advance. Does one take purely biological measures of the standard of living? Or take well-being? Or both? Or is public health merely the absence of disease? Or is the WHO picture of 'ideal health' a realistic goal? Historically, there is a big debate about how to judge progress. Is it good health or wealth? Or the distribution and interaction of both? We see public health as centrally involved in this debate. There is a battle for the soul of public health as a project. Is it progressive or repressive? Does it restrict itself to action only when the evidence is available, or should it operate through knowledge and judgement? Does it see the poor as an object of pity or a problem? Does it just study the determinants of health or confront them appropriately? These are not a new set of questions and professional dilemmas, of course. Indeed, the assumption that there is progress occurring in some idealised form should be judged warily.

The picture we paint of public health is as a core area of public policy and action, which is now torn between competing interests: professions, the State, civil society, corporations, politics and the media. We see public health also as a social movement, people uniting to demand and achieve better health at the public level. This interpretation could be seen as a purely Western one, and it could be argued that the traditions we explore here are limited by time, place and history. The European and North American conditions are not replicable. But it would be folly to reject this experience, not least since it appears to be going down a cul-de-sac, or at least having a moment of reflection about where it is going.

Ambition 5: Build public health around the fact of continuous change

The protection and promotion of the public health always have to address change. At one level, this is an obvious point: bodies grow and die as part of 'natural' life cycles. But the public health goes beyond biological processes. Whether at the economic or societal or material level, the health of the public is always altered or shaped by the dynamics of life. Today, public health articulates this philosophical reality through the language of 'determinants'. The language of 'social determinants' was introduced in the 1950s by microbiologist René Dubos. He was referring to the social determinants of 'human fitness'. Implicitly this was an evolutionary approach to human health. In this respect humankind was as susceptible to changes in the environment as are 'animals and plants'.[68] Dubos gave an example of poor 'fitness' as the rapid and continuing changes in human diet, which were set by entirely social criteria rather than by 'biological criteria', that is to say by the body's physiological needs. This changed circumstance created environmental-genetic mismatch, to be considered in Chapter 9. A rather different interpretation of social determinants, with more sociological roots,[69] has since arisen to take the place of Dubos's more ecologically related understanding (as with the WHO Commission cited earlier). In either interpretation of social determinants the public health requires an understanding of change, and what drives the relationships of people to each other and their environments.

The systems images discussed earlier are some attempts to grasp this aspect of the challenge for public health in relation to societal dynamics. Health may be advanced, threatened but certainly shaped by these dynamics. In Chapters 4 to 12, we address the key transitions that we believe twenty-first-century public health faces. These transitions might be changed by a more articulate and firm public health voice. Or the public health might be shaped by them. That plasticity of the future is what the cybernetics and systems imagery sketched earlier usefully represents.

If anything has threatened the twentieth-century approach to public health it could be argued that it was and is globalisation. At the end of the century, apparently suddenly, public health professions began to voice concerns about globalisation as a common threat.[70] No longer would they be able to assume that they could resolve public health problems within their realms of influence, whether locally or nationally. Critics had already dissected the realities of globalisation.[71] It is a misnomer, they said, a composite term for what is in reality many dynamics and trends. Many of these rightly trouble public health analysts. Many too are not that new but are merely new versions of older dynamics. Examples include the spread of cosmopolitan culture, the internationalisation of trade, the rapid expansion of private investment agreements, privatisation taking over previously public assets, the power of large corporations, the use of military might to protect strategic resource interests, and the arms trade itself. All these have been manifest before today, and have had direct health consequences.

Yet today, despite recognising these old trends in new form, we accept that there are also some new features which stretch the capacity of public health authorities. The scale of change in production systems, the global nature of supply chains, the extent and potential impact of some new technologies (e.g. nuclear), and the enormous destruction of biodiversity: all these pose qualitatively different and new threats to public health. On top of these – some argue caused by these – are the late twentieth-century massive liberalisation of trade and the effects of political weakening of the State responsibilities and barriers between nation states. Underneath, the reverse side to globalisation, is delocalisation, the trend for work, play, consumption and culture to be formed outside and almost untouched by local actors. Nineteenth-century public health was local. Today it has to operate on multiple levels, and 'the local' might not be any longer the most special realm.

The history of public health is peppered with attempts to grapple with international threats to health. Since the nineteenth century, there have been co-ordinated public health actions on issues such as the spread of infectious diseases, illicit drugs and tobacco, unsafe foods, and the spread of toxic products. The delocation of production, the emergence of long supply chains, and the intensification of high-energy production systems across the planet mean that the effects of toxins and pollution may cross borders and be of global significance. These trends mean that public health actions may not be medical at all but solely political, such as aiming for new international agreements on health, safety and standards.

Over centuries, not just communicable diseases have been spread from one country to others but non-communicable diseases too. For example, the narcotic drug trade flourished under the British East India Company in the eighteenth century, as it introduced and shipped opium from India to China.[72] Arguably, tough twentieth-century trade agreements are nothing compared to the eighteenth-century slave trade and 'golden triangle' in which goods were shipped from Britain to Africa, and exchanged for slaves forcibly taken to the West Indies, which were traded for sugar for the industrial working class.[73] The 1930s Tuskegee experiment covered in Chapter 1 is a recent manifestation of old-established economic forces of dehumanisation converted into denying good health and dignity to deliberately under-informed vulnerable groups. Figures such as the English radical Thomas Paine (1737–1809) and the French aristocrat Alexis de Tocqueville (1805–59) viewed slavery as akin to a grave infection on the American body politic, which they saw as an otherwise democratic project. Today, when the WHO deems violence a public health issue,[74] this is a welcome acknowledgement that it always was. And what historians see as social movements were also public health movements. Dignity and life expectancy go hand in hand with campaigns to promote them.

In Chapters 4–12, we go beyond the globalisation debate and propose some main transitions and trends which we judge to be critical for any decent conception of the public health. They are: Demographic, Epidemiological, Urban, Energy, Economic, Nutrition, Biological and Ecological, Cultural and Democratic. Each of these transitions shapes the potential for – and threats to – the public health. Whatever image of public health one draws from, in those we explored above, they are dealing with change. In our analysis, therefore, we place change at the heart of what is meant by public health and what any project or profession does which claims to be concerned about public health. Our case for placing these transitions, changes and systems dynamics – call them what one will – at the heart of public health requires a long view. Unravelling complexity requires long-term strategies. Our conception of public health therefore questions those who think public health comes in small, localised, short steps.

Ambition 6: Reassert public health as a democratic project

We see the pursuit of the public health as a cornerstone of the long process of the democratic project of enfranchisement. In effect, this is the unfinished and continuing legacy of the Enlightenment, the belief that people can live better, more fulfilled, happier, healthier, wealthier lives by sharing common values of dignity and collective advancement. The arguments have raged in political discourse about the relative emphases on the individual or the collective, the family or the mass, the elite or the majority, but the common democratic project of enfranchisement and pursuit of the common good sees public health as both a motor – a 'cog' in the earlier image – and an outcome.

In the foundation years of modern public health thinking in the nineteenth century, no society on earth was a democracy as the word is understood today. And yet pressures from below always mattered and yielded expenditure and action by ruling elites even when they were reluctant. Arguably, pressure from below in society was essential to secure public health action. In the nineteenth century, much that was achieved in the name of public health in Europe was cleaning up the effects of the transition to industrial capitalism, and was about protecting all classes of society from contagion and threats to the economy. Unravelling the competing interests of different social classes and interest groups is part of the history of public health. (See Chapter 12 for a lengthier account.)

Looking ahead is far more hazardous than reviewing the past, of course, but we see public health as the major contributor and defining principle for democracy. We go so far as to assert that the state of public health is a measure of success or failure for democracy. This is recognised but not often adequately voiced by modern public health practitioners. Why else promote the rights of women and children if it is not to protect and promote their health? Why else promote the necessity of reducing gross inequalities of wealth and opportunity within and between societies if it does not yield improvements in health? Public health and democratic advance are inextricably entwined. Vice versa, if health declines, this is a comment on lack of democracy. This core reality was recognised by the studies of famine by Sen and Drèze.[75] Lack of food is often not the problem; lack of 'entitlement' and aspirations is. Would the Irish famine have happened if there had been democracy? Public conceptions of entitlement define whether food is or is not made available according to need. This in turn may reflect access to information and publicity. But that is also the stuff of democracy in the Enlightenment tradition. In this sense, public health rejects fatalism (and religious notions of acceptance).

There are both narrow and wider approaches to what is meant by democracy. Social justice requires a *public* infrastructure benefiting all not just the few or elite. Democracy is about processes – *how* things are done, not just *that* they are done. That is why the public health can be such a sensitive issue. It involves judgements, and conceptions of legitimacy and acceptability. Who owns your body? Whose responsibilities shape what can and cannot be done to prolong your life or quality of life? How can collective obligations shape population health? These questions emerge from the images we have explored above.

Democracy, however, is always a wild card. The imposition of public improvements from above or conversely the denial of the worth of investing in collective measures to improve public health can occur in formally democratic systems. Likewise, public health improvement can occur under autocratic political structures. But the results of improved health automatically improve democracy by giving people, individually and collectively, hope of a better life, sufficient to begin to look above the grinding pressures of daily existence. Our argument is that public health is part of the development of democracy, and democracy is central to the development of public health.

If one follows the view of Immanuel Kant, mentioned earlier, which says that Enlightenment is centrally concerned with education and the development of personal responsibility, obligation and duty, then one can see that the broader view of democracy is not just about voting for one's own short-term interests in the ballot booth but also about the general good and infrastructure to enable both collective and individual progress.[76] By the late twentieth century, however, the world increasingly was not shaped by Enlightenment values but dominated by political and commercial power blocs. As the world's banking and debt crisis from 2008 showed, economics is shaped by and for the interests of large corporations and the financial system. The bankers' building of the consumer-debt-fuelled crisis should have been their risk. Instead, their private risk and exposure were converted into a constriction of public services, to pay off debt run up by governments desperate to save the banks.[77] The resolution of this undoubted crisis led not to a settlement of the unregulated and unaccountable workings of the financial services industry but to a public sector debt crisis. This has had the knock-on effect of reducing the public sphere, and the re-emergence of a view that public health is a drag on economic growth and that it ought to be more of a responsibility of individuals. History suggests, on the contrary, that improving public health enables economies to thrive. Our point is that thus is public health inextricably woven into notions of democracy, progress and shaping the future. It is contested.

Ambition 7: Rethink public health on ecological principles

Public health requires a framework of thinking which locates human health in the context of other dimensions of existence. Charles Darwin (1809–82) at the end of his masterpiece *On the Origin of Species* (see Box 2.1) used the metaphor of an 'entangled bank' – one can visualise him looking at riverbanks or hedgerow banks near Down House in Kent as he wrote – to try to capture the possibility of unravelling complexity yet draw out different species' functions and interrelationships.[78] The metaphor was both poetic and scientific. It expressed a theory of biological interconnection as well as progress and transitions. He used the 'entangled bank' to remind humans that their existence depends on that existence, that the laws of evolution bind all species together. All life is connected.

Box 2.1: Charles Darwin's 'entangled bank'

'It is interesting to contemplate an entangled bank, clothed with many plants of many kinds, with birds singing on the bushes, with various insects flitting about, and with worms crawling through the damp earth, and to reflect that these elaborately constructed forms, so different from each other, and dependent on each other in so complex a manner, have all been produced by laws acting around us. These laws, taken in the largest sense, being Growth with Reproduction; inheritance which is almost implied by reproduction; Variability from the indirect and direct action of the external conditions of life, and from use and disuse; a Ratio of Increase so high as to lead to a Struggle for Life, and as a consequence to Natural Selection, entailing Divergence of Character and the Extinction of less-improved forms. Thus, from the war of nature, from famine and death, the most exalted object which we are capable of conceiving, namely, the production of the higher animals, directly follows. There is grandeur in this view of life, with its several powers, having been originally breathed into a few forms or into one; and that, whilst this planet has gone cycling on according to the fixed law of gravity, from so simple a beginning endless forms most beautiful and most wonderful have been, and are being, evolved.'

Source: Darwin, *On the Origin of Species*.[79]

Public health as we see it requires ecological thinking in this Darwinian mode. By this, we do not mean that all public health is reduced to biology. On the contrary, the 'entangled bank' metaphor suggests the coexistence of different levels of life: animals, plants, soil, energy, the environment and so on, and hints at the role of humans and their reflective intellectual competence at unravelling its realities. It also voices the possibility that they can upset the nature of the bank. Darwin's genius, and Alfred Russel Wallace's (who was far more aware of ecological degradation in poor countries), was to extract one of the fundamental laws determining the coexistence of species – natural selection. Throughout both their lives, in different ways, both great men recognised that this was not the entire story but one of the keys to a house with many rooms.

We propose that public health thinking requires an ecological framework of understanding. The word 'ecology' is of course plastic, with different writers ascribing varied emphases. Its history is explored in later chapters (Chapters 4 and 10). The core meaning of ecology, relevant to public health, is that health cannot be seen as an end in itself but must be located in a web of interactions and relationships. Ecological thinking was offered in the mid-nineteenth century to explain the mechanisms of the natural world. In this, Darwin was by no means alone. The term indeed came from Ernst Haeckel (1834–1919),[80] while Wallace (1823–1913), the Darwinist co-discoverer of the principle of natural selection, actually engaged in overt public health advocacy notably addressing pollution in cities and illiberal actions of early public health administrators.[81]

Ecological thinking emerged as the common framework of understanding for Darwin, Wallace and their global network of associates, exchanging ideas by post – all without needing the internet. They took the view that life is the totality itself of the vast array of inputs and forms, the legacy of many millennia of development. Life, in this evolutionary web, became understood not as a recent phenomenon, created by a God in a monumental and unexplained act of creation a few thousand years ago, but as developed over huge distances of time by incremental change. Indeed, life is posited as a relatively recent phase on the planet, and human life an even more recent manifestation drawing upon earlier forms and species. Ecology is taken to refer to this way of thinking. Science has to be ecological, requiring human understanding of the interoperation of biotic (living) and abiotic (inanimate) processes.

Ecology can thus be both a science and a metaphor. We see the value of ecological thinking for public health as a reminder that the health of the public is contingent upon other life forms and connections with multiple other factors. All the images of health and public health we sketched earlier in this chapter recognised that public health is not an end in itself, nor self-contained. Ecological thinking has to be the framework for public health because, without it, public health is translated into a reductionist scientific schema, where one science dominates. To the biologist, the top science might be genetics. To the social scientist, it is a matter of groups and institutions. To the economist, it is price mechanisms. For us, the strength of ecological thinking is that it stops the notion of public health being dominated by any discipline or one way of thinking. As has already emerged in these early chapters, the health of the public requires multiple support. No one perspective or formula has the trump card. Ecological thinking is about weaving together multiple ways of interpreting the world and points public health towards recognition of interactions and multiple dimensions of existence.

Although Darwin thought that human existence was never detached from its biological origins, in *Descent of Man* he wrote that humans differed profoundly in one respect from other animals in that a human was 'a moral being . . . capable of comparing his past and future actions, or motives, and of approving or disapproving of them'.[82] Even the great biologist thus recognised non-biological spheres of existence. In public health, this is important. Public health is about not just bodies but what we refer to as the four dimensions of existence. It combines the world of nature and the environment, bodies, minds and institutions: the material world alongside the social world.

This book proposes that ecological thinking strengthens what is meant by public health. It does not mean that public health becomes dissipated or lost in a quagmire of multiple interests and intent. Our proposition is that what passes under the title of public health is or ought to be a combination of actions designed to shape health by operating on what we term four dimensions of existence. These are: the *material dimension*, which includes the physical and energetic infrastructure of existence (matter, energy, water), the physical building blocks which underpin human existence; the *biological dimension*, which refers to the bio-physiological processes and elements and includes not just all the animal and plant species but also micro-organisms; the *cultural dimension*, which refers to not just how people individually think but also the sphere of interpersonal relations; and the *social dimension*, by which we mean institutions created between people and expressed in terms of laws, social arrangements, conventions, and the framework of daily living generally outside of individual control. All four dimensions interlink, as shown in Figure 2.3. In this book we use these four dimensions as a 'lens' to understand the relationship between public health and societal change.

We propose that public health, as both project and practice, is about combining intervention and understanding of these four dimensions of existence. We offer them as a template or heuristic through which connections can be drawn. In the next chapter we show that to some extent public health already has a tradition of looking at health as 'Ecological Public Health', but this book explores how twenty-first-century public health requires a much more complex and sophisticated version of what is meant by Ecological Public Health. We invoke this notion, beginning here with our outline of the four dimensions above, to suggest that human health follows from ameliorating the relationship between the four dimensions of existence. Part of the value of looking at health through an Ecological Public Health lens is that it enables us to address the modern conflation of 'ecology' as nature and the natural environment with the understanding of 'ecology' as the science of looking at complexity and interrelationships. At its simplest, Ecological Public Health returns public health, so often marginalised in public policy and life, to what we see as its core task: the necessity of maintaining sound and decent conditions for good health to be protected and enhanced.

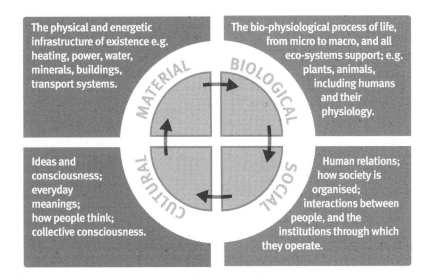

FIGURE 2.3 The four dimensions of public health

The rest of this book explores this basic proposition. In the next chapter we look in more depth at what is meant by public health by outlining five coherent models of public health which have emerged over the last two centuries. We then in Part II outline nine major transitions which shape the conditions for health today, and then in Part III we return to our core proposition and suggest how a wider-encompassing version of Ecological Public Health helps bind an interdisciplinary perspective while offering clear guidance for the tasks of the public health movement and policy ahead.

3

THE RECEIVED WISDOM OF PUBLIC HEALTH

This chapter looks at some mainstream conceptions of public health and proposes that public health has been defined differently through five major models. As we have already seen in the previous two chapters, public health is not a blank sheet of paper. It is covered by diverse ideas, images, models and definitions which compete for affections and funding. What determines which dominates? In this chapter we set out some key ideas about what public health is, how it has been defined as an intervention, and different conceptions of its role. We explore the notion that health is made by great men, women and professions, delivered by economic advance, facilitated by technical and medical innovations, and galvanised into response mode often by threats. Other ideas championed include the notion that health comes only from a return to a natural state, or requires a paternalist state, or can be addressed only as a complex interaction. Public health in other words is criss-crossed by competing interpretations and analyses. It is politically charged.

We show how the definition of public health changes over time. We start mainly in the nineteenth century, with some retrospection beyond that point. Our focus is on the state of health itself, but one where interventions are judged necessary to improve health. We start below with the Classical conception of health, with its emphasis on sanitation and environmental change to create the infrastructure for public health. But this model began to be marginalised with the growth and successes of medicine as a scientific and professional force. It is not that the infrastructural approach to health dissolved, far from it; it just became accepted as normal. And so successful was the armoury of the new sciences that public health became recast as the actions of a specialist genre of doctors who controlled a panoply of functions which collectively protect and promote health. Their main target was infectious disease and communicable diseases, the threat of which requires constant vigilance, hence the training of public health specialists today which stresses the importance of surveillance and epidemiological skills. Far less attention was given to issues of environmental pollution, little given to the determinants of behaviour, and only a small amount to economic and policy determinants of health.

Public health medicine became synonymous with public health. Yet it had relatively little to say about the determinants of health until recently. The charting of this perspective on public health extended beyond the medical world into the social sciences. But the medical version was marginalised by its own success in helping the decline of infectious diseases. This, at least, was the experience in developed countries, but not in the developing world, where safety nets are urgently needed still but lack political or financial support too often. This is a failure of institutional frameworks and of the State rather than of public health proponents.[1] This failure has not been helped by the re-emergence in the twenty-first century of a nineteenth-century view that health could be solved by individual actions. In the present century this reduces the public health function to individual actions within markets, and the role of public policy merely to one of encouraging behaviour change. In the developing world, public health advance became transmuted into a belief that economic growth would resolve health inequalities and the health problems associated with poverty.

In this chapter, we begin to unpick some of the conventional and common narratives about what public health is and more particularly the methodologies of public health intervention. We begin this by setting out a number of models or archetypes of public health. These are sketched in order to facilitate the discussion in the rest of the book, where we explore what we judge to be the core terrain on which public health action has to be displayed – namely tackling a broad range of transitions. Unless these are collectively addressed, we cannot see how the public health can be improved, protected or maintained.

From one conception, public health has improved so much – deaths in infancy are increasingly rare, and the average lifetime extends far beyond the biblical three score and ten – that to talk of rising public health threats may seem absurd to the uninformed. Such problems happen only in far-flung places surely. On the contrary, contemporary evidence suggests that there are huge challenges ahead for public health in both rich and poor economies. These threaten even some public health gains made over the last two centuries (see Part II). The assumptions of the past of ever extending life, reducing child mortality, improving the quality of life and so on have led the public health movement to an impasse where there is unwarranted faith that things can only get better and that existing foci and measures can be extended into the future.

Five models of public health

We have extracted five core models from the history and development of thinking about public health. These models are presented as 'ideal types', in the sense developed by the German sociologist Max Weber as being the essence of the ideas, an attempt to strip away the unnecessary packaging and get to the heart of how public health interventions are interpreted. We present these models within their ideological contexts. For each model, we suggest how the problem of health is conceptualised, and we give its core ideas, scope, origins, main variants, key thinkers and some criticisms. We begin also to suggest the effectiveness of each model in the landscape of public health thinking. At the end of this chapter is a summary comparison table of the different models as an aide-memoire.

Model 1: Sanitary-Environmental

This model is sometimes called the Classical model of public health, but we term it Sanitary-Environmental here for reasons given below. Its core idea is that health is determined by the external environment. In some instances, causation of ill-health and disease can be direct and immediate, literally by touch and proximity. In other cases, it may be a series of events. The Sanitary-Environmental model is often associated with the identification of health threats and disease in order to invest in their solution, be that changing the environment or ensuring access to uncontaminated sources of health such as clean water. The environment here is almost metaphorical, an 'out-there' which always impinges on health.

The origins and mainstreaming of this model largely lie in the nineteenth century, when it was shaped by the emergence of mass infectious diseases and of large conurbations. This coincidence was a challenge to the notion that the nascent sciences could transform nature and civilisation. Diseases threatened the notion of progress and the social order. And conurbations – the new teeming, noisy, polluted working towns – exercised a new relationship between technology, capital, labour and nature. The word 'conurbation' was invented by the Scottish ecological theorist Patrick Geddes (1854–1932). The growth of industrial towns, first in Britain and then quickly across Northern Europe, brought almost immediate health problems associated with their scale, relatively primitive technology and dire working and living conditions. Towns grew on the back of industrial wealth. Public health problems also emerged in ports and large trading cities.

The model is rightly called 'Classical' in some writings because giant cities were known in Classical times, long before industrial capitalism, although the term 'Classical' is usually attached to this model to imply that it is a central model in public health. Ancient Rome, for instance, had over a million inhabitants at one point, living on just over 13 square kilometres. Rome was criticised for poor hygiene at times. Lewis Mumford (1895–1990) in his magisterial *The City in History* points out that other smaller Roman cities were better run and more healthy.[2] Nonetheless Rome managed to introduce public toilets, aqueducts for water, underground sewers, paved main roads and systems for disposing of waste. These may not have been universal in the Roman Empire or indeed in the city of Rome but they were shown to be possible; the technology and case were made. Rome also created, via the nearby port of Ostia, a route through which food and the means for survival could get to the big city. But, even before it was sacked and overrun at the end of Empire, Rome was in trouble with that infrastructure. Ostia was silting up. Wars dislocated food supplies.[3] Mumford's verdict on ancient Rome was to call its management 'chaotic'. It lacked a system of control and failed to disperse technologies and infrastructure which could protect and maintain health. Addressing this deficit was what the Classical model of public health in the nineteenth century is all about.

This model of public health is often associated in the West with the Victorian past, but it should not be forgotten that it is a priority still today for much of the developing world. Indeed, in the developed world, too, there is often an appeal to this model because the infrastructure which it spawned in the late nineteenth century in Northern Europe, for example, requires updating. The drain and water systems are old and have required re-engineering in London, for instance.

Essentially, this model is about engineering the world to deliver health. We call it here the Sanitary-Environmental model rather than the Classical not only to indicate its core ideas and field of application, but also to recognise the brilliance of the nineteenth-century addition to what the Romans knew at their best. In the Victorian era, 'Classical' became 'Sanitary-Environmental'; it became bigger and better and more systematic. In the first instance the model is about building the infrastructure to enable health to be maintained. This is public health as the extensive provision of roads, water, drains, sewerage, housing, foodways, refuse and waste. It is a conception of the environment where the State regulates usually commercial behaviour. It issues licences and sets the legal parameters for activities.

This model is concerned with the environment as a physical platform for health. It is and was about: firstly, recognising the environmental nature of hazards to health; secondly, identifying the means for their minimisation; thirdly, creating new political structures to guide the public health, particularly by setting up new institutions, roles, and systems of governance; and fourthly, developing a new relationship between the (polluting and threatening) towns and the natural world and countryside.

These latter elements are often left out of accounts of the Classical model, but they deserve to be recognised. Their combination creates a modern conception of living and generates a new version of the State as a key civilising actor in a new world order. At the same time, nature is recast. It's not a state of being in itself but becomes a set of resources from which goods are extracted and to which the wastes of the town are returned. But towns are where the money is made to enable this new relationship to be forged. And towns are where the municipal grip is exerted.

The origins of the words in this model's title are indicative. 'Sanitation' is derived from the Latin *sanitas*, meaning health. Under the Classical model, the word was captured by a visual metaphor of drains and building the infrastructure for cities to be civilised, literally to be enabled to exist. The meaning of the word 'sanitary' became associated with, indeed locked into, a connotation of almost subterranean material: the hidden arteries of cities – more colon than arteries perhaps! Certainly, pipes and their capacity to bring good things – water – into towns and to move waste out became a leitmotif, a running theme. But it was also an astonishing leap of the imagination, not just engineering. The word 'environment' has its roots in Old French, via Middle English, and indicates surroundings and external conditions. This captures a core role where the public health task is to tackle the conditions which shape health and to mine the material world to do so.

Although we are stressing the utilisation of the material world for health in the Sanitary-Environmental model, it also spawned new 'common-sense' behavioural rules for everyday life. These resonate today. Dicta such as washing hands before meals and after going to the toilet, cleaning one's teeth, acts of daily domestic hygiene, may seem normal, but they were engineered into culture and often were highly contested. The role of public health actors was to shift culture, to make people behave in a way which minimised threats to health. In this respect, this model is a counterbalance and essential counterpart to the Social-Behavioural model we outline next in this chapter.

The Sanitary-Environmental model has associations with big expenditure on large-scale engineering works as well as daily habits. Very costly engineering was building new sanitary drain systems for the nineteenth-century cities. The City of London changed the shape of the River Thames in the 1860s from naturally sloping banks to the sharply edged embankments Londoners walk or travel on today. Beneath their feet are the vast drains, canalising local streams and rivers to transfer the sewerage away from the city (see Figure 3.1). The Sanitary-Environmental model is often linked with hygiene, another word with even older roots, the Greek *hygeia*.

This model is in large part municipal; it is the responsibility of towns to look after and protect health if they are to function efficiently. The word 'efficiency' is central. It links the model to the military, not least since armed forces had centuries

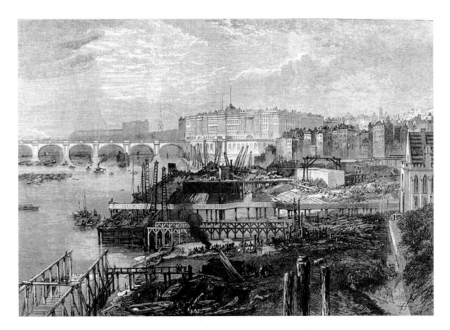

FIGURE 3.1   The construction of the Thames Embankment in 1863

of experience of the fragility of their capacities if faced by disease or lack of *matériel* or food. Certainly the British Army has at times taken the health of its forces seriously, albeit with wavering commitment. Sir John Pringle's (1707–82) 1752 *Observations on the Diseases of the Army* recognised that fevers, dysentery and jail fever were the three most prevalent and fatal diseases affecting armies, and helped to control epidemics among the ranks.[4] An 1810 study of 5,183 deaths by the Napoleonic-era British Royal Navy revealed 81.5 per cent were ascribed to illness and accidents, only 8.3 per cent were secondary to enemy action; the remaining 10.2 per cent were attributed to miscellaneous factors.[5] Of the almost 1,900 sailors who set out on Anson's 1740s expeditional voyage round the world, only 188 returned home; of the 90 per cent who died, most died from disease.[6] The American bacteriologist Hans Zinsser (1878–1940), a military sanitary inspector in the First World War and a famous writer on biology after it, documented how all wars in human history had seen death and destruction more accounted for by disease than injury on the field of battle.[7] Human history cannot be understood well without understanding the causes and consequences of human disease.

Prior to the Sanitary-Environmental model's emergence, this was accepted as normal. One of the most cited illustrations of the triumph of science over ill-health is James Lind's (1716–94) mid-eighteenth-century discovery that citrus fruit (containing what was later known as vitamin C) could solve scurvy in the British Royal Navy.[8] Not only did Lind not 'discover' this – others had noted the impact of citrus fruit before him – but Lind's success was in fact ignored for nigh on four decades, despite exposing the high percentages of sailors who died during voyages.[9] Today, this episode is frequently cited as the beginning of the process of controlled clinical trials.[10] It was, in fact, fundamentally an environmental notion of the role of food in public health. It is not so much a behavioural conception as about changing the context within which human life exists. Because disease is central to the efficient operation of military force it is no surprise that medical officers reaffirmed its importance; but often there were clashes between the simple rules for better health championed by the medical officers and the ultimate military codes which ignored them. Only later, with the publicity given to Florence Nightingale's environmental understanding of disease and bodily restoration, set out in her *Notes on Nursing*,[11] did health considerations begin to outflank the narrow considerations of military strategy.

This is still the relevance of this model today. While rich Western countries may have the infrastructure – often taken for granted – much of the world does not. Unlike in the nineteenth century, the unhealthy environments of today may be cognitive as well as physical. Advertising, for instance, is a factor in moulding food and drink tastes.[12] Billboards and advertising hoardings are physical, but their message is cognitive and social. This is the modern unsanitary environment if we were to update the Sanitary-Environmental model for the twenty-first century, which has created new combinations of threats, wastes and detritus. Within this model, the modern public health task might include the 'cleaning up' of advertising and its methods such as product placement in TV and films, and the constant barrage of messages to consume, often unhealthily. On this point, most national governments appear to be equivocal, torn between supporting advertising as an economic activity promoting consumption and recognising its consequences for health.

The Sanitary-Environmental approach to public health often can have low public appeal and votes in developed countries until something goes wrong. Then a different reflex emerges. 'Something should be done'; 'they should sort this out'. People know that actions could prevent harm, but that requires capacity and personnel, which in turn requires wealth, taxes and central services. Yet these are associated with public rather than private provision. They are common goods and services, precisely of the kind resented by neoliberal analyses of the world which stress markets, small states, and the primary relationship of individual and companies in open marketplaces. Yet, come a crisis, it is health services – all those dogged scientists with unpronounceable specialisms, working in laboratories – who are suddenly invoked to protect people from new threats. Their specialisms only exist in crises if they are allowed to develop and monitor in non-crisis times. How can we expect knowledge about germs or viruses such as influenza, or a new disease such as bovine spongiform encephalopathy (BSE or 'mad cow disease'), to exist if the experts are not there?

The Sanitary-Environmental model could be executed only if there were engineers, scientists and taxes. The dynamic depicted by this model is of expense of investment in infrastructure versus the base fears of threats such as the plague – threats which are inexorable, inexplicable at the time, promising a creeping wipe-out. In some respects, the founding motive for adoption of the Sanitary-Environmental model is the bubonic plague, whose global spread in medieval times left such a powerful legacy in Europe: deserted villages, severely reduced populations and societal weakness. As the nineteenth-century industrial towns and landscape emerged and threats to health followed, these older memories resurfaced, with their legacy of pre-scientific myths about punishment and rites. Sanitary-Environmental thinking offered a different route to tackling health than the wearing of amulets or penance for disease. Putting aside the fact that the humanistic model of nursing developed in concert with environmental considerations, a criticism has been made by the historian Christopher Hamlin that, in the form promoted by Edwin Chadwick, this approach offered a 'technical fix', attending to the 'remedial conditions of the environment' but ignoring 'the crumbling constitutions of poor persons'.[13] Another historian has argued that Chadwick's powerful, if flawed, use of statistics provided the intellectual case for 'preventive medicine'.[14] In the case of Hamlin the implication is that a more individually oriented, medically based approach might have provided a better solution. The application of the medicine of the day would have made an individual's lot far worse, however. In the other case, Chadwick was emphatically not engaged in the application of preventive 'medicine'. Prevention it certainly was, and certainly informed by medical views, but the methods were environmental not medical.

In its advanced form, the methodology of the Sanitary-Environmental model is far more than the bludgeon of big engineering based on a feeble underpinning of science, but a far closer understanding of the scientific mechanisms at the base of such engineering. It incorporates the biological to the social, acknowledging feedback effects. Given the central position in public health thinking that this (Classical) Sanitary-Environmental model has, it is remarkable how low its profile is today. The profile may be low, but the legacy persists.

Model 2: Social-Behavioural

This model differs from the Sanitary-Environmental one in that it focuses heavily – sometimes entirely – on the social and cognitive dimensions of existence as they affect health. Whereas the former model focuses (but not exclusively) on the material context and conditions for health, the Social-Behavioural emphasis is on human agency and its cognitive and immediate social determinants. It posits that the prime element for public health is information, both in the sense of facts – assumed to form rational behaviour – and in the sense of a flow to shape culture. Health is a function of information and behaviour patterns. Education and the spread of knowledge can change things.

The model emerged as a serious force in public health in the mid-twentieth century, when it was invoked as the application of a battery of social sciences, particularly psychology, to health. One root for the model, however, lies in the notion of a rational world where progress emerges through a rational process and the application of, again, rational, scientific knowledge to human improvement. The model posits itself as countering ignorance. Another root is the assumption that some products are harmful to the human condition, such as alcohol, tobacco and illicit drugs. Both of these roots coincide with prohibitionist tendencies. Some behaviours are judged good and others bad. The Temperance movement in the nineteenth century, for instance, was a social movement, rooted in Methodism and Puritanism, which identified excessive alcohol consumption as a social evil. The movement therefore set out to change behaviour, invoking moral appeal.[15] That said, autocratic powers often inveigh against cultural behaviour of which they disapprove. The British king James I wrote an early diatribe against tobacco as dangerous to health![16]

This is an Enlightenment theory. It recalls the first notions of a civilised society from the late eighteenth century, when people's manners, behaviour, social conduct and understanding of how to behave in polite society were forged anew. The model posits education and learning healthy behaviour as part of the civilising process. Before the modern period people were told how to act, how to dress, and what to think and what to aspire to, the mechanisms of enforcement ranging from instruction, to emulation, and to shame. This 'civilizing process', as Norbert Elias (1897–1990) called it, is a far longer social dynamic, bound into the endless social process of redefining social norms;[17] what the Enlightenment did was open such norms up to inspection, even if new forces – the media and brand culture – have rushed to take the place of class- or status-based patterns of life, work and consumption. Their understanding need not be reduced to a functionalist analysis, as later developed by economists, genuflecting to the Scottish philosopher David Hume

(1711–76),[18] because the determinants of social norms are always in flux. They can be deliberated upon; they can be chosen, even through collective acts of will. They raise questions about how social norms are channelled and influenced, which we discuss in Chapter 11.

The intellectual roots of this model lie in a humanistic version of the world in which the key pursuits worthy of human endeavour are freedom, empowerment and individual responsibility.[19] Education, information and reflection change lives. These are central notions in the Enlightenment thinkers on whom the model leans: the French *philosophes*, the thinkers of the Scottish Enlightenment and English liberalism, writers such as Condorcet (Marie Jean Antoine Nicolas de Caritat, 1743–94), Voltaire (François-Marie Arouet, 1694–1778), Adam Smith and his teacher Francis Hutcheson (1694–1746), as well as David Hume, J.S. Mill, Immanuel Kant and John Locke (1632–1704). To them, the task of philosophy – the uniting of knowledge, i.e. the sciences – was to map a morally defined position. The intellectual roots of this model lie in a humanistic version of the world. In Kant's account – in his 1784 essay *What Is the Enlightenment? (Was ist Aufklärung?)* – the task of any individual is to reach a state of true maturity and in so doing escape the trap of being a mere follower of advice or instruction in matters of conscience, diet or anything else. The Enlightenment was far more than about personal autonomy of course. It was a movement and set of historical processes, at the centre of which was this relationship of thought and action. The aim of the enlightened society ought to be to encourage people to make their own educated decisions.

Why is this such a powerful model in public health? And what is distinct and relevant about it?

The issue which brought this model to the fore was contraception. The first campaigns in the Anglo-Saxon world for contraception stemmed from a radical reading of Thomas Malthus (1766–1834), who for religious reasons opposed contraception. In Malthus's era, contraception was not protection as we now know it – cheap, reliable condoms or drugs or injections – but knowledge and social norms, mainly about abstention and delay. To Malthus, the attempt to control population growth was a moral question, almost in the vein today associated with the Roman Catholic Church. There is a natural order to things. He thought that sex was perfectly natural, an unusual position for the time, but was a moraliser about when to have sex. Sex should occur only within marriage, which could and should be delayed – and which for the most part was, occurring much later than today, although people died much younger. If people could delay marriage and therefore delay having children, Malthus thought they would acquire more education and achieve better lives. For the most part the medical profession and the State, for more than a hundred years after Malthus's death in 1834, remained opposed to contraception.

A different interpretation of contraception was offered by new thinkers such as J.S. Mill, who shared Malthus's views on the limitation of families but disagreed on the point of contraception. He and others saw the need for and the value of contraception. Indeed, as a young man, Mill was arrested in 1824 for distributing leaflets in favour of contraception.[20]

Mill, today viewed as a proto-feminist, thought that contraception opened the door to liberation, but his implied model of dissemination was youthful and crude. As Margaret Sanger (1879–1966), one of the pioneers of modern birth control, said in an address in 1929, 'pioneers like Francis Place and John Stuart Mill thought that all that was necessary was to scatter millions of leaflets to the masses telling them why and how they could prevent large families. A century ago, men placed great faith in the printed word.'[21] Sanger went on to say that women needed supportive advice in clinics and birth control centres. The key public health task in that sense is not the information alone, which nineteenth-century thinkers posited, but social support and a broader culture of change.

Historically, both Sanger and Mill were right. In societies where culture is shaped by religion or oppressive social norms, to argue for freedom of information is a public health act, let alone making efficient techniques available. But social acceptability is also essential, for, unless women and men feel able to control their bodies, contraception is impossible. It should be noted that in both Mill's and Sanger's times, neither the UK nor the USA was a fully functioning democracy, so the arguments they espoused – the democratisation of health information – were indeed progressive, liberating and politically radical.

The Social-Behavioural model suggests that health is framed by how little or much information humans have. In a rational, liberal world, the citizen is empowered (in modern parlance) to be able to act sensibly for health. It is hard to deny the importance of knowledge and the knowledge–behaviour interaction. A famous illustration of the knowledge–behaviour nexus is the work of the Hungarian physician Ignaz Semmelweis (1818–65). He noted, when working as director of the Vienna General Hospital maternity clinic in 1847, that survival rates of women in childbirth could be improved if attending personnel washed their hands. This is now known as 'scrubbing up' before surgery. Semmelweis introduced this new practice after statistical analysis rigorous for its day, but he received opprobrium for his views from some quarters, not least from the now revered German virologist Rudolf Virchow (1821–1902) in Berlin, who disagreed vehemently with this new procedure.[22]

It has been argued that the assault on Semmelweis set back antisepsis for years, but from our point of view this story exposes how health is subject to competing versions of 'common sense' and science, and of the delicacy of information for health. Semmelweis lost his post in Vienna and was drummed out of the city. His subsequent life was undoubtedly tortured by this injustice, and sadly he ended up in an asylum and died prematurely. What was common sense to one party was not to another. The Social-Behavioural model places great emphasis on information's capacity to transform what humans do with their senses. One cannot rely upon the senses. Practices need to be altered by rational information. Semmelweis's opponents believed that men of their superior social status could not be vectors of disease. They believed they somehow stood outside the possibilities of threat. Thus were different egos and reputations at stake through competing interpretations of facts.

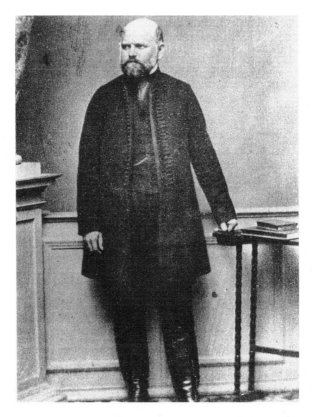

FIGURE 3.2a Ignaz Semmelweis in 1863, two years before he died

Semmelweis's legacy lies in changed clinical practice but also everyday behaviour. His ideas were taken up in Britain, interpreted as fitting the prevailing beliefs about contagion. He did not know why scrubbing up worked but that it did. He had experimental proof that his measures to change behaviour were effective. Hand-washing received its retrospective rationale by germ theory and Joseph Lister, from the 1890s onwards, again applied first to surgical techniques. But it emerges into daily life with the industrial manufacture and affordability of hygienic chemical aids and their mass marketing. Soaps, disinfectants and washing powders all began to be manufactured on vast scales. This is when modern giant corporations such as Unilever and Procter & Gamble emerged in Europe and North America. It is also the time when health products allied manufacturing capital with health through mass marketing. It is a time when advertising appealed to change behaviour. Conceptions of personal health were altered by messages that modernity is about bathing the bodies both of children and of oneself, cleanliness of the home, and women's domestic responsibilities and work.[23] The era of mass appeals to buy consumer goods to promote and protect health had begun.

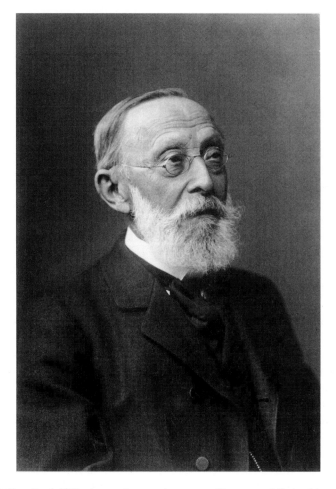

FIGURE 3.2b   Rudolf Virchow, nineteenth-century German public health reformer

The economic historian Joel Mokyr has argued that knowledge, in his terms 'useful knowledge' or knowledge that is allied to practical actions, is itself a driving force of social change in modern societies.[24] In the case of public health, this comes at the intersection of the spread of disease, modern production techniques and the establishment of marketing. The role of the family and immediate social networks around the individual are key to the Social-Behavioural model. The multigenerational family, but mostly parents and children, are the central focus to be targeted for health by any outside actor wishing change. Conservative political thinking wishes to protect the family, but sees the threats as mostly coming from the State, whereas commerce is treated with a light touch. The Left is presumed to take an inverse position. It is interesting today that the views of J.S. Mill are supported by some in their ambition to minimise the State's role, whereas what Mill was essentially arguing was that the State was in the grip of anti-democratic, authoritarian

forces. While later describing himself as a socialist and in favour of land nationalisation, Mill promoted a form of 'economic citizenship', attempting to keep in balance the respective relationships of State, the marketplace and civil society.[25]

The Social-Behavioural model maps health as the outcome of beliefs and everyday
actions which are shaped by information and changing norms or, as Winslow put it
in 1920, 'the adoption of proper rules for daily living'.[26] Thus, when in modern times
issues such as drug addiction, alcoholism and obesity vie for policy attention, the
Social-Behavioural adherents offer public health as being about changing attitudes,
mindsets and cognitive maps. In this psychological interpretation of health, there are
echoes of former mass health messages about constraining spitting in the time of contagious tuberculosis (TB). Before pharmaceuticals began to erode TB rates, streets
and buildings – particularly places like toilets and drinking parlours – were festooned
with plaques banning spitting. Exactly transmuted into modern language, this would
be called a 'nudge' according to the authors of a bestselling book of that title.[27]

In its contemporary late-twentieth- and early-twenty-first-century version, this
model has become health action with a focus on lifestyle, health beliefs and health
literacy. Education can change things. This occurs in developing countries, it is
suggested, through the teaching of basic literacy, numeracy, and subjects which
improve higher-order cognitive skills and in turn help individuals transform basic
facts into deeper knowledge that enhances risk assessment and decision-making
skills about health.[28] In other settings this mix has a moral equation at its heart:
the degree to which the individual has responsibility and the degree to which the
environment supports or undermines social and individual responsibility: hence the
enormous modern research effort into measuring the effectiveness of how best to
adjust people's cognition to behave more healthily conducted by health psychologists. The goal is defined as educating and prompting people in healthy choices for
everyday life. The role of the State and corporations is reduced benignly to facilitating that process, which remains essentially private and personal.

In this formulation, Social-Behavioural thinking sees the health 'front line' in
issues such as food labelling. Experience has shown, however, that what is supposed
to be a vehicle for information flow becomes a battleground itself. The format of
labelling becomes highly contested and entangled in arguments about how extensive labelling might be, who should control it, whether it should be delivered on a
regulated or voluntary basis, what form and presentation it should be delivered in,
and whether to believe it might even be effective in changing behaviour.[29] With
deliberate policy confusion often reigning over issues such as labelling, companies
often prefer to keep matters under their own control, espousing the ethos of corporate social responsibility (CSR) where they decide what to do. They resist being
corralled into general frameworks of action by the State. Another position they
tend to like is what is known as shared value.[30] Whereas CSR is about external
'good works', shared value is more reflective of the company's overall impact.

Today, this Social-Behavioural model promotes social marketing as a key methodology. This is the application of techniques for selling private goods to the promotion of public goods like health. If the aspiration is to generate health literacy,[31]

then there quickly appears a tension between method and purpose. Whereas health education in its original form relied upon information as a form of literacy, warning and empowerment, social marketing today relies upon the creation of branded health messages such as 'Eat five fruit and vegetables a day' or 'Don't drink and drive', and to recognise nationally approved logos which symbolise health approval, such as the UK's Change4Life, the USA's VERB and France's EPODE.[32] The latter now runs across a number of countries in Europe, Mexico and Australia, all of these focused on child weight. In modern social marketing methodology (discussed extensively in Chapter 11), old concepts of health education, with their humanistic, seemingly innocent assumptions, are seen as obsolete in a world where the drivers of social norms have a manipulative commercial edge. In one approach to social marketing, there is an assumption of individual pathology; there is often 'wrong behaviour' or the 'wrong consumers' who need to be corrected.[33] For others, there is another assumption, in this case perhaps an affected innocence, that the marketing of goods within capitalism has neutral effects and indeed that public health social marketers should work alongside large corporations, accept their funding and finesse a mutually supportive role.[34] In any case, public health emerges as merely one brand with one assumed consensual motivation among many. Already by the 1940s, cultural theorists such as Theodor Adorno (1903–69) and Max Horkheimer (1895–1973), refugee social scientists from Germany living in the USA, noted how the once-vibrant public sphere had become colonised and subverted by the 'culture industry'. If their mentor, Kant, had desired to create a state of dignified, personal autonomy as an antidote to immaturity and consumerism in this world, there was already 'nothing left for the consumer to classify'.[35] Adorno and Horkheimer's account was certainly too pessimistic then, but, in a culture where news has become primarily a form of mass entertainment and mass entertainment has become a vector for embedded advertising, their conclusions seem uncannily prescient and accurate. Their criticisms of modern culture are considered in Chapter 11.

The key profession in the Social-Behavioural model's modern form is the psychologist. For a while, there was some interest in the psychologists who attuned ideas of child development to the healthiness of the social environment.[36] This adoption of psychology's insights found political leverage in child–mother programmes such as the 1960s Head Start in the USA or, much later, the UK's Surestart in the 2000s. But this approach was about social change as much as individual change and, in a market society, consumerist decision-making, not the environment, has to be at the centre. More influential than those early social psychologists have been US cognitive psychologists Martin Fishbein and Icek Ajzen, possibly the most-cited representatives of the rational approach to behaviour. In the 1970s they proposed a simple and linear process encompassing four elements and a 'sequence of systematic relations linking beliefs to attitudes, attitudes to intentions and intentions to behaviors'.[37] It might be also demonstrated as a process belief → attitude → intention → action → behaviour.[38] In these theories of the 'self', behaviour is adapted to the current environment but it is determined by an act of conscious choice. For some people, this became the new foundation for health education thinking, and the approach currently reigns supreme in theories of health behaviour and self-regulation.

Another recent source of thinking about the behaviour in the social setting is the ecological model of interrelationships set out in the 1970s by Urie Bronfenbrenner (in Image 5 in Chapter 1).[39] The human ecology field is far older than this implies. The term 'human ecology' was introduced into sociology by Robert Park (1864–1944), a student of the pragmatist philosophers John Dewey and William James. These ideas were revived in the early 1950s by the US sociologist Amos Hawley (1910–2009). He argued that environment, population and organisation were part of an evolutionary dynamic and that the 'eco-system' served as a common denominator for bioecology and human ecology.[40] These ideas more properly form part of Ecological Public Health. What has been termed the social-ecological approach to health, as the term implies, is limited to the human–constructed environment. The natural or material environment is seen as just another influence on health. This term, nevertheless, has considerable presence in the public health field, as shown by a review of social-ecological approaches by Kenneth McLeroy and colleagues in the late 1980s.[41]

One important example of social-ecological thinking in health has been developed by Daniel Stokols and colleagues at the University of North Carolina – Chapel Hill over several decades. In the current version of the model there are 'five spheres of influence' on health outcomes, which Stokols and colleagues describe in terms of physical health status, developmental maturation and social cohesion. These five spheres are: the environmental domain, which includes multiple physical, social and cultural dimensions; personal attributes, such as genetics, psychological disposition and behavioural patterns; dynamic interdependent relations between people and their environment, which take the form of negative and positive feedback and homeostasis; the interdependence of environmental conditions within multiple settings, such as neighbourhoods, workplaces, or personal residences and life domains, these being family or group membership; and lastly an interdisciplinary approach to assessing the healthiness of settings and the well-being of persons and groups.[42] Stokols and colleagues have argued that the broadening of the environment to include the online world of the internet has resulted in distracting and discouraging people 'from confronting ecological and social challenges and joining with others in constructive efforts to resolve them'.[43]

Social-ecological thinking has also been adopted by the World Health Organization. In one influential study of violence and its causation, WHO researchers present a simple four-level model of social ecology moving from the individual, to the relationship level (group membership), to community and then to society.[44] One useful feature of the approach resides in the utility of these levels for specifying a framework of preventive actions related to a child's development stage, an approach fully consistent with the Bronfenbrenner approach. One limitation to social-ecological thinking, added in the Ecological Public Health model, is that while a broader sense of the environment is always present there is little or no attention to feedback between human activity and nature.

Other versions of the Social-Behavioural model are historically deeper and more diverse than its modern formulations imply. Entirely different schools of psychology have been invoked in the name of Social-Behavioural thinking at different times over the last century, let alone in the previous. Eugenicist social science influenced the social hygiene movement, for example.[45] Freudian psychoanalysis, dealing with the individual's apparent unawareness of his or her inner psychic struggles, shaped the development of mass marketing in the early twentieth century. In the mid-twentieth century, social psychologists were used to shape armed forces public relations in and after the Second World War. At one point, whereas psychoanalysis dominated mass marketing work, behaviourist psychology dominated clinical health work. Today, cognitive psychology dominates.

Part of the problem for psychology today is that its insights are almost too fragmented and complicated, have little tangible relation to evidence of success for changing behaviour, at least at the population level, and either are too open-ended for easy conversion into public policy or present too sobering an account of human rationality. With developments in the neurological sciences, the contemporary cognitive perspective seeks to account for psychological phenomena in terms of deterministic mechanisms, something of a return to the early origins of modern psychology.[46] Within this messy theoretical world of diverse psychologies, it is hardly a surprise that governments and their advisers desire a form of 'psychology-lite', preferably without the bothersome psychologists: hence the attraction of 'nudge' theory, the product of an economist and a lawyer, both of whom speak to the world of non-rational judgement, decision-making cues and default choices but who also desire a world in which the State doesn't do too much. We return to this issue in Chapter 11.

The Social-Behavioural model comes in a number of political variations, all concerned about the question of power and individual autonomy. One pictures the individual having power but failing to exercise it. Another sees power as within the social system which denudes the individual or fosters a false sense of autonomy. The latter position is associated with the work of the French historical sociologist Michel Foucault, whom we encountered in our image of public health as nanny or Big Brother, in Chapter 1, who was alarmed by the introduction of technologies of control. While respecting the origins of the Enlightenment,[47] he saw such technologies as manifest in the practices of public health which defined the people as a population to be regulated and controlled in the name of increasing its life, wealth and productivity. In one word, Foucault's fear was of 'biopower', control over the body, as he termed it.[48] For him and his followers the discussion of public health is not ultimately about the improvement of life but essentially a discussion of power.

Alternatively, although in some parts they join up, the conservative critique – articulated by conservative libertarianism – claims that people are all responsible for their own lives and therefore health. But it is almost an oxymoron, in that libertarianism speaks to individual freedom, while conservatism speaks to the status quo. One is aspirational and urges change, while the other is defensive and seeks to retain a firm grip on the social order. In practice, in the latter half of the twentieth century, conservative libertarianism became both noisy in public policy and active.[49] Its beliefs centred on proselytising the advantages of choice within the market. Applied to health, this became a version of public health as an outcome of private choices. It is blind to corporate power, and assumes rather naively that there are even options for all. Within public policy, this position is often corporate-funded, and one encounters it in attacks on regulation or the 'nanny state'. This variant is more of a US way of thinking, fairly recent, and associated with Chicago economics: anti-statist, against certain types of professions, but in favour of individualism.[50] Nudge is a version, but contains a paternalist aspect. Indeed Thaler and Sunstein term themselves libertarian paternalists. They view their gentle policy nudges as appealing to 'conservatives, moderates, liberals, self-identified libertarians, and many others'.[51] Other have noted that they occupy the 'uneasy middle ground between conservative and liberal politics',[52] at least as these terms apply in the USA; the political architecture elsewhere is entirely different. The implication is that the nudge is not just an aspect of economic thought or 'behavioural economics' with claims of political neutrality (although that too would be questionable) but an approach with an explicit political stance designed for a particular socio-economic setting.

One permitted amendment to the control of markets (in fact marketers, since management choice exists prior to markets) is to set what they call the 'default position', the reordering of the choices that are put in front of the customer. This is something food retailers have known for a century and would be loath to give up; they direct our choices by subtle combinations of signals, the arrangement of the setting of choice. In this version, health is a blend of one's social and financial status with the setting in which the choice occurs. Money plus information delivers health; you get what you pay for. The assumption is that the individual is responsible for health choices, while responsibility is shared with those who design the setting. Everything is to play for, but is all about changing the behaviour of the individual, while the larger questions of marketing, supply chains or socio-economic or environmental factors which influence choices are put to one side. They may even be irrelevant.

The picture we have painted here of the Social-Behavioural model is one of a fluid and changing discourse. It covers a wide variety of motivations, methods and ideological viewpoints. Centrally, however, it is about the invocation of psychological science to aid information for behaviour change. This ultimately has a problem: it is undone by the ambition of its claims: information, no matter how cleverly packaged, can define only one plane of the social world, let alone the other dimensions of existence. We return to these themes in later chapters.

Model 3: Bio-Medical

In some respects, this model is what public health has become, at least in the developed world. That status might change if the newer version of the Social-Behavioural model discussed above becomes the policy reflex and wins continuing political support. The Bio-Medical model posits medical science as the overarching way of understanding the unseen health world, which is outside and within the body. The model theorises disease and proposes explanations for how bodies succumb. These working interpretations are always subject to revision and review. As scientific knowledge grows, so the Bio-Medical model grows in sophistication. A big transformation, for instance, came with the unlocking of the power of genetics. Before that, the discovery of antibiotics transformed both medical health practice and the belief that humans could alter health rather than accept it as a matter of fate. The key players in this model are the medically qualified professions, which emerged as a serious force in public health in the late nineteenth century. Essentially, the Bio-Medical model conceives of public health as the concoction of complex measures to rebalance bio-physiological processes.

This is a model which is almost celebrated for being attacked, often by those with careers which had themselves been founded within medicine or biology. The literature is replete with critiques from various perspectives. In 1847 German physician Salomon Neumann (1819–1908) thought medical science 'essentially a social science', saying that, while this fact was not recognised in practice, medicine was but 'an empty shell and a sham'.[53] The social epidemiologist Thomas McKeown, whom we discuss below (and at length in Chapter 5), argued that the history of health improvement was not due to medicine in the main but more related to economic and material factors, particularly, following Malthus, the role of and improvements in nutrition, owing to the changed availability of food.[54] The French-born, US-domiciled biologist René Dubos, whom we encountered briefly in earlier chapters, and whose biological researches were critical to the development of antibiotics, identified a central flaw in the Bio-Medical model. It was rigid and inadequately dynamic with respect to the biological forces of evolution. It not only generated new problems within its own working environment but neglected those present in real life. Such views were partially echoed by Macfarlane Burnet (1899–1985), the Australian virologist and Nobel Prize winner for medicine. He observed that for the first time in history the deaths of children in the affluent West were no longer from infectious disease.[55] By the 1970s, with evidence of overuse of antibiotics, he opined that reliance on the wonders of medicine might be time-limited. He was an early subscriber to the fear that ecology – defined as nature's own system of checks and balances – had been 'ousted by technology'.[56] The Viennese social philosopher – and Roman Catholic priest – Ivan Illich (1926–2002) went even further than any of these. He dismissed the Bio-Medical model as entirely self-defeating. Medical interventions could create as much harm as they solved.[57] He termed this intervention 'iatrogenic' disease, doctor-induced damage.

Others pointed to how and why dualist assumptions and reductionist thinking limited the Bio-Medical model's application as a therapeutic approach and that other models were needed. The Hungarian endocrinologist Hans Selye (1907–82) argued that health was a function of mind, body and environment, and as much about stress relationships between them as bodily mechanics. Selye was criticising the Newtonian view implicit in medicine, the body as machine.[58] The US psychiatrist George Engel (1913–99) formed a similar critique, if from a different starting place, seeing health and illness as consequences of the interplay of biological, psychological and social factors, leading him to embrace systems theory and complexity theory and to formulate what he referred to as the 'biopsychosocial' model of health.[59]

Central to the Bio-Medical model is the idea that public health science advances only through improving its own understanding of how the human biological organism works. The pursuit of this knowledge may centre either on the body's mechanisms themselves or on how bodies respond to the wider material and biological environment and also, in a more complete view, how that biological environment responds to human activity. Regarding this evolutionary feedback reflex, the US biologist Hans Zinsser observed in 1935 that mankind was too prone to look at nature through egocentric eyes. 'To the louse, we are the dreaded emissaries of death.'[60] It therefore follows that the Bio-Medical model is essentially linked to the voyage of scientific discovery based upon not just the body but also evolutionary biology and our complex entanglements with other species over long periods of time and changes in habitat and population density.[61] What was previously impossible to understand can now be explained; processes replace folklore, myth and half-truth.[62]

Although there is a core to the Bio-Medical model, it is subject to variation. It is not one common understanding but two. As Winslow put it, 'The physician in the public health field practises medicine but with a difference.'[63] This version focuses, in the main, on populations. The most notable illustration of this is in the public health championing of vaccination, introduced in the early 1800s and considered in greater detail later. The second version has a more individual orientation, focusing on the particularities of individual bodies rather than on the health of social groups or collectivities. In this latter variation, key interventions have been developed such as drugs, surgery, and talk remedies, extending to the entire panoply of modern medicine. This is public health as medicine, dentistry, pharmacy or other scientific services, usually via professionalised intervention.

The history of public health medicine often reveals a tension between these two understandings, the first leading to a more multidisciplinary approach in which the bio-medical understanding is one element of the scientific and professional armoury. The second sees scientific understanding as located in the expert medical professions. The focus there is the patient–doctor relationship. In the USA, these two variants were originally more sharply enshrined than elsewhere. Although public health interventions were often medically led, they often operated with a multidisciplinary team, sometimes castigating physicians plying their trade independently for their technical and scientific incompetence and their failure to address the collective consequences of individualised medical practices. The individual practitioners returned the favour. Mobilised by the American Medical Association, they 'lobbied against public health', which meant that the number of teaching facilities was limited and jobs restricted to low-paying municipalities or the Army.[64]

For the greater period of medicine in the USA, the professional claims of many individual physicians rested on a thin scientific veneer, a problem later solved when philanthropic organisations such as the Rockefeller and Carnegie foundations funded new medical schools to champion 'scientific' but personalised medical practice. The implicit ideology there was to support efforts to pull the centre of gravity of medical science away from the collective orientation of public health, rooted in local government, and towards the individual variant of the Bio-Medical model.[65] This succeeded in the USA, although in recent years the medical profession has kept its evident tensions within itself, despite low membership of professional organisations like the American Medical Association. In contrast to other countries like France, which tends towards a single specialist organisation, the US medical profession has been able to mount enormously successful defences against what it has seen as an attack by European-type 'socialised medicine'. In fact, these more social approaches to health are often merely the pooled health insurance arrangements found in almost every other OECD country.[66]

The historian Roy Porter (1946–2002) provides an elegant summary of the growth of bio-medical knowledge and improved scientific understanding of physiology and disease processes.[67] This knowledge and understanding flowered from the nineteenth century, thanks to researchers such as Louis Pasteur (1822–95), Robert Koch (1843–1910), Marie Curie (1867–1934) and many others. Porter describes their working lives, not just as scientists but as human beings too. The growth of influence of the Bio-Medical approach is associated with clinical technical development and invention: birth callipers, X-rays, new microscopes. Inspired chance, rather than the slow step-by-step accretion of knowledge, was often the mechanism. The stethoscope was one such, invented by the French physician René-Théophile-Hyacinthe Laennec (1781–1826) in 1816. Laennec had apparently observed two children sending signals to each other by scraping one end of a long piece of solid wood with a pin, and listening with an ear pressed to the other end. He was already familiar with the technique of applying his ear directly to a patient's chest. Confronted with the difficult task of trying to diagnose a large young woman with heart disease, he felt that this would be inappropriate, so, emulating the children's game, he rolled up a sheet of paper into a tube and used that to listen for the heart. He went on to use a one-ear wooden trumpet. Thanks to his stethoscope Laennec became an expert on examining the chest, but unfortunately suffered from TB himself and died at a relatively early age. In 1852 an American physician extended the idea to produce the modern instrument. Today the stethoscope is the essential accoutrement of medical practice, at least in TV medical dramas, as we saw in Chapter 1. Other important innovations in the nineteenth century include the introduction of chemical anaesthesia, although hypnotism had already been used for this purpose. In the twentieth century, technical advances which helped enshrine the Bio-Medical model came thick and fast and were genuinely effective: insulin, anti-bacterials, cortisone – the list enlarges with each passing decade. Porter, like other historians and epidemiologists, was under no doubt that the contribution of medicine came late and was surpassed by more broadly inspired public health interventions.

David Wootton, another historian of medicine, emphasises the first aspect of this fact and reminds his readers that the Bio-Medical model has a messy history.

Far from being a long and triumphant rise of effectiveness, it is littered with false starts, failures and dire experimentation.[68] Only by the late nineteenth century does medicine emerge from being a would-be profession that asserts its value and utility to one which has a self-critical reference framework by which it may be judged externally and by itself. At that point, the Bio-Medical model emerges from obscurantism and looks at the body with fresh eyes, seeing being the beginning of understanding. In his account of Claude Bernard (1813–78), the celebrated French physician and author of *Introduction à la médecine expérimentale* (An Introduction to the Study of Experimental Medicine), originally published in 1865, Paul Hirst shows how he looked at the body in terms of its underlying processes rather than imposing a priori a metaphysical analysis of how the body ought to work.[69] The Bio-Medical model is an undeniable outcome of the Enlightenment, but it was slow to gather momentum.

Medicine today, for the most part, accepts the need to follow a critical, indeed self-critical, path. The image of the investigative doctor promoted in the TV series *House* (see Chapter 1) provides a picture of a highly intellectualised, science-biased, diagnostic expert process. The incorporation of an evidenced-based perspective on treatment, a language adopted into the model following the recommendations of the epidemiologist Archie Cochrane, enshrined the realignment of medical knowledge and technique as the route for the improvement and protection of public health. Useful knowledge must not simply be asserted, reflecting an ideology or philosophical whim, but must be demonstrated. And this must not just be done on the early basis of trial and error highlighted by Wootton but by the application of ever more sophisticated statistical techniques. The Cochrane Collaboration named in his honour represents the scientific filtration system for the separation of knowledge from dross.[70]

In the same vein, the sophistication of genetic science adds depth to the Bio-Medical model, with numerous offshoots such as genomics and nutrigenomics suggesting a new direction for medical practice. In particular, there is much attention to the notion of personalised medicine, the approach that suggests that, once people's genetic predispositions are mapped, owing to the brilliance of genetic screening, better targeting of medicines and interventions will be possible. At the same time, there is a strong bid to market genetics to the public as the search for genes or gene expressions which will unlock or explain why certain diseases take hold. Some of this is marketing, an appeal for funds from distressed families, a modern marriage of medicine and marketing. But that criticism cannot deny the astonishing effort of huge and costly enterprises such as sequencing particular genes and most amazingly the sequencing of the entire human genome.[71] But conceptually for the Bio-Medical model this is a mapping rather than explanatory process and leap. In fact, the real impact of genetics since James Watson (1928–), Francis Crick (1916–2004), Rosalind Franklin (1920–78) and Maurice Wilkins (1916–2004) conceptualised DNA is that this takes the Bio-Medical model towards an evolutionary perspective. It reminds medicine, a human endeavour, of the legacy of the long adaptation of people to the environment, with genetic pre-potential to respond to external threats and stimuli 'hard-wired in' as the metaphor puts it. Genetics makes the Bio-Medical model more complex. As many writers have suggested, this reconnects medicine as an enterprise with evolutionary biology.[72] It takes the individualism out of individuals and marks out each of us as distinctive members of a species.

Part of the power of the Bio-Medical model has been how it can be applied to so many spheres of public life. Almost everything can be turned into a disease – whether bodily or, as the *West Side Story* song has it, a 'social disease'.[73] Disease language reframes the debate and translates general social harms into disease. In doing so, it can neutralise philosophical dispute. In the USA, this has a particular hold on public discourse. 'Diseasification' (if we may coin an ugly word) even is applied in the tense debate about gun control, for example. This is notoriously a fraught area invoking constitutional rights, liberty, individualism and self-defence. The US public health movement has entered this delicate policy zone through the lens of injuries and bodily harm, highlighting how guns hurt bodies (obviously). The gun-liberty proponents have recognised the power of this argument, viewing it as having a worrying public appeal. In the words of one pro-gun activist: 'As public health and medical professionals, they see gunshot wounds not in terms of crime, self-defense, or constitutional rights, but individually as medical traumas and collectively as a "disease" which requires medical intervention.'[74] 'Diseasification' is detectable in issues as diverse as gambling, alcoholism, drug addiction, dissident youth behaviour, domestic violence and obesity. Behind diseasification lie the waiting arms of the pharmaceutical industry, searching and promising legitimate drugs to tackle or pacify the new disease. By the early 2000s, 11 per cent of women and 5 per cent of men in the USA, not hospitalised, were taking antidepressants.[75] As the psychiatrist Joanna Moncrieff observes, 'the pharmaceutical industry has popularised the idea that many problems are caused by imbalances in brain chemicals'.[76]

The Bio-Medical model is yet another product of the Enlightenment. Using its scientific and technical credentials, it has won pole position on representation of public health matters. It has undergone a long struggle to free itself of dogma, metaphysics and wishful thinking. And when it did achieve primacy it brought with it forms of social dependency, in the form of medicalisation, that early Enlightenment thinkers had eschewed. Today, its mastery of bodily matters seems technically staggering, although future generations will doubtless think current achievements primitive; such is progress. The model's success has come at a cost, however. It places particular reliance on certain disciplines and bodies of knowledge, cutting off multidisciplinary and cross-disciplinary perspectives. The enduring problem of the model is this: while far more than ever is known about disease and ill-health, medicine appears increasingly less able to find a way to deal with them. It is also often very expensive, with, as we saw in Chapter 1, estimates of healthcare rocketing in the future as the Bio-Medical model pursues ever more sophisticated methods. In major areas of public health, such as obesity, its practical impact at the population level remains negligible.

Model 4: Techno-Economic

This model centres on the view that health is a product of a particular avenue of political, economic and societal development. Health *is* development, but development is necessary for health. Health depends on society having a growing surplus of goods and the means for survival, notably food and income. Public health improvement follows from having enough wealth to invest in better infrastructure, knowledge and technology. The wealth generated leads to better nutrition, which in turn enables bodies to achieve their potential. In that sense, this model de-emphasises health and particularly medical intervention, and sees health improvement almost as a by-product of wider technical and economic progress.

From this position, public health is dependent on societies and economies achieving sufficient knowledge to be able to escape the Malthusian trap. The model asserts that it is possible to do so, and that history suggests how. Knowledge enables societies to defer the gloomy prognostications of famine from population growth. Sustained and pervasive technical progress enables humans to live better lives. In some expressions, the model almost argues that public health activity is inconsequential or of only marginal political and economic importance. What matters is the generation of wealth by technical and economic development; these characteristics ought to dominate politics and economic policy. Necessarily, as a consequence, the spread of wealth and knowledge across and within societies is a determinant of that society's health profile. This is a population and societal perspective. To some extent, it is a Whiggish view of health. It can present the improvement of health as due to technical advances paid for by economic growth, in which medicine is only one – and a definitely subservient – channel of improvement.

The social epidemiologist Thomas McKeown (1913–88), in a series of papers and books from the 1960s, controversially struck against the then pervasive view that improvements in population mortality rates were due to medical advance.[77] McKeown questioned this apparently commonsensical assumption. At the time, it should be remembered, new 'wonder' drugs such as penicillin and other antibiotics were combating previous terrors such as pneumonia and TB. The new antidepressant drugs were allowing long-stay psychiatric patients to be released from asylums. Hospitals and medical techniques were overtly cleverer and modern. Societies (in the West) were getting richer. How could this obvious connection between this technical advance and improvements in health not be made?

McKeown's point was that the decline of life-shortening diseases had begun before the introduction of these new medical techniques. Health improvements largely stemmed from people being able to eat better owing to their having bigger incomes, lower food prices and smaller family size. This argument can be directly traced back to the complex thinking of Malthus exploring the relationship between the nutritional environment and patterns of mortality rather than the draconian interpretations. Using the long and extensive data on English mortality and other socio-economic information, McKeown demonstrated that the main reasons for English health improvement in the second half of the nineteenth century were, in his own words:[78]

(a) a rising standard of living, of which the most significant feature was possibly improved diet (responsible mainly for the decline of tuberculosis and, less certainly and to a lesser extent, of typhus); (b) hygienic changes, particularly improved water supplies and sewage disposal, introduced by sanitary reformers (responsible for the decline of the typhoid and cholera groups); and (c) a favourable trend in the relationship between infectious agent and human host (which accounted for the decline of mortality from scarlet fever and may have contributed to that from tuberculosis, typhus and cholera). The influence of specific prevention or treatment of disease in the individual was restricted to smallpox and made little contribution to the total reduction of the death rate.

McKeown was aware how heretical this analysis was. He was a physician himself by training. But he was confident about his general interpretation of the evidence. He acknowledged that medicine did have triumphs such as tackling smallpox, but even there he suggested that just 5 per cent of the total reduction in English mortality in the period 1838–1900 could be attributed to smallpox. In any case, as we see later, what could and should have been a successful preventive measure was poorly managed, poorly explained, and perceived to be massively discriminatory (see Chapter 10). It created considerable opposition. McKeown argued that, from 1838 to the 1970s (i.e. beyond his initial focus on the nineteenth century), the main influences on public health improvement were also the order of their occurrence: first came a rise in the standard of living from 1840, then came improved sanitation from about 1870, and then in the twentieth century came the prevention and treatment of disease in the individual. We see here in McKeown the breathtaking perspective of the Techno-Economic model. Health is an outcome not an input. Generalised economic advance improves health, but this requires 'new scientific, educational and political circumstance which led to their introduction and continuity'.[79]

McKeown's thesis shocked and was revolutionary and to some extent triumphed, but it has latterly been damned and critically revised.[80] He was accused of playing fast and loose with the evidence and for ignoring some evidence, lacking proper clinical understanding of disease and arguing too simplistic and stark a case. The historian Simon Szreter has argued that interventions such as immunisation and vaccination have made a crucial public health difference.[81] But McKeown was not arguing against the existence of these technologies and interventions, only that they must be set in a wider context. McKeown's contribution was to present a larger thesis beyond bio-medically or sanitary-environmentally inspired interventions.

Writers, such as the economic historian Joel Mokyr in *The Gifts of Athena*, have argued that the growth of technological and scientific knowledge and its spread have been the critical factor of general progress and public health.[82] Another economist, Eric Beinhocker, suggests that this growth of knowledge is a form of 'technological evolution'. This is not a mere metaphor, he says, but a real process, involving the same principles of differentiation, selection and replication as found in biology.[83] Indeed, it is easy to slip into thinking that all that this model is about is an economic growth theory, and that it reduces public health to the kind of macro-economic theory articulated by Walter Rostow with his famous 1960s 'stages of growth' theory.[84] That theory argued that economic development had to go through a pre-ordained set of phases. Adopted by agencies such as the World Bank and International Monetary Fund, this became part of the Washington Consensus – an economic developmental model championing the opening up of markets to international investment, trade, the reduction of the role of the State, particularly taxes, and subsidy reduction.[85] The Washington Consensus both celebrated and narrowed this version of capitalism as the driver of growth and progress.[86] This is a theme we return to in Chapter 8.

Mokyr, however, is more subtle. His argument is about useful knowledge. He suggests that what makes economies prosper and civilise is the spread of knowledge or its democratisation. This enables information to go beyond the boundaries of the elite. The process thus extensifies innovation and technical experimentation. This is the process which benefits societies, he argues, with a main beneficiary being public health. Through this framework he shows how sanitary improvement could occur even while false scientific theories were in use. The classic example of that is the early-nineteenth-century belief in miasma being used to explain contagions such as cholera. Miasma mooted that disease spreads through unseen entities in the air. Although a mistaken theory, as we saw with Chadwick (see Chapter 1), it was used to justify many public health advances such as cleaning up urban water supplies and improving house design. Mokyr's analysis focuses upon the potential benefits put into action rather than the scientific validity of the action. Clearly many of the practices rationalised by miasma theory, such as vinegar spraying to combat odours, were fairly ineffective. Others such as the emphasis on ventilation may have been beneficial. Mokyr's point is that it is the utility of the knowledge which matters: how it is translated, who has the power to use it, and its dissemination. Whether it is correct or not is less important.

At one level, public health literature, public image and promise give a high pro-file to the role of technology. There is a version of the public health history which enshrines the technical breakthroughs of great women and men. John Snow's celebrated removal of the pump handle in Broad Street London (Image 1 in Chapter 1) pointed to the need to improve clean water supplies. Marie Curie (Image 1 in Chapter 1), the first person to win two Nobel Prizes – for physics in 1903 and chemistry in 1911 – discovered the effects of radium, leading to the development of X-rays. Mokyr points out that technology need not be hardware but ideas too. The advance of statistical reasoning has been critical to health success. Providing evidence is first part of the picture; another part is to persuade change to follow. Marie Stopes's role is perhaps an archetype: a proselytiser of contraception.

The Techno-Economic model has multiple motivations. One is fear of contagion, driving innovation. Another is the pursuit of profit. These can come together. The development of an entire industry centred on provision of washing and hygiene products illustrates the point, with Lever Brothers as exemplars. They emerged as a giant company – now Unilever – purveying soaps, disinfectants and personal cleansing products in the nineteenth century. Mass marketing established new norms for their use. This is behaviour change driven by the combination of technical innovation, industrial-scale manufacturing and unashamed cultural appeal. This is changing today. Few representatives of large corporations in the twenty-first century can afford to ignore, at least in public, matters like sustainability or climate change or the impact of their products on consumers and the environment. The World Business Council for Sustainable Development, which includes Coca-Cola, General Motors and a range of energy and communications companies, declaim their commitment to sustainability. The Council professes: 'We recognize the need of business to play a leadership role in fostering more sustainable levels and patterns of consumption, through current business processes such as innovation, marketing and communications, and by working in partnership with consumers, governments and stakeholders to define and achieve more sustainable lifestyles.'[87] The problem the Council identifies is that the debate on sustainable consumption has largely been restricted to the European Union and that some large global retailers are not significantly engaged.

The value of the Techno-Economic model of public health can be undermined if it is translated into being solely an economic growth argument. That is not the central proposition of the model, however. Likewise, it can reduce public health to mere technical advance. Again, that is not the model. Health is not just a matter of use versus abuse of technology. It assumes a self-fulfilling, benign relationship between the development of knowledge and its application and dissemination. One sees the model at work in the transfer of marketing techniques to public health, notably the application of social marketing and 'soft' behaviour change techniques celebrated by 'nudge' thinking, to tackle systemic health problems such as obesity. Marketing is seen as neutral. Technology is benign. The advance in technology (think of processed foods) might mean that skills in preparing fresh foods may be lost. In essence, the Techno-Economic model is an expert-oriented model which has at its heart a neutral 'knowledge growth' aspiration. The processes which lead to the production of useful knowledge determine public health.

Model 5: Ecological Public Health

The historical core of the Ecological Public Health model is the proposition that human health is dependent on how people coexist with the natural world. Modern man, said the microbiologist René Dubos, believes he has achieved almost complete mastery of the natural forces which moulded his evolution in the past, but like other living things 'he is part of an immensely complex ecological system'.[88] The state of public health is a function of the interaction of humans in their immediate environment, which is in turn affected by how they manage or fit into their total environment. The model locates humans as one among many species existing within shared space, what, as we saw in Chapter 2, Hippocrates conceived as the elements – air, water and place.[89] This space – from the atmosphere (troposphere) to seabed (aquasphere) and subterranean crust (lithosphere) – is malleable, in the sense that human actions have some flexibility in how they live with or alter it. What humans do has an impact on the biosphere, the organic basis of life with its millions of species woven together in the complex web which Charles Darwin referred to in his metaphor of the entangled bank introduced in Chapter 2.[90] And, vice versa, the biosphere forms the platform on which human activity operates. In some respects it prefigures what humans can do and ultimately provides a limit. This limit, of course, is pushed by industrial activity and, arguably, by the global development of late capitalism, spreading ways of consuming and producing which are now widely agreed to be a concern about the planet's capacities. A paradox is now emerging that economic growth which threatens the biosphere is also what has extended life expectancy and enabled more food to be produced, ways of living to enable humans to constrain the vagaries of nature, not least by medicines, as outlined in previous models. This is why, to some extent, the Ecological Public Health model builds on late-twentieth-century thinking about sustainable development. This theme is discussed throughout the rest of the book, but particularly in Chapters 8, 10 and 13.

A key theme within Ecological Public Health thinking is interrelatedness, how people fit into the biosphere, how they use and care for the natural world, how all species interact, and how their interactions have consequences, almost always with feedback loops. Ecological Public Health is imbued with evolutionary thinking. Health is not a state of existence but a continual outcome of many processes. It is not static but dynamic, and therefore often expressed in dynamic systems terms. Health is but one outcome of a series of key dynamics: material, energy, biology, metabolic processes and more.

In some respects, the Ecological Public Health model has a notion of 'fit' – how health is improved or ill-health created is dependent upon how bodily mechanisms are integrated into their environment, natural and human, made and inherited. The Ecological Public Health model sees ill-health as the result of mismanaging relationships. The notion of mismatch has been proposed as one central explanation for ill-health.[91] This argument rests upon the proposition that humanity's genetic make-up has changed little in the last 10,000 years but during the same period culture and environment have been transformed, to the point that there is now a mismatch between genetically controlled biology and everyday life. This explains, it is said, the rise in chronic degenerative disease exhibited in the post-reproductive life stage of humans today and accounting for most deaths in Western societies. This argument is pursued by some people almost to propose what might be termed an Arcadian view of health, that ill-health is the result of unnatural existence and stems from changes in society, particularly 'unhealthy industrialisation', which have brought new risks. One notes this reasoning in some alternative or complementary therapies.

The Ecological Public Health model might be posited as new thinking, a response to the current twentieth- and twenty-first-century crises of climate change, fossil fuels dependency and general environmental degradation.[92] Our argument, however, is that ecological thinking is in fact very old, and Ecological Public Health, a derivative of wider ecological thinking, just keeps being rediscovered. The general thinking about ecology and health is rooted in the evolutionary tradition not just of Darwin but of his holistic, renaissance antecedents such as Johann Wolfgang von Goethe (1749–1832)[93] and Alexander von Humboldt (1769–1859)[94] and successors such as Thomas H. Huxley (1825–95),[95] Sir Arthur Tansley (1871–1955),[96] and the Odum brothers, Eugene (1913–2002) and Howard (1924–2002).[97] In its health translation, Ecological Public Health becomes a theory about human disease patterns being shaped by humankind's impact on the biosphere, for instance in the writings of Theron Randolph[98] in the 1960s about contamination and of Tony McMichael from the 1990s to the present on disease and climate change.[99] It also becomes a recipe for redirecting modern living, with one strand centring on promoting living simple lives while criticising the anthropocentric focus of modern living. This is exhibited in a tradition extolling the co-operative elements of natural interactions, from Kropotkin[100] to Gandhi, and also in another tradition which centres on ways of living based on conservation ecology. That includes writers such as George Perkins Marsh (1801–82),[101] up to modern permaculturalists.[102] J.S. Mill, in a position barely understandable to mainstream economic thought today, argued in the mid-nineteenth century for putting environmental conservation before economic growth, as this paragraph from *Principles of Political Economy*, published in 1848, the year of political revolutions, shows:[103]

> Nor is there much satisfaction in contemplating the world with nothing left to the spontaneous activity of nature; with every rood of land brought into cultivation, which is capable of growing food for human beings; every flowery waste or natural pasture ploughed up, all quadrupeds or birds which are not domesticated for man's use exterminated as his rivals for food, every hedgerow or superfluous tree rooted out, and scarcely a place left where a wild shrub or flower could grow without being eradicated as a weed in the name of improved agriculture. If the earth must lose that great portion of its pleasantness which it owes to things that the unlimited increase of wealth and population would extirpate from it, for the mere purpose of enabling it to support a larger, but not a better or a happier population, I sincerely hope, for the sake of posterity, that they will be content to be stationary, long before necessity compel them to it.

Ecology as described here is the science of the interrelatedness of all species in the environment. In public health terms, this is translated as humans and their context. There are two broad traditions of what is meant by ecology here. The first sees ecology as interconnectedness. This notion covers thinking about topics as diverse as soil through Darwin himself[104] and the social ecology of the Chicago School of urban formation.[105] The other tradition, now dominant, pitches ecology as the means for understanding nature itself, and focuses upon the implications of humans as part of the complexity of nature.

The meaning of ecology has been debated for over a century, with the first major disputes appearing in the American journal *Science*. Was ecology primarily informed by biology or by botany? This argument is about disciplinary boundaries and professional primacy. The word 'ecology' was invented by Ernst Haeckel, who saw himself as adding to the prime thought of Darwin, Goethe and Jean-Baptiste Lamarck (1744–1829).[106] Haeckel, more than Darwin, saw human development according to the ascendance of the tree of life. For Darwin, what mattered was variation, complexity and environmental fit. The word 'ecology' was coined by Haeckel from the Greek word *oîkos*, meaning 'house', and *logia*, meaning 'study of'. 'Ecology' thus shares linguistic roots with 'economics', for which it became a substitute. Darwin used the term 'economics of nature', following Adam Smith's usage.

Haeckel was a fertile thinker, trained in medicine by the eminent Rudolf Virchow, referred to above, one of the prime movers of Germanic public health, but whose primary research interest was micro-scale sea creatures.[107] Haeckel thought – and most biologists since have agreed (although Virchow disagreed) – that Darwin's new perspective on biology provided something wholly different and fundamentally true. In wanting a term to describe this emerging form of study, one which transcended biology and botany, and indeed which could address the entire complexity of nature, Haeckel unequivocally located the term's meaning within Darwinian thought and Darwin's principle of natural selection:

> By ecology we mean the body of knowledge concerning the economy of nature – the investigation of the total relations of the animal both to its inorganic and to its organic environment; including above all, its friendly and inimical relations with those animals and plants with which it comes directly or indirectly into contact – in a word ecology is the study of all those complex interrelations referred to by Darwin as the conditions of the struggle for existence.[108]

Others have noted the limitless scope of this definition as it 'concerns the study of all forms of life over the expanse of time that life has existed on earth, and all the environmental relationships in which life is present'.[109] It has been suggested that Darwin's hypothesis was so effective outside the biological field because it was confined to it, which therefore limited the scope of ecology to the natural world, taking humans out except as observers. This view is misleading on two counts. Darwin acknowledged that the prime notion which catalysed the rest of his theory was derived from Malthus, a fact repugnant to as many then as it is today.[110] Malthus's central idea was that nature (the combination of humans, agriculture and sexual behaviour) placed limits on man, just as natural forces explained the growth and disposition of other species, as was confirmed by Darwin.[111] Malthus's views were employed by British colonial administrators and their apologists to justify official hand-wringing in the face of famine and disease such as in India.[112] As Dresner has recently remarked, what was once understood as a profoundly reactionary view, the setting of mankind's limits by nature, can be seen today as more valid and intellectually progressive.[113] The second reason, beyond the scope of the current discussion, had already become apparent in Darwin's own lifetime, namely the inappropriate extension of biological reasoning by social Darwinism and eugenics to human society.[114] Here ecological thinking was used to argue that the human world needed to be ruthlessly controlled to contain otherwise unstoppable forces, but in fact this was expressed as brutal class relations. Even today arguments continue about the relative impact of nature and nurture, which we see as a false polarity.[115]

While one contribution of biology, namely germ theory, was placed at the centre of public health thinking in the Bio-Medical model outlined above, it may be that, among other factors, distaste for these extensions of biological reasoning into society halted the application of other aspects of ecological thought to public health. Whatever the reason, at the onset of the anthropogenic era, where human population growth and economic activity are increasingly seen to threaten biodiversity, the importance of natural ecology for health is now brought firmly into view.[116] Climate change is one obvious example of a change in nature which is now seen as a major public health threat.[117] There is also wider recognition of the erosion of what is now called 'ecosystems services' and the world's 'carrying capacity'.[118] These services include forest cover, water resources, soil fertility, species diversity and habitat.[119] Evidence from the broad span of ecological sciences has contributed to the view that the erosion of humanity's relationship with other species as well as with the inorganic substrate of the biotic environment constitutes a threat to humankind's conditions of existence. This is so enormous in its implications – for economy, politics and public health – that policy-makers seem frozen and unable to chart a future. But economists such as the World Bank's Herman Daly and Tim Jackson have begun to scope an economics which better integrates humans and the natural environment (see Chapter 8).[120]

Darwin-rooted ecological thought potentially offers much more than new reasons to worry about the state of nature, about which Darwin himself had little or nothing to say. The twentieth-century biologist Ernst Mayr (1904–2005) claimed that Darwin's approach represented a new model of scientific inquiry, based upon the generation of concepts rather than the search for laws, the rejection of typologies in favour of population thinking and the importance attached to non-teleological and semi-random processes in evolutionary development.[121] Within this evolutionary model of understanding is the notion that complexity, emergence and dynamism arise out of simpler ingredients. The physicists R.B. Laughlin and David Pines have remarked that, while for the evolutionary biologist such principles are 'part of daily life', they are only now beginning to replace the scientific reductionism found within their own discipline.[122]

This is the rationale for our own proposal to view public health through four dimensions of existence, briefly introduced in the last chapter. Our view is that those four dimensions are a heuristic which enables public health policy thinking and public health practice to be more clearly charted. Ecological thinking, as in Darwin's model and Haeckel's definition, centrally addresses questions of complexity, emergence, individuality, uniqueness, interdependence and feedback – all concepts which have been established through a myriad of new ideas across the increasingly proliferating ecological field. Our proposition in this book is that these conceptual innovations are important components of the Ecological Public Health model.

Despite its Darwinian roots, the broadening of ecological thought was no simple rolling out of Darwinian precepts. As Mayr has noted, there are many interpretations of Darwin.[123] Indeed, ecology was brought into social science almost from an anti-Darwinian approach.[124] It is important to mention one simple distinction: that between natural and human, or social, ecology. Human ecology acknowledges that the human species has created a unique social world of its own whose ties to the natural world require investigation, not merely assertion via biological reductionism. It is the relationship between people and their environment which matters, and both can be viewed through an ecological lens. A century and a half since the coinage of the term, ecological thought has become extended beyond, and is often distinct from, its biological and Darwinian or Haecklerian origins.

The triggers for a fully fledged Ecological Public Health model are legion. Recognition of the sheer complexity of the relationship between people, their environment and health is one reason for renewed interest in generalised ecological perspectives. The intransigence of some newer public health problems such as obesity and so-called lifestyle diseases is another.[125] Ecological thinking offers an alternative model to health analysts dissatisfied with individualistic perspectives and linear or mechanistic thinking, as well as the dangers of biological reductionism in health.[126]

One problem of applying ecological thinking to public health hitherto has been that it has suffered from a degree of woolliness. Too often, as we saw with some in the images (see Chapter 1), analyses portray the complexity of life and health with humans at the centre. Secondly, Ecological Public Health thinking implies systemic approaches to almost all public health problems. This can easily become so immense that it daunts any action. Is it helpful to be informed that everything is so complex, even if it is true? The promise of an evidence-based approach following narrower lines of information is that it can offer both more immediate and more feasible pathways for resolving health problems. But, as journalist and writer H.L. Mencken (1880–1956) wittily once remarked, 'there is always an easy solution to every human problem – neat, plausible and wrong'.[127] A third problem lies in how ecology in public health is still mostly defined as social ecology with, at most, 'the environment' tacked on as a mediating or even ultimately external layer of influence. A fourth criticism is that, if resource limits are real, then fundamental questions are raised about the use of economic growth as the solution to deprivation, poverty and inequalities in health, which some modern public health analyses suggest are key barriers to health gain.[128]

Haeckel's original formulation spoke to the world of nature, whereas social ecology and the varying traditions in sociology and psychology address complex social influences and relationships. In our view, in the twenty-first century the Ecological Public Health model must fuse these apparently divergent perspectives: the social and the biological. That is part of what this book is about. The problem is not just the dualistic separation of natural and human ecology but fragmentations and rigidities of all kinds. What has a bio-reductionist model of health to say in an era of climate change? How can genetics fully explain obesity? How can a purely environmental approach explain the arbitrariness of life chances being set by accident of birth? Careful consideration of such questions nudges thinking towards an ecological perspective.

Historically, public health thinking is well acquainted with the interrelatedness of biology, environment and patterns of living. Interrelatedness is central to the thinking in studies such as that by George M'Gonigle and John Kirby's *Poverty and Public Health*, published in the 1930s Great Depression.[129] They showed that, in Stockton-on-Tees, England (where M'Gonigle was the medical officer of health), when people were removed from a slum area to a new housing estate their health did not automatically improve, because the fall in income and food consumption as a result of higher rent more than offset the improved living conditions. In the 1960s, a US Public Health Service parasitologist, Leo Kartman (1912–2005), saw public health as the outcome of the Malthusian challenge of how to squeeze humans, nature and environment into a vision of progress.[130] In 1969 John Hanlon (1912–88), then president of the American Public Health Association and US assistant Surgeon General, borrowed Kartman's ideas, as well as those of René Dubos. In calling for an 'ecological view of public health', he criticised 'single, specific cause and effect' thinking which was 'dangerously unsuited to deal with illnesses and disorders that have multiple causes and that arise out of an equally complex revolution in the environment'.[131] Public health thought, he declared, needed to address the complete human context, denoted as a 'multienvironment system which encompasses the physical and biotic realms and the cultural setting fashioned by his unusual cerebral capabilities'.

In Hanlon's view humans were simultaneously in a relationship with both bio-physical and socio-cultural components of the total environment, a relationship which was dynamic across both dimensions as well as within them. These relationships had evolved over 'hundreds of thousands of years'. They cast a long shadow on to the present and into the future. If in the past, because of low population and slow economic growth, human responses to the environmental conditions of human existence could be leisurely, this was no longer affordable in a period of burgeoning population growth. Hanlon said that the world was becoming increasingly 'incongruous'. One set of people could be standing 'knee deep in refuse' while others were 'shooting rockets to the moon'. In this wholly new human and natural environment humankind was bequeathing to its descendants 'waters laced with nonbiodegradable detergents and pesticides and lands littered with imperishable aluminum cans'.

In summary Hanlon was calling for a 'new basis for public health' in Ecological Public Health. It is worth citing his ambition for this perspective in length:

> The emphasis which must be given to establish such a new basis for public health is, in essence, the application of the principles of ecology to the human

circumstance. It is based upon a recognition that the health status of man is the outcome of the interplay between and the integration of two ecological universes; the internal environment of man, the biosocial organism, and the external multienvironments in which he exists. As it is with the individual, so it is with the community. Human ecology is thus concerned with the broad setting of man in his environment; that is, with all aspects of man and his nature, his interpersonal and intergroup processes associated with culture, technology, and social organisations, and the basic personality drives that are expressed in behaviour and emotion. It strives to develop a conceptual framework wherein the public health and medical needs of mankind, as individuals, in groups and as communities, may be approached not merely in a reductionist fashion – that is, viewing only a disease entity of specific etiology affecting specific organ or system – but rather in a holistic manner wherein the integrated responses of man to environmental forces find expression on a health–disease–death continuum. The human ecologic approach, of necessity and by definition, calls for an interdisciplinary effort wherein the natural, physical, and social sciences, in company with engineering, combine to study the adaptive responses of man, and especially the effects of unsuccessful adaptation on his health.

Since then, and in part associated with the vast expansion of disciplines and studies attached to the appellation 'ecological', the notion of an Ecological Public Health has, by degrees, entered the mainstream but without being articulated as such, at least in the unified and interdisciplinary terms eloquently and provocatively set out by Hanlon. A question remains as to why these ideas subsequently faded from view and if they later revived why they lacked Hanlon's beguiling acuity of vision.

Nevertheless, an ecological approach to public health is de facto expressed by the US Institute of Medicine.[132] It appears in a more limited form – since the link to natural ecology is often absent or else applied in a dualistic fashion – through the notion of a social-ecological approach to health, considered earlier as part of the Social-Behavioural model. In part the approach is enunciated by the WHO's Commission on the Social Determinants of Health[133] and through social epidemiology and eco-theories of disease.[134] The Australian epidemiologist John Last, for example, argued for the bringing together of natural ecology and human ecology in order to appreciate 'the interactions . . . on the health of all partners in the complex closed ecosystem of the planet'.[135] An ecological approach, which includes the concept of anthropogenic feedback, has been asserted within health promotion.[136] There are studies bringing a public health perspective integrating environment and health on topics such as car use.[137] The recognition that people and the environment are the nodal points for public health is there.[138] No one model has yet emerged to unify the field.

Today, the health consequences are filtered through a series of changed environmental conditions or health-shaping factors, described here as transitions, and considered in the following chapters. As we have said above, one difficulty that Ecological Public Health poses for policy processes is that it assumes complexity and feedback in interrelationships. Complexity can be used as an excuse for policy or practitioner inaction or, worse, for its trivialisation. How can food labelling be of much use in shifting food behaviour? How can people exercise more to tackle obesity when cities and lives are structured around cheap fossil fuels? The kind of quick solutions that politicians favour are not easy to find for large-scale complex public health challenges. If ill-health is the outcome of such complex interactions, then altering those interactions requires re-engineering of a large constellation of relationships and processes. The outcomes should not be expected to be quick. Ecological Public Health offers no quick fixes, only sustainable solutions.

The models and their themes summarised

Although the sections above have described the models as distinct, if overlapping, entities, each with variations and key moments, the models are all ways of looking at what is supposedly the same terrain of health. They are all reductions or abstractions of reality; a tightrope has to be walked between useful articulation of core truths and oversimplification. The models here have been offered to navigate the complexity and range of writings on public health. Figure 3.3 shows all five models. While each can be described distinctly, they also overlap. Ecological Public Health overlaps with each of the other models and draws upon them, but adds extra qualities.

Table 3.1 summarises the five models, which are used throughout the rest of the book.

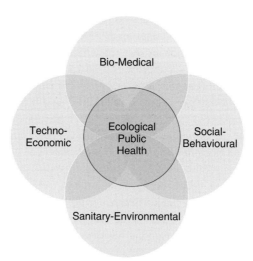

FIGURE 3.3 Five public health models

TABLE 3.1 The five models of public health summarised

Issue	Models of public health				
	Sanitary-Environmental	Social-Behavioural	Bio-Medical	Techno-Economic	Ecological Public Health
Core idea	The environment is a threat to health.	Health is a function of knowledge and behaviour patterns.	Health improvement requires understanding of biological causation.	Economic and technological growth is the prime elevator of health.	Health depends on the successful coexistence of the natural world and social relationships.
Conceptions of ill-health	Threats from the world 'out there': dirt; poor hygiene; unhealthy products.	Ignorance; lack of social support; social dependency.	Physiological malfunction.	Lack of disposable income; low standard of living.	Mismatch between bodies and the environment.
Key methods	Engineering; product quality and regulation; licensing.	Information campaigns; health literacy; social marketing.	Two strands: individual medical intervention; population interventions.	Scientific and product development; knowledge dissemination.	Systems analysis in order to manage social transitions and create healthy habitats.
Where does the idea gel?	Early cities (Roman and Arab).	Nineteenth-century professional and self-health campaigns.	Establishment of medicine on a scientific basis.	Scientific and industrial capitalism.	Evolutionary theory in the nineteenth century; sustainable development in the twentieth century.
Great moments	Provision of clean water and separation from sewerage; tobacco control legislation.	Spread of contraception; psychology-led behaviour change; HIV/AIDS information.	Medical statistics; anaesthetics; anti-bacterial drugs; vaccination.	Mass availability of hygiene products; agricultural improvements; health insurance.	Evolutionary theory.

TABLE 3.1 Continued

Issue	Models of public health				
	Sanitary-Environmental	Social-Behavioural	Bio-Medical	Techno-Economic	Ecological Public Health
Role of the State	Provision of services; funding; standards setting; town planning; pollution control.	Patron; educator; protector.	Professional accreditation; formalisation of education; medical support.	Facilitator of economic growth; legislation; infrastructure.	Co-ordination of multiple actors; protection of eco-systems.
Commercial implications	Provision of public goods, infrastructure and services.	Application of psychologies to business, education and mass marketing.	Pharmaceuticals; nutritionally enhanced foods.	Constant product technical improvement.	Ecological health becomes a driver of economic activity.
Appeal to civil society	Protecting the public.	Informing and empowering the public.	Evidence-based health gain; access to expertise.	Spread of wealth improves the standard of living.	Long-term security for future generations.
Professions involved	Planners, sanitary engineers, housing specialists, public health doctors.	Psychologists; marketers; health educators.	Doctors; dentists; pharmacists; biological scientists.	Economists; technologists; marketers.	Multiple; all who identify with sustainable development.
Main criticisms levelled at the model	Leaves out individuals; limited impact on 'modern' lifestyle diseases.	State interference; reduces health to cognitive factors; underplays cultural determinants.	Cost; reactive not proactive; narrow disciplinary base and concepts of prevention.	Perverse impacts of economic growth.	Too long-term; requires systems change; hard to initiate; downplays individual room for manoeuvre.
Current status of model (early twenty-first century)	Mainly seen as applicable to developing countries; low visibility.	Incorporated into consumerism, e.g. via 'nudge' theory.	Increasingly focused on genetic predispositions; personalised medicine.	Public–private partnerships; CSR; shared value.	Increasing awareness of macro-environmental change.

In the following chapters, we set out some major traditions of thinking, and outline some transitions or large-scale processes of change that we consider to be essential for any conception of public health. Public health or ill-health is the outcome of how these transitions are conceived, addressed and themselves changed. Our view is that public health is not a process but the outcome of processes. Twenty-first-century public health has to continue to address these transitions. This requires Ecological Public Health thinking.

PART II

The transitions to be addressed by public health

Introduction to Part II

> The influence of Darwin upon philosophy resides in his having conquered the phenomena of life for the principle of transition, and thereby freed the new logic for application to mind and morals and life.
>
> *John Dewey, 1910[1]*

John Dewey was born in 1859, the year of the publication of Darwin's *Origin of Species* and died in 1952, just before the announcement, by Francis Crick and James Watson, of the discovery of DNA. He was one of the first philosophers to take full cognisance of evolution or apply the term 'transition' centrally to an analysis of society. An even simpler word can also be used: 'change'. Dewey located the need to understand change, and the need *for* societal change, in the forces driving transition in nature. For Dewey, as for Darwin, there was no destination, no goal, in nature, only continuity of growth and continuity of change, which meant for him that mind, consciousness and knowledge must be expressed in the same language of continuous change as evolutionary theory. According to one account of Dewey's views, anyone trying to establish a hard line between mind and body, or between the mental and the physical, risks reverting to a 'pre-Darwinian' way of thinking.[2] One no longer needs to apply such rigid dualism in thought. In our terms, Dewey is stating that one cannot sidestep ecological thinking. This is the reality.

As we have shown in previous chapters, a core notion within public health – however defined – is also the notion of change. The ground on which health depends is subject to endless change. Life, said the microbiologist René Dubos, 'is an adventure in the world where nothing is static: where unpredictable and ill-understood events constitute dangers that must be overcome, often blindly and at great cost'.[3] It seems obvious, although the implications are not. As a result of change, the actions of those seeking to protect public health will vary, as circumstances and conditions dictate. Accordingly, public health proponents have to be nimble in their thinking, prepared one moment to push for institutional change, the next for societal or technical change, and always for change in knowledge. Public health is thus wrapped around the reality of change. The difficulty in grasping the role of public health knowledge is fourfold. Firstly, knowledge is accumulative; more is known about life today than a century ago. Secondly, knowledge can be fallible; it is itself changeable, being always interim. Thirdly, knowing more does not necessarily mean that courses of action are clear or everlastingly correct. Fourthly, greater knowledge also means there is competition for policy supremacy.

Many writers on public health acknowledge the importance of 'context' or 'influences' on human behaviour and health, as though these factors are external to the body or its state of health. As we have argued in earlier chapters, we are troubled by this implicit model of there being a core and periphery to public health, seeing it to be yet another component of what Dewey called the 'compartmentalism of life'.[4] He warned some eight decades ago that the compartmentalism of life, experience and human outlook took a number of institutional, political, economic and aesthetic forms and characteristics, not least the apparently static separation of society into classes, fractured by enormous socio-economic differences. Although a proud citizen of the USA, he was highly critical of his country's social class system. Although biological evolution was purposeless, for Dewey human development was full of purpose, which is why he devoted much of his life to developing the philosophy and practice of education. Academic discussion of compartmentalism continues today, even if the language of class is seen as obsolete by some and given less emphasis (although the world financial crisis from 2008 re-injected it into mainstream political discourse). People working in public health understand this point very well. Almost universally in the anglophone countries they refer to 'organisational silos' or governmental 'departmentalism' as restricting effective public health action. Wherever public health people gather, they frequently vent frustration at institutional or professional distinctions which block or obscure the essentially cross-cutting nature of health and influences upon it. Public health is intellectually omnivorous. It inevitably enters into diverse territory and fields of knowledge, even if some dominate, as we noted in the discussion of models of public health in Chapter 3. That is why it is essential to understand the key dynamics of change, now addressed in Part II. The transitions we explore here are the grounds on which the public health task has to be forged, although a stronger public health perspective alters both how the transitions are perceived and the room for manoeuvre.

Dewey spoke of the 'principle of transition'. In Part II we look at actual transitions, and we examine the different intellectual compartments through which each societal transition is expressed. All of these transitions shape both health outcomes and the possibilities of public health interventions. We are not alone in finding transitions and change as intrinsic to the notion and practice of public health. In the main, public health analysis highlights just two transitions: the Demographic and the Epidemiological Transitions. Here we give many more, which we believe to be of equal significance. Our list is longer: the Demographic Transition; the Epidemiological and Health Transition; the Urban Transition; the Energy Transition; the Economic Transition; the Nutrition Transition; the Biological Transition; the Cultural Transition; and, finally, the Democratic Transition.

Our focus on transitions, having a purpose in examining processes of change overall and breaking these changes into manageable elements, is therefore not new. The output and list is, although in the form given in Part II it is similar to the narrative model proposed by the physicist Murray Gell-Mann, a Nobel Prize winner for physics. His was an analysis of the world and life seen as a complex adaptive system.[5] He spoke of a minimum of seven transitions for analysis: a Demographic Transition, looking to the means to obtain a roughly stable human population worldwide and in each broad region; a Technological Transition, to methods of supplying human needs and satisfying human desires with much lower environmental impact per person at a given level of conventional prosperity; an Economic Transition, to a situation where growth in quality gradually replaces growth in quantity, and where extreme poverty is alleviated; a Social Transition, to a society with less inequality, and where large-scale corruption is defeated and human activity regulated through law; an Institutional Transition, to more effective means of coping with conflict and with the management of the biosphere in the presence of human economic activity; an Informational Transition, in the acquisition and dissemination of knowledge and understanding; and, finally, an Ideological Transition, to a world view that combines local, sectarian, national and regional loyalties with a 'planetary consciousness' and a sense of solidarity with all human beings and, to some extent, all other living beings.[6] His was big thinking indeed! Our choice of transitions has some overlap but also differences. Our purpose and focus were set by a desire to establish a framework for Ecological Public Health. Our task was framed by our focus on health. Gell-Mann's was all life, essentially a major updating of the Enlightenment.

No transition can be seen in isolation. It is their totality that matters, and that gives modern public health its complexity, but it need not paralyse action or thought. For us, an intellectually coherent way of connecting these multiple transitions is to see them as cutting across the four dimensions of existence outlined earlier: the material, the biological, the cultural and the social worlds. Each of these transitions we describe now has a discernible impact on the four dimensions of existence. Vice versa, the four dimensions of existence are altered by the transitions. We are thus positing a complex, multi- and inter-dimensional model of public health by addressing these transitions. In each of the chapters that follow, we set out the core idea, how and when it was identified, some key thinkers and champions, developments in the idea over time, and why it matters for public health. In Part III, we draw out the implications for Ecological Public Health.

4

DEMOGRAPHIC TRANSITION

The term 'Demographic Transition' describes the change from a societal regime based on high birth rates and death rates to one of low birth and death rates. It is a remarkable change in human history. The term 'demography' is derived from Greek: demos meaning people and graphikos writing. It describes a process which was recorded by mostly Western societies in the nineteenth century as they industrialised, and other countries since. This reflects a rise in standards of living, which removed the pressure on men and women to have many children, plus the expectation that they might live longer. This was made possible both by new techniques of fertility control and changed aspirations for life, and the freeing up of culture from religious and traditional guidance. The Demographic Transition is a notion that thus refers to a highly complex set of changes, social, technical, economic and cultural, all unleashed by rising wealth. It takes only a moment's reflection to realise how the situation it describes indicates a societal departure from all human history hitherto.

The germ of the concept was originally floated in 1929 by the American demographer Warren Thompson (1887–1973), although the term 'transition' in the context of demographic change was first employed by the French demographer Adolphe Landry (1874–1956).[1] Landry first published the notion of the 'transition démographique' in his 1934 book *La révolution démographique*.[2] The use of the word 'revolution' as a metaphor signifies his recognition that what was being described was shattering, placing it on the scale of change alongside that of political or industrial revolutions. Landry depicted the later phases of the process as a function of changing individual aspirations set against the economic and productive potential of society. In other words, the new productive base of society unleashes social and cultural change on a new scale. It opened up new variance between societies; some lived in the old pattern, while others entered the new. The anglophone equivalent to Landry's first exploration was by Frank Notestein (1902–83) and Kingsley Davis (1908–97) a decade later.[3]

The term is now a core part of the demographer's lexicon internationally. Unsurprisingly for such a grand claim, it has attracted both assent and criticism. The term may be current, but it is regularly unpacked and revised. No longer is it always seen as a single and unified process towards a common end state, although that remains the case for many users of the concept, but rather an assemblage of transitions, usually covering separate aspects of the observed processes, be they fertility, mortality or migration.[4] The Demographic Transition deals with life and death, and therefore one might expect that the concept would be a central plank in the public health architecture. In fact, with the exception of public health considerations of fertility, the term and debates about the Demographic Transition remain mostly within the disciplinary field of demography. In public health, a rival term, the 'Epidemiological Transition', was substituted, which is dissected and summarised later (see Chapter 5).

The language of the Demographic Transition is modern and twentieth-century. It is a magisterial account of large-scale change, but the concept would not be viable were it not for the new sophistication of social statistics inherited from the Victorians and their forebears. Indeed, the study of demographic change was well established before Landry coined the term. Early investigations of mortality, for example, were conducted in Britain by John Graunt (1620–74) and William Petty (1623–87).[5]

One of the first attempts at explaining population change also pre-dated what the literature describes as the Victorian love affair with the 'statistical idea', the unleashing of mathematics and social concepts on to the shape of populations and the administration of societies and natural life. Adam Smith's 1776 *Inquiry into the Wealth of Nations* can be taken as a key point of entry into the modern analysis and debate about population. Smith summarised his own views thus: 'the most decisive mark of the prosperity of any country is the increase of the number of its inhabitants'.[6] Smith here is not speaking of the total number of inhabitants in a country but rather their rate of growth. It is rate of growth, aligned with growing economic prosperity, which represented societal progress. It is an important attribute for Smith, a key member of the Scottish Enlightenment. We return to his theory of social change later when discussing the Economic Transition (see Chapter 8). For the moment it is useful to consider how it was interpreted by those who followed him, notably by Thomas Malthus, also a political economist, and by other contemporary writers on economic growth and population.

To illustrate his case Smith had observed that in Britain and other European countries the population had hardly doubled in 500 years, whereas in North America, although not as rich as Britain, it was 'more thriving' and doubled every 20 to 25 years. One of the factors which boosted Britain's North American colonies was not the birth rate but immigration. However, in overall terms immigration was not an important distinction; Smith was arguing that a buoyant economy was required to support a rapidly growing population. His underlying reasoning was that North America had something which was in short supply back in Europe: land. To use a current notion, he was arguing that North America had achieved a greater 'carrying capacity' than Britain or Europe and could thus support rapid population increases. It had what they lacked: highly-quality, virgin land and an expanding frontier.

In Britain there was a more complex picture of population change being established, involving, on the positive side, improving agricultural production in the countryside and, on the negative, greater risks from the diseases of urbanisation, industrialisation and squalor. It has been suggested that infectious disease may have represented about 40 per cent of all deaths in England and Wales in the 1850s and may have exceeded 50 per cent in towns and cities.[7] The situation in the colonies was often poor, many settlements closing because of disease, but not as intense overall. In British cities lacking the resilience to disease afforded by the improved nutrition of the Americans, a variety of circumstantial contextual features may have afforded some extra protection. The social anthropologist Alan Macfarlane, for example, proposed in the 1970s that 'chains of circumstances' had the effect of raising survival rates. Factors might include the drinking of tea or the home brewing of beer. Such changes, he posited, could explain the Demographic Transition occurring in countries as diverse as England and Japan.[8]

The link between economic growth and population change and health has been subject to intense debate. It has been proposed that economic development, the generation of wealth alone, might not be the principal driver of population change let alone of other improvements in the quality of life or health. The Demographic Transition is an expansive intellectual territory of contested fact and debate. As historian Simon Szreter has remarked, the 'human record . . . shows no necessary, direct relationship between economic advance and population health'.[9] This may be true. In the period from slavery to state socialism and through the neoliberal period of the Washington Consensus, the means of economic advance matters as much as its depth and scale. Adam Smith, as we have already seen, had argued that the indicator of prosperity was not necessarily the accumulation of capital but the rate of population growth. Yet here is one among many modern analysts suggesting little or no relationship between economic performance and health, when the founding father of modern economics took a different benchmark: that rising population, based on better health, was *the* indicator of prosperity. This divergence of perspective shows how the question of population carries social assumptions, all of which may be valid.

Without getting stuck in an academic quagmire, is it possible to paint a 'big picture' of the relationship between population and prosperity, enough to be helpful to clarify the public health project? From the late Middle Ages (and with this age of 'data' one has to be cautious), there appears to be a remarkable, if puzzling, association between them. The economic historian Angus Maddison (1926–2010), setting out a panorama of world economic changes, suggested a close link between per capita gross domestic product (GDP) and population growth.[10] Until the early 1800s the world population and economy grew slowly, varying from one part of the world to another. The really big increase in world GDP began in the early 1800s, led by the UK, and this is precisely the period when more rapid population growth also began. From this time until the end of the millennium, world GDP grew around ten times. The world's population in 1800 was around 813 million, and by 2000 it had reached around 6 billion. Into this picture, famines, epidemics, wars and, much later, changes in fertility patterns introduced blips and reversals. Nevertheless it would be quite mistaken to suppose that average height and average longevity, which at various times have been taken as useful measures of health (or, another term introduced later, the 'biological standard of living'), exist in a linear relationship with economic development, yet *some* relationship appears to be present. The question is: what is that relationship and what drives it? The attempt to put this question on a firmer footing is often associated with the name of the Reverend Dr Thomas Malthus. As Landry pointed out in the 1930s, Malthus was not the first to consider the possibility of the existence of an economics–population equation, but his name is the one that is inevitably cited.

First published anonymously, Thomas Malthus's *Essay on the Principle of Population*, published a couple of decades after Smith's *Inquiry* – and much influenced by Smith's book – evolved a more defined and certainly more controversial analysis of the relation between prosperity and population.[11] Malthus's *Essay* betrayed an explicitly polemical intent: it was drafted to counter what he considered to be utopian arguments of the day, the idea that human progress could be advanced through politics and could ignore the material limits imposed by nature and human behaviour. It was for this reason, for example, that Malthus, in his extensive researches around Europe, disapproved of free healthcare in Sweden, because it promoted population growth without addressing food scarcity, but approved of Norway's promotion of agriculture and education, because the former boosted production while the latter was likely to reduce family size.[12] Although Malthus took over from where Adam Smith had left off, and used similar examples, he offered a more refined, and certainly more controversial, explanation. Many writers have denounced him as being plain wrong, yet Malthus's analysis has remained a starting point for much demographic inquiry, as well as being a benchmark of ecological crisis. This suggests some power of endurance for his ideas.

Maddison's work suggests that global population size has increased around six-fold since 1800. Given that Malthus is usually associated with population crises and risks of famine and starvation, his predictions appear wildly in error. He died before Queen Victoria had ascended the throne, and the first edition of his work was published before the first British population census had certified the real population of the country. What makes Malthus's perspective current is his model of analysis for pre-industrial societies, while his theory of limits, as well as the analysis of attempts to circumvent limits, remains controversial.

The bigger question of whether Malthus's specific analysis is still relevant for industrial and post-industrial times is more uncertain. He thought industrial capitalist society unwelcome. His analysis was of more or less 'steady-state' societies, albeit with a modicum of growth due to improving technology. If the case is that technological change has for ever suspended ecological limits – the modern counterpart to Malthus's critique of what he thought was utopian political theory – then his theory is surely obsolete. Yet his framework of thinking remains troubling, not least because of the arrival of late-twentieth-century and twenty-first-century concerns such as climate change, water stress, oil dependency and food crises. But for public health it is useful to consider what Malthus actually said about population change, rather than his neo-Malthusian followers or his denouncers. He offers a rich theoretical framework for the Demographic Transition (and as we see other transitions). In Malthusian terms, does the Demographic Transition represent a societal escape from the food, land, population and health nightmare or does it simply describe an unusual growth period placed within two different phases: low growth followed by high growth followed by low growth? From this perspective, the Demographic Transition might be bookended by, if not low growth, then the re-emergence of steady-state societies.

Malthus's theory

'Demography is a science', wrote Jean-Claude Chesnais, the French demographer, in 1992, 'in which general theories are rare.'[13] The exception he cites is that of Thomas Malthus: hence the value in a return to Malthus to see what value this much-criticised representation of economic thinking has to say about the present.

Malthus presents what might be termed a 'bioeconomic' thesis, a theory trying to grapple with interrelationships. It was that agricultural surpluses beyond the maintenance of subsistence consumption were channelled into population growth. Malthus travelled extensively around Europe collating a wider net of information than England to test and modify his core notion. He found that countries having higher land productivity could sustain larger populations, given the level of socio-economic development, and that societies with more advanced farming techniques could also sustain higher population densities, although he described some limits. For example, much earlier than in Europe, China, with its then advanced agricultural technologies, could increase farm yields. Even so, Malthus reasoned, China had failed to increase the standard of living above subsistence. He also recognised that importing agricultural commodities – through trade or Empire – would provide a solution to restricted land availability, although, in the case of Britain, he reasoned that, because this would make the country dependent on foreign suppliers and on the vagaries of insecure trade, the productivity of British farming would decline. He changed his views on whether to support protectionism or free trade in the heated British debate on the issue. Initially, he supported free trade but within two years switched to backing British farmers.[14]

Malthus's theory integrated features of conditionality. When population size grew beyond the capacity sustainable by available resources, it would be reduced by 'preventive checks' (such as intentional reduction of fertility) and by 'positive checks' (such as malnutrition, disease, wars or famine). This is sober theory. Malthus thought that public health interventions, such as Jenner's vaccinations for smallpox, might make a difference in raising population survival rates, although he added the rider that measures which increased population would only increase pressures on the food supply. Thus, central to his thinking was an 'incessant contest' between population growth and food sufficiency. What became known as the Malthusian trap has remained a more or less constant reference point for all economic studies of pre-industrial agricultural economies.

Malthus's ideas, thus presented, appear perfectly logical, if forbidding, although recognisably limited to societies which experience limited productivity increases: in effect, all human history hitherto. However, to say the least, Malthus's expectations were overtaken by events. Almost from the time he completed the first edition of his *Essay*, population trends began to rise. Why did this happen? Friedrich Engels, collaborator with Karl Marx, thought he had the answer. In reply to the political economists of scarcity – Malthus had been dead for a decade – Engels remarked:

> The productive power at mankind's disposal is immeasurable. The productivity of the soil can be increased *ad infinitum* by the application of capital, labour and science. According to the most able economists and statisticians . . . 'overpopulated' Great Britain can be brought within ten years to produce a corn yield sufficient for a population six times its present size.[15]

Although an industrial revolution was ongoing in his time, in fact the industrial sector of the economy was then relatively small compared to agriculture, and the actual increase of economic productivity was fairly low. Agricultural productivity was growing. Many studies suggest that improvements in farming had raised nutritional standards, but, without the increase in agricultural imports achieved later in the nineteenth century, the considerable population rise that ensued was not matched by increases in food. Recent analysis has argued how fortunate it was that Britain (and the rest of Europe) benefited from an inflow of grain from North America as well as the outflow of migrants.[16] Without this, it is unlikely that the rapid and sustained increase in population and thus the Demographic Transition would have occurred.

Malthus thought that better health and education might lead the poor to reduce fertility voluntarily, especially if accompanied by appropriate policies. It was only through moral restraint – that is to say, the postponement of marriage and children – that humanity would be able to increase its patterns of health and well-being, he argued. For his own moral and religious reasons, Malthus actually opposed contraception; this was ironical given that his own theory suggested a role. A consequence was that post-Malthusians moved in two directions. Some were associated with reactionary, 'do-nothing' policies in the face of famine and disease, while others argued for rising living standards and female liberation. Although the term 'neo-Malthusian' was in use in the early-twentieth-century English-speaking world, it was already deemed 'repulsive' to many members of the international birth control movement.[17]

What is now looked back on as neo-Malthusianism, the support of birth control, was de facto a part of the public health movement, since the promotion of contraception was seen as part of the means of lifting up the material and social conditions of women and children. As we noted in Chapter 3, John Stuart Mill, future author of *On Liberty*, when an 18-year-old young man, was arrested for distributing birth control pamphlets in 1824. In his *Autobiography* Mill spoke of Malthus's ideas as a 'great doctrine', but he completely reversed its conclusions. It was 'originally brought forward as an argument against the indefinite improvability of human affairs, we took up with ardent zeal in the contrary sense, as indicating the sole means of realising that improvability by securing full employment at high wages to the whole labouring population through a voluntary restriction of the increase of their numbers'.[18] In a similar spirit the Malthusian League was formed in 1877, by the freethinker Charles Bradlaugh (1833–1891) and the feminist Annie Besant (1847–1933). This was public health policy advocacy, freedom to publish birth control literature without penalty (Besant lost custody of her children in her fight with the authorities) and freedom to discuss contraception, then also denied. This was territory inhabited by radicals but also curiously by more conservative economic individualists, a cause of continuing friction.[19] While the population of Britain rose dramatically in the early nineteenth century – often cited as the evidence for the falsity of Malthus's theory – what was less obvious was that the birth rate was already falling as an increasing number of families of both the middle and the lower class began to practise simple forms of birth control.[20]

The language and concept of the Demographic Transition, which points to industrial and post-industrial society differences, suggests a thoroughly modern outlook and the entire jettisoning of Malthus's simple and clear model. On the contrary, Malthusian thinking, for a while at least, remained in the mainstream before fading, only to return in the 1970s and again in the early twenty-first century. In 1920 the biologist Raymond Pearl (1879–1940), former head of the US Food Administration's statistical service, explicitly followed Malthus in predicting that the physical boundaries of the USA and limits imposed by agricultural productivity would limit future US population growth. A population of 200 million (it was then around half that) would require, he claimed, the importation of half the then current number again of calories to sustain this level of population.[21] In the 2010s, in contrast, the population of the USA exceeds 300 million people, and between 20 per cent and 30 per cent of its agricultural production is exported not imported. The growth of agricultural productivity has continued to exceed and contradict Malthusian predictions.

Nevertheless Malthusian prognostications continued into the following generation. Warren Thompson's 1915 doctorate at Columbia University, New York formed the basis for a new disciplinary focus on population studies, yet it was little more than an exegesis and updating of Malthus's ideas. In his conclusion Thompson remarked that there was 'no essential difference in the struggle going on to-day in most of the countries of the western world and that going on at the time of Malthus'.[22] He did also acknowledge that cultural conditions in developed countries had materially changed. Attention to these 'cultural conditions' vastly expanded in Thompson's studies thereafter.

In his 1929 article on population,[23] Thompson classified the countries of the world into three groups: (1) countries with high birth rates and high but declining death rates, facing the prospect of rapid population growth; (2) countries with declining birth and death rates in certain socio-economic strata, with the rate of decline in death rates outstripping the rate of decline in birth rates; and (3) countries with rapidly declining birth and death rates, with fertility declining more rapidly than mortality, resulting in a declining population growth rate. Thompson assumed that these three groups were representative of historical stages. By limiting his scope to contemporary demographic regimes, Thompson offered a truncated evolutionary scheme. He described neither a fully fledged pre-transition regime nor a post-transition regime. Thompson had less to say, however, about the causes of demographic change than Adolphe Landry and his successors Notestein and Kingsley Davis subsequently.

In the mid-1940s, building on Thompson's work, the sociologist Dudley Kirk (1913–2000), economist Frank Notestein and sociologist Kingsley Davis generalised the Western demographic experience on broadly similar lines. Notestein had argued that the mortality decline was the result of economic and scientific change.[24] In high-mortality countries, fertility was kept high by religious and cultural mechanisms which, in the face of modernisation, suffered slow decay. In particular, economic development spawned individualism and rationalism, undermining the traditional supports of high fertility. Over time, elaboration of the Demographic Transition thesis shifted to the consideration of fertility rather than mortality. The triggers for this shift, it has been suggested, were the re-colouring of the political map of the world after the Second World War and the theoretical changes released by modernisation theory, a component of sociologist Talcott Parsons's structural-functional analysis.[25]

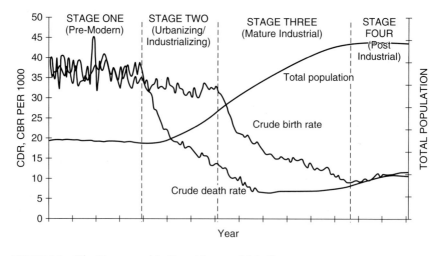

FIGURE 4.1   The Demographic Transition model in four stages

The Australian John Caldwell applied the notion of 'modes of production', borrowed from Marx, to develop an understanding of what he termed the 'mortality transition'.[26] With this notion, he argued that a shift in the morality governing family life – in particular, a higher valuation of the conjugal relationship and of investments in children – leads to a dismantling of high-fertility reproductive regimes. Fertility decline was thus triggered by a shift of emotional changes within the small (nuclear) family, itself a social structure in response to broader economic and cultural changes. Caldwell introduced the notion of a Health Transition, which he saw as an alternative to Omran's Epidemiological Transition (discussed in the next chapter), which he described as being essentially more about mortality than health.

Looking back over four decades of Demographic Transition studies, Dudley Kirk observed, perhaps self-critically, that his field was 'short on theory, rich in quantification'.[27] The Demographic Transition was primarily descriptive. Its value, if it had any at all, might be only the accuracy of its descriptive powers. Malthus, in contrast, had initially provided a theory, but its apparently faulty predictions on population limits pushed it to the sidelines. Jean-Claude Chesnais, representing the French tradition of Landry and no doubt unnerved by the American occupation of a European field of thought, observed that demography had become instead caught up with a vast panorama of fragmented complexity, ranging across culture, health, the economy, social organisation and hierarchy, education, gender, politics 'and so forth'.[28] (One wonders what he left out!) Thus he made a plea to return to a holistic and historical perspective of demographic change in order to discover 'the true mechanisms' at work. But, if it hadn't been found already in years of study and field research, and if not in Malthus, what?

The Demographic Transition and public health

The above account of the notion and reality of the Demographic Transition suggests considerable complexity. We note, too, that although notionally about population change it actually ranges across our four dimensions of existence, grounded on the material, malleable about the biological, and invoking but implicit rather than explicit about both the social and the cultural. Yet demography emerges as a field attempting to comprehend the multifarious drivers of change without an overt social theory of change. Like all the transitions we review here, it is subject to considerable input from diverse disciplines, sources and ideologies. These are hard, to use a modern word, to 'unbundle'. There might not be one transition but many. The availability of modern birth control techniques changes the picture as well as the hand of the State, as with China's one-child policy launched in 1979. Demographic trends may seemingly take account of the religious proscriptions of birth control, but then again populations may blithely ignore them.

We think it is more fruitful for public health analysts to reconsider Adam Smith's original point – that the indicator of economic success is the rate of population growth. From an extended Malthusian perspective – one that looks at the ecological basis of sustaining life in an era of climate change and planetary stress – many questions are raised by the Demographic Transition. Is it good or bad for public health? That depends on perspective. Shying away from such deep philosophical implications, many demographers have preferred to stay with detail, looking at how specific factors can shape life expectancy and population health and size. Small variations in fertility can produce major differences in the size of populations over the long run. As John Cleland and colleagues have stated:[29] 'It's fertility, not mortality, that drives the future trajectory of world population. There's a huge amount at stake. Quite colossal, and it depends on minor trends, minor differences in what happens to fertility.'

Such a conclusion could not have been evident until relatively recently, and demands excellent data. In 1798, the year Malthus published, the typical woman had between seven and eight live births in her lifetime, several would have died in childhood, with the survivors living fewer than 40 years on average. Populations in towns and cities did much worse. Around this time, the world's population reached 1 billion. What happened then was remarkable. One hundred years later the global population stood at 1.6 billion. In 1968, the world population reached roughly 3.5 billion people. In an essay widely interpreted as a revival of Malthusian thought, Paul Ehrlich's *The Population Bomb* warned that, given such a rate of population growth, famine was inevitable; hundreds of millions of people would die.[30] Although this book was a huge publishing success, with almost 2 million copies sold, this specific warning did not come to pass. Rising agricultural productivity staved it off. Once again it appeared that, in this aspect at least, Engels was right. Since the publication of Ehrlich's book the world population has doubled again, to exceed 7 billion people.

Contrast the slowness of the first billion with that of the seventh. Now the speed of growth appears to be decelerating. According to the UN Population Division, the eighth billion is projected to take 13 to 14 years, slightly longer, and world population is due to reach 10.6 billion in 2050 and a possible 15.8 billion in 2100. Figure 4.2 shows the rapid rise of recent decades, with high, medium and low projections. Much of this increase is projected to come from the high-fertility countries, 39 countries in Africa, nine in Asia, six in Oceania and four in Central and South America.[31] In most cases they are also the poorest countries in the world. Not surprisingly, these high-fertility countries have lower-than-average life expectancy rates, at around 56 years. Still, their population is expected to increase from 1.2 to 4.2 billion people by 2100.

One of the factors widely agreed to augment population growth in the future is the constant increase in life expectancy among the better-off countries. In 2005–10, the average person on the planet could expect to live about 68 years, but in 2095–2100 that life expectancy is set to increase to 81. The pressure on the earth's resources is undeniable. In his reappraisal of the thesis of *The Popula-*

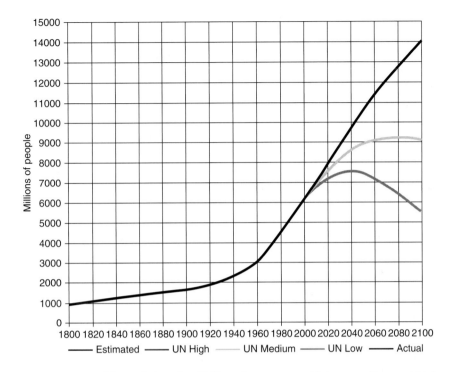

FIGURE 4.2 World population rise, 1800 to the present, with low, medium and high prospects

Note: Before trend divergence the trend is actual, after then it is estimated. The continuing black line is the high estimation, the other two are medium and low.

tion Bomb some four decades after his book's publication, Paul Ehrlich, with his wife Anne, said that the fundamental point of the earlier book was still 'self-evidently correct'. This was for reasons which were substantially the same as those argued by Malthus two centuries before: 'the capacity of Earth to produce food and support people is finite. More and more scholars have realised that as our population, consumption, and technological skills expand, the probability of a vast catastrophe looms steadily larger.'[32] The projected growth of population shown in Figure 4.2 could be greater again because it fails to take into account future advancements in medicine. Or conversely, to echo Malthus, the threat of natural or human-created disasters, unforeseen mass epidemics, or food shortfalls leading to worldwide famine could effect drastic reductions. Which direction the lines on the graph take (high, middle or low), and for what reasons, has a level of importance that cannot be overstated.

What is the value of the notion of the Demographic Transition for a twenty-first-century conception of public health? Firstly, it focuses on a key element of humanity's ecological and material challenge: how to juggle the enormous tasks of feeding people, making the economy work to enable decent quality of lives, and managing planetary conditions. Secondly, it suggests that it is inevitable that theories are needed to interpret evidence and reality if one takes a population rather than an individual perspective on health. Thirdly, it reveals variations in the conditions facing humanity in different parts of the world, and also reveals how people's intimate choices – how and when to have children – are shaped by forces beyond individual volition. Over the twentieth century the question of finite limits to population growth sporadically disappeared only to return again and again. Larger populations use more resources; ageing populations unbalance patterns of economic dependency between generations. Reviled and rejected, the figure of Malthus still casts a shadow over humankind's growth and level of population.

5

EPIDEMIOLOGICAL AND HEALTH TRANSITION

The term 'Epidemiological Transition' is attributed to the American-domiciled but Egyptian-born Abdel Omran (1925–99). In seminal papers from the late 1960s, Omran argued that there was an observable sequence of disease patterns linked to economic and societal development. This notion captures how patterns of disease and morbidity shape population health. The word 'epidemiology' comes from the Greek words *epi*, meaning 'on' or 'upon', *demos*, meaning 'people', and *logos*, meaning 'the study of'. The Epidemiological Transition implies changes in the distribution and the determinants of mortality and disease. In Omran's various accounts there are transition points from one state, or stage, to another. The term is now frequently cited in the public health, not just the specialist epidemiological literature, and has acquired wider resonance. An alternative term, the 'Health Transition', originally proffered by John Caldwell, according to historian John Riley 'links changes in mortality to those of morbidity, or sickness, and to the modern decline of fertility'.[1] The term 'Health Transition' is easier on the ear and, by putting morbidity into a more central focus, claims to offer greater clarity and relevance to modern public health. The question is whether this alternative title is that different to the term and model offered by Omran or whether it is an extension or modification.

Tantalisingly, Omran himself suggested a cultural dimension and set of dynamics to perceived stages in population disease patterns. This cultural element in the Epidemiological Transition has not fully been adopted and amplified but in our view deserves to be. It was one motivation for our inclusion of a lengthy account of the Cultural Transition (see Chapter 11). Omran recognised that a process of cultural modernisation occurs, alongside energy and economic changes (see our Chapters 7 and 8). As an Egyptian witnessing the extraordinary change to the post-Second World War Muslim and developing worlds, on which he wrote extensively, he was acutely aware of the need to make sense of social change as it is reflected in and alters health patterns. This is an intellectual challenge which we try to address in this chapter by identifying the many processes within the Epidemiological Transition, and how they connect and affect public health. Although it appears that Omran's analysis is limited to forms of disease, his interest was in the opening up of understanding about the shaping factors of disease. As he acknowledged, it draws on some of the insights of the British epidemiologist Thomas McKeown (see Chapter 3). Omran makes the case for disease to be understood in broader population terms rather than just the physiological manifestation of microbiological (or microbial) processes. He thus made a conceptual pathway from infectious diseases to what are now referred to as non-communicable diseases, anything but infectious disease.

Omran's initial notion

Omran's 1971 model of the Epidemiological Transition provides a historical account and analytic framework with which to assess the extraordinary advances in health made in industrialised countries since the eighteenth century. His use of the term directly recalls the Demographic Transition, on which it is partly based and from which it was developed. The concept was a product of what he called 'population epidemiology', which he presented as a new field alongside the work on population presented by demographers, sociologists and economists. The substantial point of difference from these others, in his view, was the incorporation of disease patterns, with the implication that demography and disease were essentially matters of public health and not just the mapping of population trends.

As with some other transitions recounted here, Omran's model is a theory of stages. In this case there are three, later extended to four. In its first formulation, all societies are posited as experiencing three 'ages' in the process of modernisation. Firstly there is the 'age of pestilence and famine', which roughly corresponds to the formation of urban settlements, during which mortality is high and fluctuating, with an average life expectancy under 30 years. Then there is the 'age of receding pandemics', during which life expectancy begins to steadily rise, from under 30 to over 50 years. And thirdly there is the 'age of degenerative and man-made diseases', during which the pace of the mortality decrease slackens but continues to extend, and where the disappearance of infectious diseases increases the visibility of degenerative diseases, while man-made diseases become more and more frequent. Omran later suggested that the form in which the Epidemiological Transition occurred was itself shifting. Nineteenth-century England and Wales, for example, exhibited what he termed a Classical Transition, characterised by change from high mortality plus high fertility to a state of low mortality. Japan in the early twentieth century illustrated a speedier decline in mortality, which he called an Accelerated Transition. And in developing countries in the late twentieth century a new Contemporary Transition was witnessed characterised by slow and unsteady decline in mortality, high fertility rates, and rapid population growth.

There are many questions the thesis raises and thus, like the Demographic Transition before, it has become something of a lightning rod for epidemiological researchers worldwide. In many accounts of the epidemiological pattern of a particular country Omran's model is briefly stated and then the researchers seek to define local variance from Omran's descriptive pattern. In Western countries it is often the last phase – degenerative diseases – which has received by far the greatest comment. Is the epidemiological pattern true for all societies? Underlying this and other questions, there is the question of the general and precise reasons for such changes. As a descriptive big picture it is captivating, but while there is undoubted veracity in his description there are also many loose ends. Certainly, the model is a mostly positive vision for the future: a world in which people are living longer if compromised by chronic or degenerative diseases.

While Omran's first presentation cites studies around the Demographic Transition as his primary influence, his account of the influences on epidemiological change two years earlier referred to a broader set of 'macro transitions'. It is this intertwining of transitions which explains why the Epidemiological Transition was offered. These are shown in Table 5.1. Here there are four additional forms of the transition presented. They include, besides the Demographic Transition, a Societal Transition (given his reference to sociologist David Riesman, it would have been more accurate to name it a Cultural Transition, as we do later), Economic Transition and Energy Transition. The implication might be that all five forms of

TABLE 5.1 Omran's summary of macro transitions in the West from pre-industrial to modern times

	Macro transitions in the West		
	Pre-industrial	Early Western	Modern Western
Demographic Transition (Thompson and Notestein)	High-growth potential.	Transitional growth.	Incipient decline.
Societal Transition (D. Riesman)	Tradition-directed society.	Inner-directed society.	Other-directed society.
Economic Transition (C. Clark)	Primary economic sphere (agrarian).	Secondary economic sphere (early industrialised).	Tertiary economic sphere (industrialised).
Energy Transition	Primitive, manual agriculture.	Early Energy Transition.	Developed Energy Transition.
	↑↓	↑↓	↑↓
Epidemiological Transition (A. Omran)	Age of pestilence and famine.	Age of receding pandemics.	Age of degenerative man-made disease.

transition are mutually supportive. Also, by implication, the precise form of Epidemiological Transition is explained by cross-cutting factors and understandings. The transition, he intriguingly argues, is 'ecobiological' (by which he meant the interaction between biology and the environment), alongside the socio-economic, the psychological, and the medical and public health. Although population epidemiology is presented as a new field, the implicit logic is cross-disciplinary. He draws upon a long tradition of thinking that we have already sketched in our chapters so far.

Where, however, is the starting place of this intellectual panorama? Malthus, we saw, was the historical stepping-off point for the development of Demographic Transition theory. The epidemiologist John Caldwell posed the question as to why Omran's concept had such strong impact on the public health community. He too made the connection to Malthus, pointing out the similarities between Omran's thesis and Malthus's 1798 *Essay on Population*. Like Malthus, Omran firmly stated a number of propositions which were descriptively brief with limited references or evidence. He republished his argument several times, although unlike Malthus he limited his additions largely to applying the thesis to the United States and suggesting a fourth stage. Malthus too had been interested in the interplay between nutrition and disease. In Omran's case he suggested that infectious pandemics would be replaced by 'degenerative and man-made diseases' without explaining what was meant by the latter; only in 1983 did he specify that these included 'radiation injury, mental illness, drug dependency, traffic accidents, occupational hazards'.[2]

In fact the link to Malthus is even stronger. While Omran's account is frequently interpreted as a mode of speculative theorising around the shift from infectious to chronic diseases, principally as an outcome of industrialisation and rising prosperity, this was not his primary intention at all. On the contrary, Omran's essay was part of his broader, indeed lifelong, effort to reorient international health institutions, such as the World Health Organization, towards incorporating a population control within their public health strategy. Omran's principal concern was the transition from high to lower birth rates in the developing world and how this beneficial trend in human affairs could be further promoted. This idea is certainly Malthusian, or more correctly neo-Malthusian (as described in Chapter 4), in that it argues for enhancing the technical and cultural power of communities, more particularly women, to promote health and well-being. This is certainly not the usual understanding of Omran's thesis as propounded by many epidemiologists even if they think it.

The causes of mortality decline

As we saw in Chapter 3, critics of the Bio-Medical model of health advance were beginning to influence public debate from the 1950s. Not all were critics at the margins of the medical establishment. In the late 1970s, Richard C. Lewontin, professor of population sciences at Harvard University, frontally attacked his country's medical care system, which despite an 'exponential growth in funds for medical research' had failed to have a significant impact on the mortality for 25 years, he alleged.[3] Among the British critics of medicine as the prime source of public health advance, introduced in Chapter 3, the most celebrated is probably Thomas Mc-Keown, a Northern Ireland-born, Canadian-trained epidemiologist whose critique of the assumed health impact of medicine on public health emerged in the 1960s. McKeown's critique became one of the most influential and certainly, for medical colleagues, the most controversial. Partly, this was a function of his perspective. He took a much longer historical view than others. The ensuing debate around his work – multi-stranded though it was, as we show below – has continued to keep McKeown's thinking a source of debate in public health today.

As we saw in the account of the Bio-Medical model, to question the role of the medicine, even from the inside, was hardly new. C.-E. Winslow, the public health theorist and microbiologist, had enunciated high-strength criticisms of its role in the USA in the 1940s.[4] Like Winslow, McKeown was of a generation deeply influenced by the economic depression in the 1930s and by the dire situation facing the poor and unemployed and the often limited and cynical official response to their plight. John Pemberton (1913–2010), a member of the social medicine movement, who had provided medical support to a 1933 hunger march, observed how it was 'remarkable' how the mainstream of the medical profession, 'with a few exceptions, was not more concerned about the effects of poverty on health'.[5]

By the mid-1950s, the post-war economic boom was in motion in the West. The Second World War had triggered tremendous medical advance, one example being antibiotics (see Chapter 10). Such advances established the view that the Demographic Transition was the result of a long, cumulative and progressive chain of medically managed breakthroughs over the previous two centuries. Improvements in health seemed to parallel improvements in medicine. Certainly life expectancy at birth went up (see Figure 5.1). This common-sense interpretation incorporated the advantages gained by the establishment of medicine and the clinic in hospitals in the eighteenth century, and the application of smallpox inoculation and vaccination since the early nineteenth century, as well as the remarkable impact and general progressive improvements in scientific medical knowledge. The connection between the growth of medical science and changed demographics seemed intuitively unassailable. The Demographic Transition and advance of the Bio-Medical model were apparently one and the same thing.

It was this common-sense and inherently complacent interpretation that was McKeown's principal target. In a series of articles and books, he set out an alternative reading of history. Health improvement, for which he took the 'modern rise of population' as a proxy, owed little, he said, to medical advance.[6] Reversing this medico-centric view, he even suggested that hospitals had produced if anything only a negative effect. For most of their recent history, patients' lives had been compromised by the risks of infection in hospitals. In modern parlance, they became pools of infection and cross-contamination rather than sites of protection. In overall terms, he argued, medical measures had little effect on mortality before around 1935. Most controversially, McKeown set off a debate which

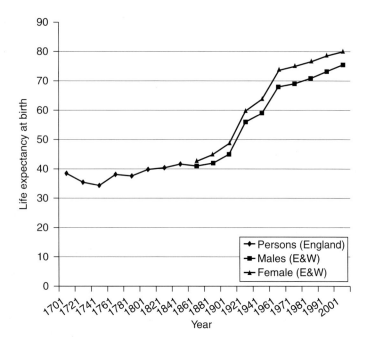

FIGURE 5.1 Life expectancy at birth, England/England and Wales, 1701–2000

continues to today that much of medically inspired public health had played a more limited role than customarily thought. Even public health engineering or sewage disposal, which were environmental improvements, only became significant in impact from around the 1870s, described within our Sanitary-Environmental model (see Chapter 3). His reasoning was that these interventions primarily influenced water-borne illnesses such as cholera, responsible for just a small portion of the total mortality decline, while it clearly had no influence on airborne diseases such as TB, which then accounted for a substantial proportion of disease and mortality.

In McKeown's view, the societal change which produced the most important impact was the general improvement in living standards; this is why we included him in our description of the Techno-Economic model (see Chapter 3). Among the factors shaping these general economic and social conditions, the most significant in his view was the improvement in diet and nutrition. In this thesis, McKeown arguably ascribed to nutrition more significance in public health and policy than anyone since Malthus at the turn of the eighteenth and nineteenth centuries. Malthus, as we saw, looked at food through the lens of population nutrition. In the twentieth century, a social class perspective had begun to emerge, not least through the pioneering work of the likes of Seebohm Rowntree (1871–1954), whose studies of his home city of York, England underlined the social class differences in consumption.[7] A modern nutritional science perspective – rather than sociological – had emerged with the work of people such as John Boyd Orr (1880–1971), who took nutrition into the centre of the public health enterprise, by arguing for a twentieth-century agricultural revolution to produce more food, lower prices and enable poor house-holds to eat better. For this he won not the medical but the peace Nobel Prize in 1949. McKeown added a different argument: that nutrition was the variable which explained differential progress within societies. The implication was that improved diet increased host resistance to airborne infectious diseases, especially TB.

The McKeown thesis was to be highly influential. It has been suggested that it aided the construction of the 'new public health', the new or at least extended paradigm for public health action articulated in the 1970s and 1980s.[8] The now widely used expression 'the determinants of health' began to be applied in Canada as a response to the McKeown thesis and the landmark 1974 Lalonde report for the Canadian government, which argued for a shift to prevention in order to stem rising health costs.[9] McKeown was one of the cited background influences for that report, which was an important restatement of the Chadwick argument that invest-ment in prevention pays dividends for society as a whole. It is not surprising, there-fore, that McKeown has also been judged to be central to what has been described as the 'social environmental approach' to public health.[10]

The thesis has also been subjected to serious testing. It was alleged that Mc-Keown had misinterpreted historical events and relied on faulty technical and data analysis. As one critic put it, he suffered from 'bland obliviousness to historical fact'.[11] Not only had he misunderstood historical demography but his critique of medicine had sidelined the effectiveness of general public health measures, attrib-uting too much to the improving standard of living and to nutrition in particular. McKeown also received much personalised criticism, being accused of medical nihilism, recklessness, insufficiently acknowledging the role of preventive public health, sanitary and local government services or the public health movement's powers of advocacy, and much else besides.[12] Most wounding of all perhaps was the suggestion that his ideas were attractive to neoliberal economists wishing to undermine public health investments as part of a drive towards instituting market-led growth. Within the USA it has been argued that McKeown's ideas received support from those who opposed providing free medical care. According to Ryan Johansson: 'After all if medical care did not matter to health and longevity, then government had no obligation to provide it to those who could not afford it.'[13] Such an inference would not be possible from anything but a headline reading of McKeown's work.

Another central criticism of McKeown, made by the historian Simon Szreter, is that he overplayed the role of nutrition and underplayed the role of public health services. Setting aside the main line of sanitarian advance, sanitary engineering or housing control measures, the more medically inspired public health interventions may have been of variable impact. Medically recommended patient isolation did play an important role in reducing the spread of smallpox however. In Leices-ter, England, isolation of the infected individual had first been systemically used by the Board of Guardians to combat smallpox since the 1870s. Measures had included disinfection, quarantine of contacts, and mandatory notification of cases. This approach became an alternative to vaccination which neither the town nor its people were willing to accept. These measures indeed seemed to work, with selective vaccination also being introduced from 1901.[14] This hybrid approach foreshadowed smallpox elimination campaigns from the late 1960s, to considerable success. Leicester was unusual however. It developed its own measures in a local setting, established in defiance of official advice, but later amended, establishing itself as an exemplar of good practice. Leicester in effect showed the benefits of an imaginative approach in the face of Bio-Medical orthodoxy. We look at vaccination in greater depth later (see Chapter 10).

Szreter's critique, argued one of the defenders of McKeown, showed that he was 'extremely anxious to minimize the importance of nutrition'.[15] In this regard McKeown's assessment of the role of nutrition was strongly backed by the studies of the US economist Robert Fogel. His studies of changes in human body size and physiology and the relationship between economic and bio-medical processes over three centuries provided new evidence about the effect of nutrition on changes in mortality and chronic disease, placing particular emphasis on the role of nutrition in building physical capacity and shaping people's capacity to work during Britain's Industrial Revolution. Fogel, who received the 1993 Nobel Prize in economics, compared Britain with the nutritional circumstances of the colonial and post-colonial USA and the much poorer situation in France.[16] Before the middle of the nineteenth century in England (and later in studies of the USA), he argued, under-nutrition had led to weakened immune systems and increased vulnerability to infectious diseases. Poor physical growth resulting from poor nutrition increased not only the risk of death from contagious diseases but also the likelihood of chronic disorders in adult life. This fact was obscured by the separation in official statistics of cause-of-death data on chronic diseases from that on contagious diseases. This phenomenon, said Fogel, was not disease-specific but was related to the development of the immune system and of other organ systems, as well as general physical growth. In terms of the apparent attack on public health interventions, McKeown did grant them far more importance than medicine, although later historical work filled in the benefits that had been missed.

The debate over the McKeown thesis is rich in detail and still raises copious theoretical questions today. In this sense what appears to be an otherwise dead debate still has life and relevance for twenty-first-century public health; it is about the search for what improves health. The essence of McKeown's distinctive contribution may have become obscured. One defence of McKeown's overall thesis by Gretchen Condran, a US epidemiologist, argues that some of the critics misunderstood the central intellectual value of his thinking. 'Minor critiques of his numbers and methods', she notes, do not undermine his general thesis, which offers a different, more humane approach to medical practice, encouraging it to focus 'on eliminating the underlying environmental sources of disease, revealed by examining the trends and variations in disease patterns'. In particular his key notion 'that many of our current medical problems will not be solved by clinically treating one patient at a time' was hard to fault or dismiss.[17]

A different point is that McKeown showed that multiple factors were at play which were outside the orthodox understanding; he was searching for the entangled bank. His lasting contribution therefore may be that he threw the imaginative net of thinking and evidence further and wider than those before him.

The Canadian public health thinker Robert Evans has applied a kindred line of argument to the medical and public health situation of Cuba. Here was a country with 'first world' patterns of health though a 'third world' economic base. Rather than seeing 'medical and non-medical determinants as competitive', Cuba, despite extremely limited economic resources, has attempted to develop a health system merging medical and preventive measures. Cuban doctors are trained in both an environmental approach to health and a medical one.[18] Perhaps this mix is the ideal McKeown strove for. Political realities aside, the outcome of the McKeown debate goes wider than the role of medicine or the particular contribution of nutrition, although we return to his legacy when discussing the Nutrition Transition (see Chapter 9).

Is the Epidemiological Transition a worldwide phenomenon?

McKeown's thesis was essentially historical in focus. Without downplaying the importance of nutrition for health, the wealth of data and evidence that other factors play a part in determining health is surely irrefutable. If McKeown was looking into the past, Omran's far more general proposition of a pattern of development appears to say more about the future. If the most developed societies followed this path, it is inferred, other 'developing' societies might follow them. This too is the implicit suggestion of the Demographic Transition and – as we see later – is found in other transitions. But even accepting the validity of the historical assessment about Britain or other European societies or North America, how accurately does this describe the situation elsewhere on the globe?

The answer given already is that it was never going to be that simple. Most of the populations in the world live in less favoured circumstances. When previously isolated populations come into contact with new sources of infection, or new imposed patterns of living, as during the period of European colonial expansion, changes in disease environments have a major impact on indigenous populations which may be felt up to this day. It has even been suggested that such major episodes shape the path of social, economic and institutional development far into the future.[19] Environments change even if economic growth is lacking, let alone the democratic spread of wealth. Modern analogues to past processes of colonisation and the spread of foreign-sourced infectious diseases might today be processes such as the impact of foreign direct investment or the spread of alcohol, tobacco and particularly the processed foods industries.[20] The global success in tackling some infectious diseases such as smallpox has been accompanied by improving life expectancy overall, but inhabitants saved from smallpox may now be suffering chronic or degenerative diseases from the changed lifestyles.

Mortality is an important indicator, but, as mortality lessens, other indicators such as morbidity become more important, Omran proposed. Not that mortality

Raymor + Lang (2012)

Ecological Public Health

WHO - leading killer

has given up its usefulness as an indicator. The leading global risks for mortality in the world according to the WHO are high blood pressure (responsible for 13 per cent of deaths globally), tobacco use (9 per cent), high blood glucose (6 per cent), physical inactivity (6 per cent), and overweight and obesity (5 per cent).[21] Overall this is a dramatic global change from 100 or even 50 years ago. Of course, some diseases are more concentrated regionally, nationally and sub-nationally. Indeed it is possible, as we see below, for a society to disclose both high rates of infectious disease and increasing rates of chronic disease on a pattern found in richer countries.

The Epidemiological Transition developed from an analysis of Britain. Using the example of the US, an alternative to Omran's fourth stage has been proposed by Jay Olshansky and Brian Ault. This has been characterised as rapid mortality declines in advanced ages 'that are caused by a postponement of the ages at which degenerative diseases tend to kill'. This they named in Omran's style as the Age of Delayed Degenerative Diseases, which they describe as a stage for the potential elongation of life expectancy beyond eight decades.[22] This is accurate for many societies, not just North America and Europe but also Japan, which has better health patterns generally, including relatively low rates for obesity, as well as the highest life expectancy of all OECD countries.[23] Its spending on healthcare is less than half of that of the US. European societies too are experiencing an unprecedented increase in the number of elderly people yet falling birth rates.[24] While older groups may be living longer, healthier lives in some societies – the USA is one – younger age groups are becoming less healthy, in particular through diet-related diseases such as obesity and accompanying diabetes. The picture is therefore a variegated one, even within a one-country context. The impact of and explanation for obesity, and measures for tackling it, are considered later (see Chapter 9 and 13). If the Epidemiological Transition remains of value, it therefore needs further amendment or adaptation.

Thomas Gaziano and colleagues have usefully employed this amended model to examine how the Epidemiological Transition might be linked to the changing profile of cardiovascular disease. They claim that, although countries tend to enter these stages at different times, the progression from one stage to the next tends to proceed in a predictable manner and with predictable cardiovascular consequences.

Although the circumstances are quite different, a similar trend of differentiation and segmentation by socio-economic group is occurring elsewhere. In the USA a key factor is age, although other factors may also apply. In Accra, Ghana, wealthy communities experience higher risk of chronic diseases, while poor communities experience higher risk of infectious diseases; lower-income groups experience a double burden of infectious and chronic diseases.[25] In the South Pacific islands, conversely, changes in the economy have brought with them behavioural changes alongside changes in nutrition and the shift to more sedentary life modes.[26] These new shaping factors for health are sometimes called 'diseases of lifestyle' or even more loosely 'diseases of affluence'. The first term is often poorly defined, if it is defined at all; and while a source for the concept can be found in the ideas of the psychologist Alfred Adler (1870–1937) the term is also used by marketers and entertainment periodicals.[27] What is insufficiently clear in its use is the degree to which the life is chosen or whether it is an artefact of culture which is almost automatically adopted, given age, gender or other demographic quality. Culture matters, but the common aspect to behaviour-related diseases is the clustering of health burdens in lower socio-economic groups.[28] Poorer groups appear particularly exposed to the double risk of infectious and chronic degenerative ailments.[29] The identification of a new pattern of double or even triple burdens of disease for particular socio-economic groups poses an urgent challenge for public health. It calls for a rethinking of the language and intellectual categories through which this blend of multiple determinants and outcomes is represented.

The rethinking of epidemiology?

As patterns of disease have seemingly shifted from causation linked to the physical environment, to biological factors and more recently to the mixing of environmental, biological, economic and cultural factors, the means for understanding the relationship between society and disease has expanded accordingly. The Epidemiological Transition, in effect, required a transition in epidemiology. One of the main contributors to the clarification of medical thinking about disease was the English epidemiologist Geoffrey Rose (1926–93). Rose successfully illuminated the difference between the type of thinking about diseases which began from medical premises and thinking which started from a population perspective. The former, he argued, led to an effort to determine individuals at greater risk, an approach Rose called the 'high-risk strategy'. The latter led to measures aimed at the entire population, what he termed the 'population strategy'. He clearly spelt out the assumptions implicit for each approach. Rose himself pointed out that the purpose of mass environmental controls had been to produce a mass population effect. The modern analogue, he suggested, might be to alter the 'norms of behaviour' shaping public health outcomes, although he acknowledged that such efforts had so far been of limited success.

In his essay 'Sick Individuals and Sick Populations', Rose argued that one of the limitations of contemporary epidemiology is that it drew from medical thinking about diseases derived from looking at the differences between individual patients. A problem with this approach was that the more widespread a particular cause, the less it could be explained by the distribution of cases. Thus the hardest cause to identify would be the one that was universally present, as it then has little or no influence on the distribution of disease. Following the case variation approach led to a paradox: 'We might achieve a complete understanding of why individuals vary, and yet quite miss the most important public health question, namely, "Why is hypertension absent in the Kenyans and common in London?"'[30] Generally, it would be more accurate to say that both infectious and chronic diseases have declined but that older forms of chronic disease linked only to nutrition have been replaced by newer forms. These also have a nutritional basis. In the past, disease patterns were shaped by diet-related diseases and specific nutrient deficiencies such as pellagra, rickets and beriberi, as well as protein-energy malnutrition.[31] To these today we add diseases of malconsumption such as obesity and diabetes.

Rose's main pointer for public health action was to focus on the population. There will always be variations within and between populations, but the task of public health is to move entire populations in a healthier direction. This implication turns epidemiology into a political movement for changing disease causes, yet retains that impetus as based on medical and statistical evidence. Naturally, this approach produced its own, implicitly political response. Bruce Charlton, an evolutionary medical researcher, has observed that in offering a radical prescription for societal change Rose's approach entails 'an explicit programme for increasing government influence on every aspect of life for everyone'. He criticises Rose's concept of health as 'meaningless except as a tool of political rhetoric', while he judged the overall approach 'unscientific', citing Rose's admission that only infrequently could preventive policy offer watertight evidence or 'reasonable confidence' in the diagnosis and the link between diagnosis and necessary action. Charlton's recommended alternative guidance was 'if in doubt: do nothing', in effect perilously close to objections offered by *The Times* to the preventive proposals of Edwin Chadwick more than a century before (see Chapter 1).[32]

To be judged unscientific is especially damning, especially since the self-image of much of epidemiology is that it represents, as one epidemiologist has put it, 'the science of public health'.[33] Putting aside the implied slight to anyone working in the public health who is not an epidemiologist, this raises the question of what science represents in public health. Is science identified by the use of statistical techniques? This was the gloss introduced in Chadwick's day and underpinned the claims of his report. Is it constructed from rigid associations between cause and effect? This was the implied claim of Bio-Medical epidemiology. In a situation of dynamic feedback and changes of the same infective agent or virus over time this is no longer credible.[34] Today it has been argued that the social dimension of infectious disease requires a much broader perspective.[35] Attempts to develop this more 'ecological' picture of environmental and group interactions brought forth the early criticism of 'ecological fallacy', the attribution of inferences about individuals from the studies of groups.[36] This is a 'mindset' and set of methods the Australian epidemiologist Tony McMichael has countered.[37] Or is it a much broader span of thinking using many methods, quantitative, qualitative, systems-building, modelling, and more, based upon investigation, imagination and willingness to scrutinise accepted explanations? The philosopher of science Karl Popper (1902–94) had originally claimed that Darwin's framework of assumptions was tautological, that is to say not testable in the terms he, Popper, had specified for separating science from non-science. He later issued a 'recantation' (his word), saying that he had changed his mind about 'the testability and logical status of the theory of natural selection'.[38] In effect he had changed his views about what a science is rather than about Darwinian thought. Questions about what science is or is not are as difficult as those about what is or is not art. If the only credible scientific theory of the origin of life fails the Science Test, what does it say about much humbler efforts? Given the enormous span of complexity in comprehending disease causation and in designing responses to it, not just in the case of NCDs but also with many infectious diseases, it is quite unlikely that what many think is the ideal specification for scientific analysis, that of invariant and unilinear causation in conditions of testability, is going to be available or feasible. By implication, this changes and radically expands the framework of science.

Rose's thinking has been developed by Professor Sir Michael Marmot and colleagues at the neighbouring University College London (UCL) Department of Epidemiology and Public Health which has become a world centre of such thinking. In a series of studies initiated by Rose, but developed much further, they have argued that social status and social-psychological factors have a direct impact on health outcomes, with lower-class employment showing worse disease patterns and life expectancy.[39] The UCL studies have regenerated a serious public health critique of contemporary affluent societies and are returned to later (see Chapter 8). They have picked up the 1930s tradition of public health activism concerned about socio-economic inequalities. The starkest expression of this revitalised thinking has come from the work of Richard Wilkinson and colleagues, who have suggested that a large range of social ills can be linked to the level of inequality within societies. This is a new social relativist approach to epidemiology. It has been enormously influential and controversial within epidemiology and, with the publication of *The Spirit Level*, in public policy debate worldwide.[40]

By stating the importance of social psychological dynamics within public health, these thinkers reassert an old debate within social science, associated with the work of the French sociologist Emile Durkheim on suicide rates in societies.[41] This is a debate about social cohesion, self-respect, the level of social support for individuals and groups within wider society, and how such features independently shape public health outcomes, over and above individual psychological dynamics. Another earlier strand of thinking about society and disease is, of course, the overtly radical political tradition of analysing disease put forward by Marx, Engels and, in the sphere of ecology, Alfred Russel Wallace. They too all saw societal inequalities as fundamental drivers of health outcomes. More recently, a 'neo-materialist' view of health inequalities has been proposed by an international group of epidemiologists, drawing on this earlier radical tradition of thought. It has parted ways with the modern supporters of the more socio-psychological, or for that matter cultural, interpretation of health inequalities, championed for example by the WHO's Commission on Social Determinants of Health.[42] The policy implications of this neo-materialist view are clear. Inequality itself has to be addressed, say its proponents, who argue for more equitable distribution of resources or investments in public assets used by poorer communities. The implicit argument here is that, when there are material factors determining health inequalities, the only policies which can address health inequalities are those which alter and equalise the material world. An alternative to the neo-materialist view, the suggestion that inequalities can be dealt with by investments in 'social capital', is given short shrift by the neo-materialists.[43] This later issue is considered more closely in Chapter 11.

The key point for our argument in this book is that discussion of the Epidemiological Transition, and the persistence of health inequalities, among other matters, is always theory-laden and seems inexorably to draw upon and/or move into socioeconomic terrain. This is partly why we propose our four dimensions of existence – material, biological, cultural and social – as the inevitable and correct multilevel framework for public health. Here, in this chapter, we have witnessed how scientific epidemiology requires social science.

Alongside the discussion of the Epidemiological Transition is an ongoing – and possibly irresolvable – debate over the underlying causes of disease and ill-health. In a sense this is an argument about the priority list of shaping factors, ranging from nutrition to sanitation. Some of this debate sparked by McKeown is tortuous, at times obscure and, as we have seen, replete with *ad hominem* accusations about motives and mischaracterisations of arguments. In short, this is a status not unknown in heated academic discourse! Yet the McKeown thesis remains a towering contribution and appeal to public health thinking. It calls on anyone invoking the Epidemiological Transition to think beyond the individual and beyond the role of medicine or public health interventions. Although McKeown thought living standards and nutrition to be the priority explanations, other factors were not dismissed; they merely played a different role at different times. A case can be made that medicine, *contra* McKeown, plays a bigger role than ever before. But what role could medicine possibly play in dealing with the new non-communicable diseases like obesity? The answer so far is very little.

This chapter has suggested that public health needs panoramic views of the 'shaping factors' on health, long after the events themselves. We learn from the Epidemiological Transition, as from the Demographic Transition in the preceding chapter, that progress has to be judged as a collective or societal phenomenon. But public health cannot be reduced to these two first and much cited transitions, if only because, as we have seen, they quickly enter social, political and moral terrain, while claiming to remain on medical and professional solid ground – hence Chariton's jibe cited earlier. Key measures for progress may not be the health of the average or the better-off but the status of particular social groups within society. They are the social canaries in the cage. For Omran, the key issue was women and fertility. For Rose, Marmot, Wilkinson and Pickett, it is the health gap between rich and poor. This too is debated. Does this turn public health into a moral domain? What measures and actions can be derived? Does public health become the health conditions of the new material circumstances of largely urban living? These are questions to which our quest to clarify public health now turns.

6

URBAN TRANSITION

The Urban Transition is a phenomenon which is frequently labelled as 'urbanisation' – from the Latin *urbe* ('city' or 'town') and *urbanus* meaning 'pertaining to the city'. Here we use the term 'Urban Transition' to highlight that the long shift in human populations from rural to urban existence poses qualitatively new challenges for public health. While urbanisation seems a modern idea, linked to the modern growth of cities, the idea that health and habitat are interrelated is very old. Certainly, human beings, and their domesticated animals, are unusual among animal species in having most of their deaths caused by disease. This reflects a change in human environmental conditions from the Neolithic agricultural revolution of some 12,000 years ago which brought people into close proximity with domesticated animals and with each other. To speak of an urban impact on health, therefore, is to have a coherence which is not captured by or subsumed within the notion of the Demographic Transition. As we show in this chapter, many writers have pointed out that the shift to urban existence has definable characteristics. We see the Urban Transition as posing new threats and opportunities for the quality of life and the public health. Sometimes these are extended and improved, sometimes drastically curtailed. The role of public health champions often makes the difference between good and bad urbanisation. The invisibility of public health which concerned us in Chapter 1 is largely due to the legacy of public health pioneers who recognised the threats from early urbanisation, and then acted, as we see below, but have subsided into unwarranted obscurity in public health.

Our argument is that in the twenty-first century, as the Urban Transition spreads worldwide and deepens with the emergence of mega-cities, it is highly likely that a new wave of public health action and champions will be required to civilise what otherwise could become the globalisation of urban ill-health. Within public policy, there is an ambivalence about the Urban Transition. It is loved by some as progress while feared by others as creating mass threats. Public health actions are the pivot on which the outcome emerges.

UN Habitat, an agency of the UN, now firmly states that a global process is under way which it terms 'global urbanisation'.[1] This describes the shifting form and impact of humankind's settled living, be this in small settlements or in larger conurbations such as towns and cities, as well as slums and sprawl. Analysts now agree that a fundamental change in human experience has become the majority reality. This Urban Transition makes extraordinary demands on resources (energy, water, food, chemicals, atmosphere, biodiversity), on physical infrastructure (demand for roads, houses, sanitary arrangements), on economic relations (the need for jobs, cash exchange, trade) and on culture (new social relations, changed family structures, new identities). In the urban milieu, human contact is compressed; new institutions are required or emerge, such as property ownership; and, most importantly, populations constantly move. In the Urban Transition, public health encounters new problems of scale. UN Habitat now posits that virtually the whole of the world's demographic growth over the next 30 years will be concentrated in urban areas, a stark contrast to all previous human history (see Table 6.1). In this, it is

TABLE 6.1 Urban population projections, by region (2010–30)

Region	Urban population (millions)			Proportion of total population living in urban areas (%)			Urban population rate of change per year (%)	
	2010	2020	2030	2010	2020	2030	2010–20	2020–30
WORLD TOTAL	3,486	4,176	4,900	50.5	54.4	59.0	1.81	1.60
Developed countries	930	988	1,037	75.2	77.9	80.9	0.61	0.48
North America	289	324	355	82.1	84.6	86.7	1.16	0.92
Europe	533	552	567	72.8	75.4	78.4	0.35	0.27
Other developed countries	108	111	114	70.5	73.3	76.8	0.33	0.20
Developing countries	2,556	3,188	3,863	45.1	49.8	55.0	2.21	1.92
Africa	413	569	761	40.0	44.6	49.9	3.21	2.91
Sub-Saharan Africa	321	457	627	37.2	42.2	47.9	3.51	3.17
Rest of Africa	*92*	*113*	*135*	*54.0*	*57.6*	*62.2*	*2.06*	*1.79*
Asia-Pacific	1,675	2,086	2,517	41.4	46.5	52.3	2.20	1.88
China	636	787	905	47.0	55.0	61.9	2.13	1.41
India	364	463	590	30.0	33.9	39.7	2.40	2.42
Rest of Asia-Pacific	*674*	*836*	*1,021*	*45.5*	*49.6*	*54.7*	*2.14*	*2.00*
Latin America and Caribbean	469	533	585	79.6	82.6	84.9	1.29	0.94
Least developed countries	249	366	520	29.2	34.5	40.8	30.84	3.50
Other developing countries	2,307	2,822	3,344	47.9	52.8	58.1	2.01	1.70

posing the possibility that the Demographic Transition might even now be folding into the Urban Transition.[2]

Contemporary discussion of the Urban Transition starts with what historians refer to as the early modern phase, the few centuries pre-dating industrialism. In England, the first industrial country, the fraction of the population living in settlements of more than 10,000 people increased from 7 per cent to 29 per cent in 1500–1800. Cities like London, at one point the largest city in the world, required an expanding hinterland of food production and resource provision. This pre-industrial phase was characterised by rising productivity on the land, with the share of the workforce engaged in agriculture falling from about 75 per cent to 35 per cent.[3] Some rural labour also sailed away to the new colonies, but the majority formed a steady export to the city, balancing rural labour demand and supply[4] and forming a new pool of labour in the towns. This movement of people and things to the towns broke the old social order and allowed new economic relations. It broke up long-established modes of thought, a shift which the German sociologist Ferdinand Tönnies (1855–1936) characterised as from 'community' to 'society'.[5]

Tönnies was not alone in detecting the new mental architecture emerging in and from the Urban Transition. But, if culture was changing, other features remained the same. The British sanitary reformer Thomas Southwood Smith (1788–1861), for example, argued that the physical infrastructure remained antiquated. 'We still have epidemics – and why?' he asked, only to give the answer: 'Because in all our towns there are large portions of the people who live in a state essentially the same as that which existed in the middle ages. The conditions are similar; the results are similar.'[6]

Southwood Smith, an infectious disease specialist and a friend of Utilitarian philosopher Jeremy Bentham (whose body was left to him in his will for dissection), was one of the principal movers in the new Health of Towns Association, created in 1844 in Britain. Southwood Smith, like other Utilitarians, was no enemy of capitalism but did see himself as part of a force for social change.[7] Characterising the political economic cycles of production and consumption as one of 'Nature's beautiful adaptations', he announced that human happiness must 'necessarily continue to increase because the main conditions on which life and health depend have experienced, during the whole of the present century, an expansion and improvement, on which no former age presents a parallel'.[8]

The solution to the disintegrating aspects of urban life for Southwood Smith was sanitary action. Whether giving evidence to a Committee of the House of Commons in London or lobbying for reform of children's employment or housing improvement, he represented one of a new breed of practical-minded scientific agitators who 'preached, argued and cajoled' in order to bring their cause and its remedies to public and political attention.[9] Appointed a medical member of the British General Board of Health, he produced reports on quarantine (1845), cholera (1850), yellow fever (1852), and the results of sanitary improvement (1854) went hand in hand with praise for the industrial and commercial revolutions then defining British society. Southwood Smith represents that now hidden body of public health change agents who enabled urban life and capitalist exchange to coexist.[10] We have more to say about the need for new versions of such social change agents in our final chapter (see Chapter 13).

There were alternative perspectives to the kind of policy accommodation which Southwood Smith championed. One saw the Urban Transition as ruthless exploitation, depicting the new industrial cities and rapid urbanisation as the central explanation for the degradation and alienation of human existence. Karl Marx, a leading exponent of this ultra-critical position, based his immediate knowledge of city life on his friend Friedrich Engels's studies of the Manchester urbanisation experience. Manchester, Engels wrote, had entered a phase of 'primitive accumulation' which exposed an epic collision between economy, nature and biology. The health conditions of the city spiralled from bad to worse owing to the essential dynamics of capitalism, he argued, not just a mismatch of old and new. Engels concluded that 'everything which here arouses horror and indignation is of recent origin, belongs to the industrial epoch'.[11] In any case an explanation at the level of household or neighbourhood went only so far. It ignored the role of factory conditions and the poverty born of inequality. Accumulation of profit necessitated a degradation of the human experience for the mass urbanised working class then emerging. This was much commented on and analysed by Henry Mayhew (1812–87) and Charles Dickens (1812–70) in England and visually in both France and Britain by Gustave Doré (1832–83).

Manchester, indeed, did provide an example of an unhealthy city, but even while its ill-health was being documented it was being exported and replicated elsewhere. In the USA, which we saw earlier was once defined by Adam Smith as the very model of a prosperous society, early urbanisation 'did not go well from a public health perspective'.[12] As in Britain, there was a substantial health penalty for US urban living. Mortality rates were 30 per cent higher in cities than in rural areas. Similar health problems, associated with poor infrastructure for water and sanitation, were noted in otherwise dissimilar places. Was the prognosis inevitably gloomy? Ironically, Marx, who castigated capitalism as the cause of ill-health, also thought that capitalism's Promethean productivity was the potential solution if tamed by radical political change. Urban existence could be improved; squalor and poverty were not inevitable.

Sanitarians believed that disease was spread by miasmas, in effect putrefaction and its attendant bad smells, a theory promoted by Southwood Smith, Chadwick and many others, including the leading cellular biologist of the age, the German sanitary reformer Rudolf Virchow. The cholera epidemics of mid-nineteenth-century London provided the opportunity to explore this theoretical viewpoint using new statistical methods. In Chapter 1 we saw that John Snow – replete with the image of the Broad Street pump – is celebrated today as the medical scientist who solved the mystery of cholera transmission and in so doing became the founder of modern epidemiology. Snow argued, in opposition to miasmatic theory, that cholera was a communicable disease which spread when humans swallowed food or water contaminated by previous cholera victims. In contrast to Snow and his almost saintly elevation to hero status, the epidemiologist William Farr, statistical superintendent of the General Register Office and a member of the Committee of Scientific Inquiries in 1854, who was seen as much more authoritative on cholera at the time, is barely remembered today. One obvious reason is that Snow's analysis was later seen as a better fit with newer scientific conceptions of cholera, although it was only after Louis Pasteur developed techniques for growing microbes that it was possible for Robert Koch to culture and isolate the cholera 'comma' bacillus and demonstrate a new scientific proof that the disease was water-borne.[13] Ironically, the Italian biologist Filippo Pacini (1812–83) had described the cholera bacillus in 1854, 30 years before Koch, but his work was unknown to either Farr or Snow. It has since been suggested that the difference between the two was that, while Snow had arrived at his views through conviction, Farr was on his way to a similar understanding but through a more open-minded route of investigation. Farr, it has been suggested, was keener than Snow to weigh a larger list of social, environmental and biological factors and more willing to explore new ideas.[14] If this characterisation is true, it is Farr, not Snow, who is a better role model for the current era. In any case, the mortality levels in Britain's industrialising cities did not improve significantly until the 1870s and 1880s.

Scientifically speaking the early sanitarians may have been wrong, the economist Richard Easterlin has written, but their policy conclusions were nevertheless 'correct'.[15] This point requires some qualification. Historians argue about whether the early investment in infrastructural improvements had a positive effect on the standard of living in the long term, but there is wider agreement that the short-term impact was negligible or even negative.[16] Improvements in sanitary technology such as the flush toilet or water closet made the situation strikingly worse often by delivering human excreta into sources of city water supplies.[17] In the late nineteenth century, the primary sewer outlets of many American cities emptied in close proximity to water intakes, meaning that the cities with the most extensive sewer systems had the greatest potential to pollute their water sources.[18]

Although the miasma theory could not scientifically explain the urgency of separating clean from polluted water, it could certainly explain the necessity for public parks. Beginning in New York, but later right across the US, Frederick Law Olmsted (1822–1903), for part of his career the head of the USA Sanitary Commission, successfully argued that the large public parks would have both an 'air purifying' and a 'decorative' value; forested and open green spaces could allow city dwellers to breathe clean air.[19] Olmsted understood that good sanitation required well-drained land, well-circulating waterways and well-designed sanitary facilities, reflecting his knowledge of the sanitary movement. Olmsted and his colleagues offered an early model of Ecological Public Health, unifying natural and human ecology, meaning for him the promotion of easier circumstances of co-operative living, through the 'green' reorganisation of shared space, but he also understood that technical change alone was not enough to sanitise the Urban Transition. Social changes were required too. What was most prominently needed was a radical shift in perspective by elites resistant to change. Every step of the way, it appeared, such elites resisted what they saw as unnecessary interventions until crises 'made them inescapable'.[20]

What followed in Britain and Germany – the latter which became the world centre of the hygiene movement – was a broadening of sanitary interventions, from public baths to the availability of heavily marketed soap, albeit often, in the case of Britain, with a barely disguised tension between the promotion of public health and the seizing of commercial advantage.[21]

Understanding the Urban Transition

In interpreting the Urban Transition, few social scientists have provided a better analytic grasp than the American writer Lewis Mumford (1895–1990). Mumford's picture of urbanisation is by turns historical, ecological and philosophical, but always profoundly interdisciplinary. In all these respects he was influenced by the now largely forgotten Scottish ecological and social theorist Sir Patrick Geddes (1854–1932). Geddes, originally trained in biology by Darwin's younger colleague T.H. Huxley, moved from biology to botany and thence to sociology and town planning, assimilating or establishing clear schools of thought in each discipline en route. Unusually for the times, Geddes made the journey from the biological to the sociological analysis without imposing an authoritarian biological outlook. Although he was interested in eugenics, he was not ultimately seduced. He was interested in the fluidity and evolutionary elements of ecological thinking, as applicable to urban existence. That Geddes is barely remembered today, although he was the co-founder of the British Sociological Society (now Association), may be due to this interdisciplinary, unconstrained and free-thinking perspective. He was deeply imbued with utopian and evolutionary thinking.[22]

Mumford observed in a 1956 essay that a 'natural history' of urbanisation had yet to be written.[23] In his later and famous work *The City in History*, 600 pages long, he attempted to provide just that.[24] The earlier essay offers the brevity that the *magnum opus* lacks. In it he sets out three historical stages of the Urban Transition. Although Mumford's book included 'city' in the title, it was clear from his account that he believed that cities and urban development were distinctive categories and phases of the transition. In the first phase, the chief characteristic of urban settlements, irrespective of size, was their integration with their agricultural surroundings. This today might be called bio-regionalism. It followed that the number and size of cities varied with the amount, availability and productivity of their proximal agricultural land. The location of cities was thus limited to valleys and flood plains like the Nile, the Indus and the Hwang Ho. Mumford diagnosed four natural limits to this phase of urban development: the nutritional limit of an adequate food and water supply; the military limit of protective walls and fortifications; the transportation limit for the movement of objects and people; and the power or energy limit set by water, wind and the use of animals.

In Mumford's second phase, what he termed 'the industrial city', these limits ceased to hold. These cities developed as energy systems, based upon extraction of food and fuel from the countryside. Thus Mumford spoke of wheat cities, rye cities, rice cities and maize cities, and characterised rising urban centres according to their source of energy, particularly with the switch to coal power. In this second phase, he suggested that 'growth takes place by colonization', exerting political control not necessarily annexing the physical reality.[25] The more complete the urbanisation, the more definite the release from natural limitations. The more independent the city seems, the more onerous it becomes for the territory it dominates. Cities, in a word, are colonial powers and social entities.

The next phase, from a word coined by Geddes, was the conurbation. This was urbanisation taken to a new degree and new form. Urban areas, hitherto distinct, politically and geographically, combined to form dense population masses on a new scale, forming a new configuration as different as the city itself was from its rural origins. His view of this latest phase was harsh:[26]

> The extension of the industrial conurbation not merely brings with it the obliteration of the life-sustaining natural environment but actually creates, as substitute, a definitely anti-organic environment; and even where, in the interstices of this urban development, land remains unoccupied, it progressively ceases to be of use for either agriculture or recreation.

Mumford was critical of organic possibilities of urban culture becoming subservient to more mechanistic and technocratic rhythms of urban life. He thought that the Urban Transition could develop positively, although many permutations were likely. Britain was a model in this respect for him because it was that country which had suffered the worst excesses of industrialism yet generated among the best attempts to chart an alternative civilising course. Mumford called for an urban and industrial pattern that would be 'stable, self-sustaining, and self-renewing', in contrast to 'the blind forces of urbanisation' which he found at least in England in early urbanisation and in the Ruhr Valley in Germany. He thought that this direction for urban futures required the balancing of city populations and regional resources to maintain a high level of development across all elements necessary for decent communal life: social, economic and agricultural progress. The philosophical background to Mumford's urban thinking lay not just with Geddes but with writers such as the Russian émigré and early ecological theorist Prince Peter Kropotkin (1842–1921), whose observations of urban–rural synergies celebrated the necessity of balance.[27]

Twentieth-century town planning translated this thinking into the reality of British garden cities, championed by Sir Ebenezer Howard (1850–1928), whose celebrated work *Garden Cities of Tomorrow* was originally published in 1898 as *To-morrow: A Peaceful Path to Real Reform*. As the title showed, these early critics of urbanisation believed that a better integration of urban and rural space could generate viable mutuality. Recent writers have extended this concept with what they call 'techno-cities', planned and developed in conjunction with large technological or industrial projects.[28] (We see such thinking unleashed in modern

China today.) These urban thinkers, while not directly focusing on public health, saw the value of harnessing urban development as the production of a better quality of lives. They had a broad notion of the health of the public. Mumford, indeed, warned Europeans of what could happen if they followed the US love affair with the motor car. In *The Highway and the City*, he prophesied what has happened, the domination of the car over urban quality of life, segmenting human relationships.[29]

Urbanisation in the developed world

The Urban Transition varies by intensity and place through different means and changing technologies. In North America, prior to colonisation, the indigenous people held that the land with its flora and fauna was part of the common domain under the control of the supernatural. Land and resources were not considered alienable property. The colonists introduced their own political economy over land as they moved west. It must seem curious for Americans, if the fact were widely known, that both the agricultural and the urban lines of their country are determined by the English game of cricket, for it was the length of the cricket pitch, 22 yards, which became the measure of America. The explanation lies in the fact that 22 yards was the length of the original measuring chain devised in 1620 by one-time Oxford divinity student Edmund Gunter (1581–1626). Gunter's ambitions went beyond the measuring of cricket pitches to land surveying generally, and his chain became standardised throughout those parts of the world influenced by the British. A Federal law was passed in 1785 that stated that all official government surveys must be done with a Gunter's chain, which resulted in each similarly measured parcel of land acquiring an identifiable map address and thus allowing it to be sold unviewed in distant financial centres like New York.[30] Division and owner registration in this manner captures and stores a critical component of its nascent capitalist economy – ownership relations. Common systems of measurement and the standardisation of ownership right meant that the march of capital, labour and land was seamlessly integrated. Unfortunately, this was not to be the fate of cricket. England's leisurely game was replaced by 'all-American' baseball in the mid-nineteenth century, albeit with rules devised by English-born Henry Chadwick (1824–1908), sanitarian Edwin Chadwick's half-brother![31]

This system of measurement was neat. Armed with chains and theodolites, surveyors divided up America for farmer, wagon, railroad and, much later, the automobile. But no system of measurement by itself was able to constrain the forces thus unleashed. Today compact Manhattan vies with the sprawl of not only Los Angeles but also its own suburbia. For public health, a key distinction lies between those urban areas which operate public transport systems and those reliant on private vehicles, and between those which encourage walking and cycling and those where pedestrians are looked upon with suspicion and discouraged. What the automobile gave Americans, before most other countries in the world, was point-to-point travel which railways could not and which buses could do only by making people wait and which were dispensed with when people's incomes increased. The automobile permitted the filling in of suburban forms along railway tracks and in the process extended far beyond those railway lines, making access by other means than the automobile difficult. With the building of freeways, suburbs and regional business points, shopping malls and the like became as accessible as, or more accessible than, the central city area, marking the beginning of the central city's decline. Once under way, this process has proved difficult to reverse. Houston in Texas, built on the petroleum industry, today possesses just one line of light railway track among a vast sea of urban freeways. Its impact is mostly decorative. Turning back the automotive tide is not entertained. The question for such cities is how they will chart a future course for personal transport in the light of coming increases in the cost of petroleum.

Jane Holtz Kay, an architectural and planning critic, has described this world as the 'King of the Road' lifestyle, where American culture feeds the aspirations of developing countries to adopt this way of life as progress.[32] The spread of motorised modes of transport suggests that people leap at the opportunity to be driven by hidden energy. Figure 6.1 gives the global picture of the rise and rise of motorised transport, showing how in the twentieth century people shifted from animal or human power in the form of walking or riding bicycles to motor-bikes, buses and cars, reliant on fossil fuels. It is estimated that car ownership worldwide will triple to 2 billion people owning cars by 2050, according to the International Energy Agency and OECD.[33] The same prognoses anticipate that movement by trucks or lorries will double, and air travel will increase fourfold.

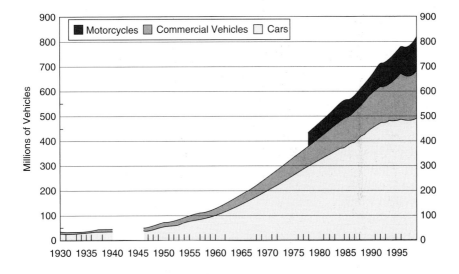

FIGURE 6.1 The rise of motorised transport, 1930–2000

Energy analysts are troubled by the energy requirements of this rise in motor-ised movement. Transport accounts for about 19 per cent of global energy use and 23 per cent of global CO_2 emissions. On current trends, transport energy use and CO_2 emissions will rise by nearly 50 per cent by 2030 and more than 80 per cent by 2050. If the implications for climate are serious, the health implications – from pollution to transport-related deaths and injuries – are potentially dramatic. The issue of work-related transport deaths is considered in the Economic Transition (see Chapter 8). Shifting passenger travel to more efficient modes is part of the picture, but the other part is urban design, the move to less car-oriented cities, as has occurred in some parts of Europe, and making it easier to walk and cycle for short trips. Major areas for improvement are the transport systems for goods. As the International Energy Agency has stated drily, 'strong policies are needed'.[34]

The automobile as twentieth-century cultural siren has been explored in many novels, from Kenneth Grahame's Toad figure in *Wind in the Willows* (see Chapter 1) to Ilya Ehrenburg's prophetic Russian 1929 novel *Life of the Automobile*, which begins symbolically with the first death from a car. The road movie is a Hollywood staple. Today, the car not only defines public space, hindering social interaction, framing what is dangerous, but also pollutes. UN Habitat has summarised the fuel consumption and associated greenhouse gas emissions of some big cities (see Table 6.2).[35] These figures suggest considerable variation of impact, reflecting the level of public infrastructure. The car shapes how and whether people can build exercise into their daily lives, dictates experience in the city and is a cause of accidents and ill-health, ranging from chronic obstructive pulmonary disease (COPD) to noise-related stress.

Besides this account of car-led urbanisation, there have been attempts to sketch a broader understanding of the relationship between human movement and habitat.

TABLE 6.2 Ground transportation, fuel consumption and GHG emissions, selected cities

City	Gasoline consumption (million litres)	Diesel consumption (million litres)	GHG emissions (tonnes CO_2 equivalent, per capita)
Denver (US)	1,234	197	6.07
Los Angeles (US)	14,751	3,212	4.74
Toronto (Canada)	6,691	2,011	3.91
Bangkok (Thailand)	2,741	2,094	2.20
Geneva (Switzerland)	260	51	1.78
New York City (US)	4,179	657	1.47
Cape Town (South Africa)	1,249	724	1.39
Prague (Czech Republic)	357	281	1.39
London (UK)	1,797	1,238	1.18
Barcelona (Spain)	209	266	0.75

In the early 1970s the US geographer Wilbur Zelinsky suggested that changes in human mobility occurred in a series of stepped transitions mirroring that of other transitions we have already considered.[36] Phase one ('premodern traditional society'), before the onset of urbanisation, implied very little migration. Phase two ('early transitional society') involved 'massive movement from countryside to cities . . . as a community experiences the process of modernisation'. Phase three ('late transitional society') corresponded to what he referred to as the 'critical rung . . . of the mobility transition' where urban-to-urban migration surpasses the rural-to-urban migration, where rural-to-urban migration 'continues but at waning absolute or relative rates', and where 'complex migrational and circulatory movements within the urban network, from city to city or within a single metropolitan region', increase, and non-economic migration and circulation begin to emerge. Phase four ('advanced society') entailed the 'movement from countryside to city . . . but is further reduced in absolute and relative terms, [and] vigorous movement of migrants from city to city and within individual urban agglomerations . . . especially within a highly elaborated lattice of major and minor metropolises' is observed. Phase five ('future superadvanced society') is characterised by the following: 'Nearly all residential migration may be of the interurban and intraurban variety . . . No plausible predictions of fertility behaviour and . . . a stable mortality pattern slightly below present levels.' Zelinsky's often-cited model was based on the urbanisation experiences of currently developed countries (but particularly the USA) up to the late 1960s, although his assessments about mobility in prehistory appear somewhat speculative (given that humankind managed to spread itself worldwide without the assistance of maps and wheeled transport).

The Urban Transition analysts collectively describe a 'plastic' process where there is a long overhang of past decisions (or non-decisions) stretching into the future. Investment in particular patterns of mobility freezes the potential for alternative modes of moving in towns, yet the twenty-first century requires more sustainable models of migration, transportation and urban development. The urban experience has been moulded by past investment, shaping public health today. This is true not just of mobility but of physical infrastructure, such as water, roads and foodways, and of social infrastructure, such as housing, parks, public libraries, opportunities for social interaction, and healthcare. Jane Jacobs (1916–2006), an acute observer of urban change, set out such parameters for what she called the 'liveable' city.[37] Los Angeles with its endless urban sprawl and suburbia represented for her atomised and mechanised existence, at one pole,[38] with London or Toronto as more organic, complex and integrated existences, at the other. The discourse on urban change, she thought, ranges from public to private, individual to the collective, external to internal. All is in tension, which public health investment can resolve in some places but which it cannot in others and in which the energy cost of servicing cities is a rising factor.

In the latest phase a new problem of the urban form begins to emerge as retail capital concentrates. In this later phase of urban economic development retail activity becomes concentrated in larger and larger economic units and retail distribution moves to online (internet) sales. In a trend which began decades before, small grocery chains make way for larger grocery chains, and high street or main street shops, often individually owned or in small or otherwise unviable chains, close as retail malls located on cheaper sites replace them, and they in turn are replaced by companies which, by sheer volume, are able to undercut them. This is a dual process, a further concentration of capital in companies like Wal-Mart, the world's largest retailer, in the USA, Tesco in the UK, Woolworth's in Australia (which had disappeared in the USA, where it originated), and their equivalents elsewhere, and a change in physical form, the demise of local shopping. In the wake of this process comes the destruction of small capital, in the form of money, physical plant, vacant store fronts and other buildings, and for that matter excess labour.

Such changes might appear to be just a technical process in the reformulation of urban living, one kind of economic organisation supplanting another. As the geographical and economic theorist David Harvey has argued, changes in urban form need to be understood as one of the rhythms of capital accumulation.[39] In examining responses to such changes Harvey has critically observed that environmentalism often summons up images of some rural, communitarian vision of the past. 'The pervasive and often powerful anti-urbanism of much of the contemporary environmental-ecological movement', he says, 'often translates into the view that cities ought not to exist since they are the highpoint of the plundering and pollution of all that is good and holy on planet earth.'[40] As has been suggested at various points, an Ecological Public Health perspective is based on understanding change, not wishing for the past. The more practical answer to this critique is simply the reality of urbanisation. If the reality of urban life in the rich, developed world appears difficult to manage, that of the developing world is far more perplexing, as we now see.

Urbanisation in the developing world

Cities such as London, Toronto or Paris no longer represent global urbanisation. In these centres, concentration of wealth, knowledge and power allowed for specialisation, which contributed to technical, cultural and social innovation and, after early periods of chaotic environmental and health challenge, the cities were civilised by rising levels of economic and social prosperity. The rise of mega-cities such as Lagos, Cairo, Mexico City, Mumbai or Sao Paolo provides more accurate archetypes for twenty-first-century urbanisation. In the first half of the twentieth century, the population of Lagos, former capital of Nigeria, grew slowly at around 3–4 per cent per annum. It has been mooted that this slow growth is explicable by mass sterility in the wake of the high level of infectious disease.[41] Be that as it may, from 1950 population growth leapt to over 18 per cent, settling to a 14 per cent rate of growth in the early 1970s. Lagos state, the hinterland included, now numbers 18 million people.[42] Despite Nigeria being Africa's largest oil-producing country, the urban area of Lagos is characterised by sharp inequality, widespread poverty amidst substantial wealth, and persistent and widespread corruption. The difference in other African cities is a matter solely of degree.[43]

As yet Lagos falls into second place as a growth phenomenon to Cairo, although it is predicted to grow beyond it.[44] The official size of the Egyptian capital was around 11 million in 2010, but the greater Cairo area contained upwards of 17 million people. The problem with such estimates is that they are only very approximate, a consequence of the vast increase in informal settlements. Since the 1970s the majority of new housing was built without planning permission on formerly agricultural land. A critical consequence for health is that without accurate figures or stable definitions of tenure and occupancy it is not possible to plan for the health needs of populations which are now effectively the majority part of Cairo. As one typically despairing German technical study concluded: 'How many schools and health centres does each area have and how many are needed? Which ones are missing basic infrastructure such as water and sanitation? What are the characteristics of their populations?'[45] If the causes of Cairo's informal growth lie within the country's specific geopolitical history, then this localised specificity of explanation is repeated in every case of urban growth throughout Africa. In the case of China, the world's most populous country (but likely to be overtaken by India), the story of urbanisation has its own dynamic, the difference from Africa being that in its case urbanisation is linked to a startling record of economic growth. The proportion of the Chinese population living in urban areas increased from only 20 per cent in 1980, to 27 per cent in 1990, and reached 43 per cent in 2005. By the middle of the twenty-first century, China's urbanisation rate is anticipated to reach 75 per cent. In the space of just a few decades, it has been suggested, China will complete an Urban Transition that took the West hundreds of years.[46]

In some respects, the rapid rise of mega-cities, both in African and Chinese variants, does reflect the extension and globalisation of the conditions of 1840s Manchester: at its worst unplanned, unregulated and chaotic, and abundant in public health victims as well as criminality of omission and commission. But Manchester was also the location of countervailing social forces arguing for public protection, health investment and co-operation, not just ruthless competition. Civic pride as well as self-educated working people's organisations transformed and humanised the brutal initial Urban Transition of Cottonopolis's ceaseless industry into a trading city marked more by its grand textile warehouses and championship of economic liberalism and global outlook. From its transformation and similar stories of cleaned-up cities came Sir Benjamin Ward Richardson's 1876 depiction of *Hygeia, a City of Health*, a book dedicated to Sir Edwin Chadwick in his 'pre-eminent position as the living leader of the sanitary reformation of this century'.[47] Richardson (1828–96), an anaesthesiologist, physiologist and medical researcher, but also sanitarian and campaigner, could not have been less like Chadwick in personal disposition, but he shared the aspiration of a healthy city. It was to be clean, secure, orderly and health-enhancing, a foundational idea and durable beginning for the soon-to-emerge town planning movement.[48] In such places cities did become the framework for a new society, an expression of social justice and social needs within a fiscal and legal framework. In contrast, in many parts of the developing world, local elites have discovered new ways to insulate themselves from new-style poverty and chaos. The result is gated developments, imported servants, and even plans for 'floating utopias', say Michael Davis and Daniel Monk.[49] These contrasting economic directions are equally manifest in the developing world's mega-cities. Already, public health researchers are documenting the health impact of this new fourth stage of the Urban Transition, beyond Mumford's three.

Conventionally, it has been argued that urbanisation inevitably raises GDP, yet the consulting firm McKinsey has argued that mega-cities might break this connection and become the laggards of economic development.[50] There are two pictures of the future. One is based on growth with short-term negative health and environmental effects which could be resolved by economic buoyancy. The other is urbanisation with chaotic economic growth, limited investment in infrastructure and the domination of the informal economy. In the latter, slums proliferate and a large proportion of the population remains workless or locked into the informal economy. For some intellectuals and development agencies in the West, as a result, the argument is about the benefits of political and financial aid, with some arguing for and others against. Other issues are corruption – 'bad government' – and the apparently patronising role of international experts.[51]

In China, people in urban areas may have on average better health than their counterparts in the countryside. The urban dwellers are younger and have access to healthcare. Globally, the urban picture is also one of worsening self-reported health.[52] There is a tension between physiological health and mental health (in our terms the biological versus the cultural). According to UN Habitat's *Global Report on Human Settlements 2011*, 43 per cent of the urban population in developing regions live in slums; in the least developed countries, that proportion rises to 78 per cent.[53] Among the 1 billion people who live in informal settlements, one-third of households are headed by women. Environmental degradation and a rapid decline in the quality of life are reported as the results of this rapid urban growth. Air pollution, lack of sewage disposal, and lack of potable water are among the most pressing environmental and health problems in such urban areas of developing countries.

The health outcomes and impact of chaotic urbanisation at its worst are well recognised by developing countries. That is why Cairo so appropriately hosted the 1994 UN International Conference on Population and Development. This called for renewed efforts to transform the now common experience of cities undergoing the Urban Transition. The Conference called for birth control, sustainable development, human rights, improved circumstances for women and mothers, and much more.[54] All this, however, represents a public health agenda which could have been written half a century earlier. The immensity of the mega-cities' challenge for public health still somehow has not been faced. At the global level, a fledgling UN body, UN Habitat, was created in 1978 to begin that policy journey. It started, however, with thin resources and backing, but grew along with the recognition that the global trend to urbanisation was now unstoppable. Its second major world gathering, Habitat 2 in 1996, signalled long-overdue official recognition, with 171 countries adopting the final document with its 600 recommendations and 100 commitments.[55]

This belated political acceptance that the Urban Transition needed to be faced, not denied, was reflected in the adoption of the shorter and more focused eight UN Millennium Development Goals in 2000. These had a clear public health theme running throughout:

1. Eradicate extreme poverty and hunger.
2. Achieve universal primary education.
3. Promote gender equality and empower women.
4. Reduce child mortality.
5. Improve maternal health.
6. Combat HIV/AIDS, malaria and other diseases.
7. Ensure environmental sustainability.
8. Develop a global partnership for development.

These failed to capture public imagination. Nor have they generated the immense capital and human resources needed as mega-cities come to dominate vast slices of human existence. The rosy picture of the Urban Transition is that urban settlements are the source of wealth and health. This version of urbanisation offers policy-makers a rationale to support exchange of goods and ideas. Towns represent progress and modernity. They are where the previously rural population can change, if not exchange, identity. Yet now cities are where vast amounts of greenhouse gases are emitted, and where the products which exacerbate environmental damage are designed and consumed. Mass consumption is driven by urban patterns of economic activity: the pursuit of the new, ever-changing technology, ceaseless use of building materials, and so on. All these activities, concentrated in urban areas, generate what in modern policy analysis are termed 'footprints'; they literally have an impact on the earth.

Ecological blight, poverty, inequality and health risk are inseparable. In Greater Lagos, only 9 per cent of its 10 million residents have access to piped water. According to the WHO, almost 137 million people in urban populations worldwide have no access to safe drinking water, and more than 600 million urban dwellers do not have adequate sanitation. Densely populated cities with poor sanitation provide favourable circumstances for emerging diseases. They also reveal the potential importance of domestic animals in the ecology of disease and the formation of new virus strains with pandemic potential, as shown by the severe acute respiratory syndrome (SARS) or the recent H1N1 influenza epidemics.[56] Can urban elites seal themselves off from such risks? In Edgar Allan Poe's (1809–49) short story *The Masque of the Red Death*, first published in 1842, Prince Prospero seals himself and his rich friends into the abbey of a castle in order to protect themselves from a deadly pestilence – the Red Death – that is ravaging the countryside. To distract themselves from the suffering and death outside their walls they organise a lavish costume ball into which the Red Death, disguised as a costumed guest, enters and claims the lives of everyone present. Poe's tale presented one of the enduring images of the disguised and shapeless spread of infectious disease, the image of the plague (see Chapter 1). While privileged groups think they have built protective walls separating themselves from risk, somewhere a doorway remains open.

Demographers argue about when humanity became a majority urban life form. Was it in the late twentieth century? Or is it only just happening? Does it matter? The point is that urbanisation also contains the twenty-first-century threat of such massive environmental impact that human history is put on the endangered list. The scale of the Urban Transition is, we believe, one of the key realities to be addressed by twenty-first-century public health agencies. How can urban existence be wrapped around a zero-carbon economy? How can mega-cities feed themselves without ever widening ecological zones of influence? How can they reduce and reuse their waste? How can they recycle water rather than pollute it? How can they provide energy?

Whereas early-twentieth-century Chicago ecological analysts such as Robert Park (1864–1944) and Ernest Burgess (1886–1966) struggled with their challenge of addressing the impact of waves of migrant labour,[57] barely worrying about the continued growth of the US economy (the worry was soon to arrive), today twenty-first-century Lagos or Mumbai has to address the possibility of a permanently low-work, casualised economy. If this is so, immense blocks will be put on to consumer aspirations which have been fanned over recent decades for economic wealth. Will there be a city which takes a different path and carves out a low-impact economy while spreading a better quality of life? These questions are what Adam Smith would be posing today were he to return, we believe, not the facile reiterations of contemporary neoliberalism which urge ever more resource-guzzling consumption and which reinforce human progress as possessive individualism. A new approach to the Urban Transition requires Ecological Public Health indicators as well as a political and institutional mechanism for their achievement.

Although cities existed in the ancient and medieval worlds it is the scale of the shift to urban forms of living that justifies the expression 'Urban Transition'. Just as the sanitary measures of the past were an attempt to make the ancient cities liveable, so it was the almost identical measures applied in the fast-growing cities of Europe and North America which transformed the patterns of health of the nineteenth century. The massive contrast today is between the cities which grew from these times and the developing country mega-cities, which grew rapidly only in the last half-century without, in many cases, a planned or managed process of expansion. It is in these cities, it has been suggested, already operating at the margins of viability and experiencing horrendous health inequalities, that the potential health crises of the future lie.

The story of urban stress is not just about the concentrated habitation of poorer countries, some of which experience rapid economic growth, such as in China or India, and some of which do not, as in the case of major African cities. Areas of urban sprawl in otherwise rich countries, where the private motor vehicle has made journey patterns viable, are increasingly threatened by the changing cost of energy, in particular petroleum fuel. The post-'peak oil' era will makes the economic basis of this mode of living fragile, affecting not only transport, but also all the economic sectors reliant on petroleum from healthcare to agriculture. The impact on the urban form is likely to be profound. In the developed world the challenge is to shift from high-energy to lower-energy transport. In fact, this might be a forced migration rather than a chosen one.[58] In developing countries there is the opportunity to make investments in more sustainable forms of transport early on.

By the second decade of the twenty-first century, urban areas had become home to 50 per cent of the world's population, and accounted for 60–80 per cent of energy consumption and 75 per cent of global carbon emissions.[59] What the United Nations Environment Programme has referred to as the 'greening of cities' required, it argued, a mixture of public health, energy, transport, physical hazards, consumption and environment measures. Greening a city, making its sustainable for the future, required an Ecological Public Health perspective. Addressing health meant also addressing energy use. It is to the issue of energy, far broader in scope than petroleum or transport fuel, that we now turn. In this present chapter, we have seen again how a transition raises basic questions for public health about the nature of social progress and why human lives require the better handling of the four dimensions of existence. We have seen, too, how the Urban Transition, like the two discussed before it, drew upon various models of public health, particularly in this case on the Sanitary-Environmental and Techno-Economic models.

7

ENERGY TRANSITION

Possibly one of the most remarkable changes in the twentieth century, with a direct impact on public health, was the emergence of a new form of society based on apparently plentiful forms of energy. This has altered the role of the human body by literally replacing human and other animal energy with fossil fuel energy. This produces a pathway of physiological metabolic effects. In this chapter we explore the features and implications of this astonishing transition. It has led to a normalisation of a particular type of economy and way of living which by the late twentieth century had become almost entirely dependent on non-renewable energy. As has been written, '[w]ithout modern energy systems, society as we know it today would cease to exist'.[1] The far-seeing social philosopher George Herbert Mead (1863–1931), speaking to his students at Chicago University in 1909 on the revolutionary implications of Darwin's evolutionary theory, observed that 'the conception of Energy' and its connection with 'the economic history of Europe' gave it an importance 'which places it on a par with that of evolution'.[2]

We here use Grubler's term of the 'Energy Transition' to locate what others in the academic literature sometimes refer to as the Socio-Metabolic Transition.[3] We prefer to use 'energy' rather than 'metabolic' because it is more immediately understandable. The account we give in this chapter explores two strands of thinking which need to be addressed by twenty-first-century public health. One focuses upon the energy source itself and its place in the wider energy system. The other focuses on the human body as a locus of energy. In the first, the feedback loops are mostly toxicological – the effects of dioxins, lead, NO_x, SO_2 and more. The pathways there are mostly environmental; the consequences also mostly ecological. In the second, the feedback loops are physiologically metabolic, creating an entirely new class of human diseases, now recognised and labelled as metabolic. These include diabetes and obesity.

Energy is the power to do something. The Energy Transition, simply described, is the series of steps from traditional, usually renewable energy types such as biomass, water, wind and muscle power to much higher-output fossil energy sources such as coal, oil and gas, known from earlier centuries, and new mineral sources such as nuclear power unleashed in the twentieth century. The Energy Transition is not just about energy per se but about the changes in society which both help explain and also result from changes in energy use. Helmut Haberl and his colleagues have written of a shift between three fundamentally different 'socio-metabolic' (i.e. energy) regimes: hunter-gatherers, agrarian societies and industrial society.[4] Van den Bergh and others have also described the Energy Transition in terms of minor, intermediate and major Energy Transitions.[5] Given that for most of human history energy use was low, probably around 1–2 per cent of that used per person today, the major Energy Transition appeared in roughly the eighteenth century (in the West) and is ongoing almost everywhere today.

From the standpoint of modern comforts, the Energy Transition appears to have been overwhelmingly positive. Energy abundance – for lighting, heating, transport and the like – has freed an ever-increasing portion of humanity from darkness, freezing cold, unbearable heat and much more. The vagaries of seasons have been apparently conquered by ubiquitous energy sources. People can take long journeys for granted and easy communications as cheap. Shakespeare's Puck boasted he could put 'put a girdle round about the earth' in 40 minutes. Despite space flight, humanity can emulate Puck. Telephones send voices round the globe in milliseconds. It is possible to think of these advances and advantages as the province of the late technological age, but in fact the vast bulk of technologies underpinning modern society were invented before the First World War.[6] The electric motor, a major user of electrical energy, is a device which underpins almost every possible aspect of modern society, yet it was first invented in the 1830s.

While energy abundance has made possible huge improvements in public health, it has brought damage and risk, the latter often projected far into the future. Although the electricity which drives electric motors, lights houses and works computers is a 'clean' form of power, the principal means for producing it is still coal, a dirty fuel now known for its direct climate change impact. Coal also has direct impacts on health, causing major respiratory, cardiac and neurological effects.[7] Coal's environmental consequences range from mining spoil (waste) to acid rain.[8] Although coal has been a central feature of public health concern for centuries, we seek here not to demonise it but to acknowledge that the huge use of coal is merely part of the wider Energy Transition. The mining, transportation and use of oil, gas and nuclear power also have their own, well-documented health and environmental consequences.

Some of these health consequences are indirect. Petroleum made possible the internal combustion engine and hence the motor car, a powerful aid to the movement of both bodies and goods, as we saw in the previous chapter. It is implicated in the reduction of physical activity and the global phenomenon of rising population weight and obesity.[9] The spread of obesity then compounds the reliance on petroleum, by discouraging people from using their bodies to get, say, to the shops, if they have recourse to a car; a vicious circle of mutual dependency with ill-health effects has been created.[10]

This rise of non-renewable sources of energy has been much commented on and continues to be controversial in both political and scientific debate. The impact of energy on climate is now a supremely important issue, threatening human quality of life itself. The impact of energy emissions on climate change is considerable. From a pre-industrial value of 270–275 parts per million (ppm), atmospheric carbon dioxide rose to about 310 ppm by 1950, and atmospheric CO_2 concentration has risen from 310 to 380 ppm since 1950.[11] Although scientists are overwhelmingly in agreement, the veracity and implications of human-created climate change are contested by so-called 'climate change deniers'. Only infrequently do public health arguments about fossil fuels and climate change take centre stage in these public policy arguments.[12]

Although energy politics troubled the twentieth century, not least as powerful countries fought over sources of oil across the globe,[13] the Energy Transition needs to be located as occurring over a longer period, within evolutionary time scales. Some decades ago, even before the statistics of climate change were being debated, the economist Nicholas Georgescu-Roegen (1906–94) painted a picture of human energy use as disturbing and bleak as anything written by the Rev Dr Malthus. Economic growth, said Georgescu-Roegen, not only plundered energy past in the form of fossil fuels but also mortgaged the future of energy use. At some point, he argued, the laws of physics dictate that economic development will peter out and the human species will be put on the slow road to extinction.[14] Georgescu-Roegen put the Energy Transition into a longer biological evolutionary framework:[15]

> Some organisms slow down the entropic degradation. Green plants store part of the solar radiation which in their absence would immediately go into dissipated heat, into high entropy. That is why we can burn now the solar energy saved from degradation millions of years ago in the form of coal or a few years ago in the form of a tree. All other organisms, on the contrary, speed up the march of entropy. Man occupies the highest position on this scale, and this is all that environmental issues are about.

The Energy Transition and public health

The Energy Transition, it has been stated, is not just about energy but about society. As we saw with other transitions, Britain was the first society to shift from a primarily agrarian model to a primarily industrial model and in so doing provided an archetype for the rest of the world. In 1820, the year the OECD has suggested as a transition point in economic development between agrarian and industrial capitalism in Britain, 94 per cent of world energy came from biomass. One hundred and eighty years later, at the end of the second millennium, fossil fuels accounted for 89 per cent of all energy use.[16] In Darwinian terms, this is the blink of an evolutionary eyelid, but the impact on humankind is already profound.

Before the coal era, the central motors of the economy were water, wind, wood and animals, alongside the labour power of humankind. In the eleventh century, when the victorious Norman French audited their new English dominion for their victorious King William in a report known as the Domesday Book,[17] there was one watermill for every 50 households. Water continued to provide a key role in agriculture and industry (for textiles, mining and metals) until late in the nineteenth century.[18] Britain's industrial phase Energy Transition however was fed by the mass availability of coal. Already by 1700, England produced the vast bulk of the coal in Europe.[19] Even so, charcoal remained the fuel of choice, being more pleasant to use, especially for cooking. Coal was originally limited to small industrial processes requiring higher levels of heat, such as blacksmithing and lime burning. In the late Middle Ages, coal and charcoal sold at about the same price for the level of heat given but, with increasing population, demand outstripped supply. Britain's forests were almost entirely depleted by 1800, and the black riches of 'the Subterranean Forest', as coal was known to be, took their place.[20]

The increasing use of coal, it has been suggested, was prompted by rising labour costs which created the incentive to invent ways to substitute capital for labour in production.[21] The rising use of coal then fed back into technological changes within the wider economy. Coal production provided the spur for the development of the steam engine and shaped the rising cotton industry, processing imported cotton.[22] Although its use varied considerably between the main areas of energy need – heating, power, transport and lighting[23] – such was the trajectory of increasing demand that the Victorian economist Stanley Jevons (1835–82) thought that Britain's vast reserves might run out.[24] British coal production peaked in 1913 at 287 million tons annual production. By the end of the twentieth century it had fallen to 34 million tons. These changes were not driven by declining availability alone but also by other factors including political choices and cost differences with other energy sources. There were parallel labour market changes. In an industry noted for being labour-intensive, inefficient and undercapitalised, the number of British coal miners peaked in 1920 at 1,250,000 and had fallen to a mere 9,000 by 2000.[25] Throughout the twentieth century, Britain's industrial base dwindled and, by the end of the century, it was importing low-sulphur coal and also gas, which were substituting for previously domestic sources of energy.

The British coal industry based on deep mining, however, left a lasting legacy of health consequences.[26] The direct health effect is shown in coal workers' pneumoconiosis, or black lung disease. This is coaldust-induced lesions in the gas exchange regions of the human lung. But the health effects of coal spread far beyond mining communities. Although the effects of pollution had been noted in Britain centuries before – indeed the burning of coal had once been forbidden in London – the science of the health effects of hazardous air pollutants dates from 1872. This was when *Air and Rain: The Beginning of Chemical Climatology* by the Scottish chemist Robert Angus Smith (1817–84), the world's first inspector of energy pollution, was published.[27] Smith showed himself to be an independently minded chemist. He was trained by the notable Justus von Liebig (1803–73). Unlike other early chemists, Smith refused to act in the courts on behalf of polluters, siding with the victims in an honourable public health manner.

The towns and cities of the UK were Smith's natural laboratory. While coal pollution had been noted and experienced for hundreds of years,[28] urban levels of pollution sharply increased from around the 1840s with the Urban Transition (see Chapter 6). Smith's interest was in industrial pollution. Coal use for domestic heating in towns spread an ever-present and thickening pall of smoke over Britain's cities. Mirroring other sanitarian campaigns, several attempts had been made to introduce laws to require owners of furnaces to reduce smoke emissions. The Smoke Abatement and then Alkali Acts brought Smith into a lead role for the establishment of a system for pollution control. The legislation was poorly written, however, established on principles of pragmatism, and difficult to enforce. Smith and all the inspectors who followed him were under intense pressure to fall into line with dominant industrial interests.[29] In most respects Smith, as a follower of Edwin Chadwick, took a pragmatic view of his relations with industry. Like Chadwick, he sought to stimulate improvement by appealing to long-term interest. Excessive air pollution represented wasted fuel, he thought. In many cases, such rational pleadings were resisted by industrialists, who were 'curiously blind' to the potential benefits that might accrue to them.[30] From the 1880s foreign industrial competition allowed British employers to pose the regulators with a stark choice: either unregulated pollution or factory closures.[31] Although subsequent legislation improved the scope of control on emissions, the regulatory system became increasingly inactive, even complicit. Local authorities and central government were both reluctant to take the lead in delivering controls, blaming each other for inaction.[32]

In relation to the health consequences of the Energy Transition public health science had failed its first major test. Whereas sanitary reform had met with success despite limited and indeed initially erroneous scientific understanding, as regards pollution the going was far tougher. The implication was, perhaps, that the science of pollution and its health effect was far less a consideration than the power and economic importance of its adversaries.

The physical visibility of the Energy Transition was so obvious that it is recorded in the paintings of Claude Monet (1840–1926), the French Impressionist. From his rooms at the elite Savoy Hotel on the Thames Embankment, Monet painted the London sky an acid brown-yellow, thus capturing the state of sulphurous smoke-filled air. This pollution persisted for decades until, in 1952, after years of official inaction, an appalling level of pollution was noted, now known as the 'Big Smoke'. This was an impenetrable and deadly smog which spread across London. Up to 12,000 people were recorded to have died as a consequence; many times that number were incapacitated.[33] The British Parliament was embarrassed into action.

Such delays between evidence and public health intervention are all too common. Part of the reason for this, as we explore later (see Chapter 13), is the difficulty of 'proving' causation when there are powerful vested interests which can question it and engineer delay. Very few diseases are pollutant-specific, which is why the literature now talks of risk levels. Exposure may be due to a range of factors, making it very difficult to assess the health burden attributable to specific risk factors. Moreover, pollutants are rarely present in large concentrations, so the effects on health may be neither immediate nor obvious.[34] Underlying the hazy link between coal-related pollution and health damage was economics. Coal pollution entailed much the same blend of policy issues as water and sanitation – cost and priority – but energy in the form of coal was a central driver of the British economy. Regulation for public health benefit was always going to be troublesome, and subject to political trade-offs.

In the twenty-first century, London fogs and smogs (the word coined for smoke plus fog in 1905 by a Dr Henry-Antoine Desvoeux) are a thing of the past. London Fog is now the brand name of an American raincoat! Emissions from coal globally, however, continue and are greater than ever. Proponents of coal-fired energy transmission argue that modern coal burning is now 'clean', with the emissions of particulates captured by sophisticated filters. To be more accurate, the pollution emitted is now, for the most past, invisible. Its invisibility, according to one modern account, means that action to curtail its impact is limited.[35] The visibility of its presence may have been addressed, but not all of its impact.

The global Energy Transition

Beyond Britain the Energy Transition progressed more slowly. In the case of Scandinavia and Canada, the demand for energy was met by harnessing their massive potential for hydroelectricity. Use of biomass as energy in the Netherlands, for example, fell to less than 50 per cent of energy input from 1864, from the late 1920s for Sweden, and from the late 1930s for Italy and Spain. In Austria, in the 1830s, when the switch to coal had already occurred in Britain, humans and working animals were still providing around 85 per cent of the mechanical energy. A century later biomass had faded almost completely from Western European energy use and policy attention.[36] It has returned in the guise of biofuels, which were promoted as 'green' energy by the USA and European Union to counteract strategic dependency on politically volatile sources of energy (oil from the Middle East and gas from the former Soviet Union).[37]

The United States, with vast coal reserves, overtook Britain as the world's industrial powerhouse in the late nineteenth century. In the early twenty-first century, around half of all US sources of electrical power were still coal.[38] This proportion is set to decline, as 'new regulations, intended to reduce the damage to public health from industrial pollution include tighter restrictions on toxic chemicals in power plants' waste gases, on water use and the disposal of coal ash'.[39] The character of disputes over the use of coal, public health on one side and the impact on employment, investment and energy availability on the other, differs hardly at all from that of disputes in Britain a century or more before. The accolade 'workshop of the world' has now passed to China, whose energy use far exceeds that of Britain at any time in its history. Table 7.1 gives the changes in coal use of major users over recent decades. The pace and scale of this change is remarkable. In 2006–08 China's share of world coal use rose from 38 per cent to 43 per cent.[40] The result of such rapid change has been rising experience of localised atmospheric pollution,

TABLE 7.1 Energy: coal consumption

Rank	Country	1980	1990	2000	2005	2006	Percentage of total
1	China	305.1	529.9	667.4	1,095.9	1,191.3	38.55
2	USA	388.6	483.1	569.0	574.2	567.3	18.36
3	India	57.1	107.8	169.1	222.0	237.7	7.69
4	Japan	57.6	76.0	98.9	121.3	119.1	3.85
5	Russian Federation	n/a	180.6	106.0	111.6	112.5	3.64
6	South Africa	43.5	71.3	81.9	91.9	93.8	3.04
7	Germany	139.6	129.6	84.9	82.1	82.4	2.67
8	Poland	101.6	80.2	57.6	55.7	58.4	1.89
9	South Korea	13.2	24.4	43.0	54.8	54.8	1.77
10	Australia	26.1	37.0	48.3	52.5	51.1	1.65
11	United Kingdom	71.1	64.9	36.7	39.7	43.8	1.42

comparable to that faced in Britain a century before.[41] The public health effects of this transfer of manufacturing capacity from the West to the East are being steadily documented, helped by far more sophisticated methods than were available when the West industrialised a century or more earlier.[42] The stark reality remains however similar for both past and present Energy Transitions. Economic demand pushes health considerations into second place. China, unlike the West earlier, is beginning to invest hugely in renewable, cleaner sources of energy. Today it has the largest wind and solar energy industries in the world. While its vast river dam projects may be contentious outside, this push for 'cleaner' renewable sources is less remarked.

There is perhaps only one major and outstanding difference between the USA or China now and Britain a century or so ago. What Monet captured in paint a century ago was *local* pollution; nowhere else in the world matched it. Today the Energy Transition is worldwide with worldwide effects. In Britain, the pollution problems were partially resolved by deindustrialisation (and hence relative decarbonisation) and the desulphurisation of energy production (using imported coal and gas). But this is a new energy 'colonialism', with energy use being displaced and hidden by transferring it abroad from the West. The emergence of sophisticated product life-cycle analysis is now exposing how the West is exporting the pollution caused by its consumption to far-off places. This poses new public health challenges for governance: who has the responsibility and capacity to tame ill-health effects caused beyond national boundaries? In Europe, policy formation and regulation that cross borders have been helped by regionalisation in the form of regional controls through the European Union, a legal entity which binds former separate states into shared responsibilities. Intergovernmental negotiations over climate change emissions, however, tend to be slow at the global level, with political battles between economic and health interests to the fore.

Sight and smell give an additional charge to public health arguments. One way of visualising the global effects of energy and pollution is to see them from space, or more conveniently on an IMAX cinema screen. Witnessed from the international space station, the night-time surface of the earth resembles a fine coating of luminescent powder, light pollution effects which follow humanity's success in extending the day into night. This occurs because light (energy) has been rendered relatively cheap. In 1800 it required nine hours of human labour to afford a 100-watt bulb to run for an hour. Today the equivalent labour time (in the developed world) has been calculated as less than one second.[43] Moreover, the spread of energy for night-time lighting is unequally distributed. From outer space, only some areas of the globe are bright, while others remain in darkness. This mirrors energy use. The oceans and mountains of course are one reason for darkness, along with low population density, but the variation also indicates energy wealth.

Biomass still constitutes one-half of domestic energy use in most developing countries and as much as 95 per cent in lower-income countries. Around 2.4 billion people rely on biomass (wood, dried dung, crop residues, etc.) as their main source of domestic energy for cooking, heating and lighting.[44] More than 1 billion people in industrialised countries, around 20 per cent of the world's population, consume nearly 60 per cent of the total global energy supply. Around 5 billion inhabitants of developing countries consume only 40 per cent.[45] Inequalities between countries are also reflected within them. Rich and poor consume differently everywhere, but, as rising energy prices filter into the price of food or the cost of basic commodities, the impact is felt most clearly among the poorest.[46]

Given the climate change association with profligate energy use and pollution, can one argue that less developed societies are the way forward? Is progress to be a return to a biomass past? If so this would be a nostalgic and somewhat romantic view of poverty. It would also be to ignore the significant health problems caused by the burning of low-quality biomass, which particularly affects women and children in developing countries.[47] According to the WHO, indoor smoke in high-mortality developing countries is responsible for an estimated 3.7 per cent of the overall disease burden, making it the most lethal killer after malnutrition, unsafe sex and lack of safe water and sanitation.[48] Questions of sustainability also apply, with the potential eradication of wooded areas and forests being accelerated if there is a continued reliance on biomass. The shift to cleaner, sustainable power sources, often feasible and cheap through technology transfer such as improved stoves, is therefore a worldwide requirement. Poor countries, whose quality of life would be improved by better and more energy, and rich countries, whose energy footprint ought to drop, both need new energy policies based on sustainability. This vision of the future is made more complicated by the scientific recognition that the full effects of the Energy Transition are not just a matter of heat and light and their consequential pollution. Energy and health researchers now note the complex interactions and impact of multiple sources and forms of pollution, all associated with the Energy Transition.[49]

The world faces a conundrum. Higher energy use is associated with better quality of life, health improvement and wealth. Yet that same energy use is now directly associated with threats to civilisation and sustainability, notably through climate change.[50] Mainstream economists remain convinced that the path of the Energy Transition will continue. It defines progress. Yet the cost of tackling the consequences now mounts.[51] The OECD calculates that CO_2 emissions will rise from 29.7 billion tonnes in 2007 to 33.8 billion tonnes in 2020 and 42.4 billion tonnes in 2035, an increase of 43 per cent.[52] World CO_2 emissions, which were 12 million tonnes in 1820, had risen to 6,611 million tonnes by 2000.[53] While 'traditional' biomass sources grew in use fivefold between 1820 and 2000, the use of 'modern' sources (such as oil, gas and nuclear) rose 700-fold in that same period. In the OECD states, total energy consumption is projected to rise from 73.4 quadrillion British thermal units (q-Btu) in 2007 to 76.9 q-Btu by 2035, while energy use in non-OECD member states is projected to rise from 111.1 q-Btu to 184.9 q-Btu in the same period.[54] The global rise in energy use is projected to occur across all major sources of energy: liquids, coal, natural gas, renewable and nuclear (see Figure 7.1).

Energy, evolution and Ecological Public Health

The picture being presented by energy analysts of importance for public health is thus sober. Firstly, there is an inexorable rise in energy use. Secondly, there is a long process of what Roger Fouquet and colleagues have called substitution, in which new forms of energy replace the old (see Table 7.2). In the long process Fouquet

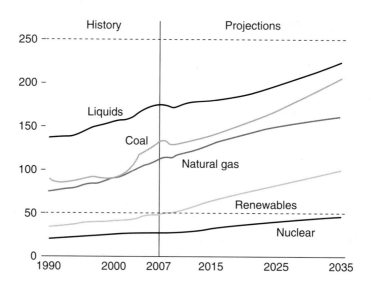

FIGURE 7.1   World marketing energy by fuel type, 1990–2035

outlines, a permanent search for new sources occurs.[55] Thirdly, there is rising evidence of the Energy Transition's harm to both the environment and human health. And, fourthly, there is an apparent lock-in of energy use to economic development, not least in consumerism as pleasure. This coupling is what now troubles economists who are beginning to worry about how to address just the environmental impacts of the Energy Transition. One school of thought argues for decoupling, by pursuing new forms of energy with lower-impact forms. Others argue for a simplification of economies. Still others propose a focus on nuclear energy, which is claimed to be low-carbon when up and running but requires huge capital and carbon costs to create. Still others deny there is a problem at all, but events like the nuclear meltdown in Japan after the 2011 tsunami ought surely to be corrective. It helped generate Germany's remarkable commitment to abandon nuclear energy altogether and to promise to forge a non-nuclear energy system.

The narrative about the Energy Transition suggests that human use of energy is intimately caught up with the evolution of life on earth today. Almost all sources of energy – and thus of life itself – are solar in origin. Biomass is directly or indirectly

TABLE 7.2 Some energy substitutions and transitions

Substitution (original → new)	Service where energy is applied	Approximate period (innovation to dominance)	Approximate period (diffusion to dominance)
Residential woodfuel → coal	Heating	1500–1800	1580–1800
Iron woodfuel → coal	Heating	1709–90	1750–90
Manufacturing woodfuel → coal	Heating	1300–1700	1550–1700
Residential coal → gas	Heating	1880–1975	1920–75
Ox → horse	Power	900–1600	1070–1600
Animals → mills	Power	700–1350★	1000–1350★
Animals → steam	Power	1710–1920	1830–1920
Steam → electricity	Power	1821–1950	1920–1950
Fossil → mineral/nuclear[++]	Power	1930–present	1950–present
Fossil → modern renewable (hydro/solar/wind/wave)[++]	Power	1960s–present	1990s–present
Horses → railway	Land transport	1804–60	1830–60
Sail → steamship	Sea transport	1815–90	1830–90
Railways → combustion engine	Land transport	1876–1950	1911–50
Candles → gas	Lighting	1800–50	1810–50
Candles → kerosene	Lighting	1850–1900★	1860–1900★
Gas → electricity	Lighting	1810–1935	1880–1935

Notes:
★ Peak share, as it did not become the dominant source of energy.
[++] Additions by present authors.

produced by green plants in photosynthesis, a process which secures the energy input for almost all food chains in the earth's eco-systems.[56] Modern fossil fuels are only yesterday's biomass, albeit compressed from hundreds of millennia. The connection with evolution is clear. Humankind's command of fire marks a point of differentiation from other animals, recognised by Rudyard Kipling's character Mowgli in *The Jungle Book*. Command of fire pulled humankind away from its original ecological niche (that of a 'large, mobile omnivore'[57]) to a situation where it has no ecological niche at all, and indeed is threatening the niches of others. Fire made cooking possible, and thus humans evolved to eat cooked diets, including meat.[58] Cooked food was safer, was easier to eat and digest, and enabled the routine consumption of larger amounts of energy than raw food. The evolutionary physiological and social consequences ranged from diminishing jaw size to speed of food consumption, enabling time horizons to change.[59]

Energy concepts featured large within Victorian evolutionary theory. Biologist Jean-Baptiste de Lamarck (1744–1829), physicists Ludwig Boltzmann (1844–1906) and Carl Gottfried Neumann (1832–1925) and most influentially Herbert Spencer (1820–1903) all drew attention to the central role of energy capture and utilisation in living systems. Spencer, not Darwin, introduced the expression 'survival of the fittest'.[60] His ideas may be deeply unfashionable today, but Spencer's view on energy as the principal driver of increasing environmental and social complexity remains intriguing.[61] In the 1920s, Alfred Lotka (1880–1949), an American epidemiologist and member of the American Public Health Association, added an energetic conceptualisation to the Darwinian notion of natural selection.[62] To see natural selection as an energy system, argued Lotka, implied that increasing evolutionary complexity was matched by increasing energy complexity.

A similar idea was presented in terms of cultural evolution in the early 1940s by the American anthropologist Leslie White (1900–75). White argued that the development of energy and cultural evolution were but two sides of the same coin. 'Culture', he argued, 'is a kind of behaviour. And behaviour, whether it is man, mule, plant, comet or molecule, may be treated as a manifestation of energy.'[63] White meant by energy 'the capacity for performing work'. Societies which captured more energy and used it more efficiently possessed an evolutionary advantage and hence were more advanced than other societies. White's ideas were grounded in Alfred Lotka's reformulations of Darwin and Ludwig Boltzmann.[64] White even proposed a formula, $E \times T \to P$, where E is the amount of energy harnessed per capita per year, T is the quality efficiency of the tools employed in the expenditure of energy, and P is progress and cultural development. Energy use thus provides a measure of society's technological and hence cultural progress. White was making such arguments against the background of the rejection of evolutionary thinking in American social science.[65] His approach was emulated by another, later social anthropologist, John Bennett, whom we discuss within the Ecological Transition (see Chapter 10).[66]

If White associated improvements in the technology of energy capture and efficient use with cultural progress, the Romanian but American-domiciled economist Nicholas Georgescu-Roegen (1906–94), a one-time president of the American Economic Association, spelt out its more negative implications. His approach was entirely theoretical, indeed conceptually profound. It entailed two central elements, a materials balance approach based on the finite quantity of material available on earth, and a thermodynamic approach based on the fact that production lowers the amount of energy available in a closed system.[67] This latter observation restates the second law of thermodynamics. According to this law, the production process changes a certain amount of energy and matter into heat, thus transforming irreversibly low entropy into high entropy. The result is the irreversible downgrading of energy over time.

In reviving the idea of environmental constraints on economic activity (in fact the essential laws of physics), Georgescu-Roegen resuscitates the ghost of Malthus, suggesting that even a 'steady-state' economy cannot mitigate the impact of entropy or energy downgrading. The evolutionary solution, if there is one, must therefore lie with 'de-growth'. For reasons explained earlier, this represents a full-frontal attack on industrial, or for that matter post-industrial, society and the form that international capitalism took throughout the twentieth century.

This 'thermodynamics paradigm' has been criticised as constraining complex societal and human constructions to the physical properties of matter. It has been accused of being a 'theoretical *cul-de-sac*'.[68] Attempting to steer a course through this ideological let alone economic minefield, Herman Daly, former economist at the World Bank, has offered the model of a steady-state economy. In so doing, he essentially revived the model of John Stuart Mill in the mid-nineteenth century. Another ecological economist grappling with this fundamental question of energy and progress was Kenneth Boulding, another former president of the American Economic Association. He proposed the possibility of a growth economy within a closed ecological system. He suggested that the economic system may grow for a time but only within a larger eco-system which is finite, non-growing and materially closed. The picture here is of the world as 'Spaceship Earth', merely a larger form of the tiny world of the astronaut or cosmonaut of the late 1960s, where all their needs must be carried with them or recycled. Daly employed a somewhat modified metaphor. For all these energy-conscious economic thinkers, the crisis of economics is that man-made capital is filling up ecological space by generation and waste of energy.[69] This debate continues.[70] The most positive view is that a new wave of technical advance will cut a path towards a healthier energy future by a shift from unsustainable to sustainable energy. Humankind's future, if it is to extend into the future without environmental chaos in its wake, unwittingly returns to Leslie White's evolutionary prospectus. Progress depends upon an energy-efficient society.

The Energy Transition discussed here appears primarily to be about the material world, in our conceptualisation, but as we have shown it leaks into the other dimensions of existence. Aspirations for better and healthier lives drive energy use. Once people are used to an energy-abundant society, they appear loath to renounce it. Health consequences follow whichever course is taken. Energy is also old biological activity. The pursuit of cleaner 'sustainable' sources of energy might illustrate the continuing role of the Techno-Economic model of public health.

8

ECONOMIC TRANSITION

In the previous chapter, we explored how energy was fundamental to a modern (possibly any) notion of economic development. Further, we noted the re-emergence of debates about progress and economic activity in an era being circumscribed by rising concern about the environmental impact of unfettered burning of fossil fuels. This raised an intriguing debate – explored further in this chapter – about whether material prosperity was the same phenomenon as prosperity, and whether material wealth is automatically synonymous with health for the public. This is part of a deeply philosophical debate about whether social progress, growth-based economics and health advances can be mutually reinforcing. Human labour, access to capital, and the role of land as the primary source of wealth (by dint of it 'holding' the ecological stock of the planet) are all woven into the huge changes exhibited over the last 200 years of human history. In a sense, the notion of the Economic Transition is very simple, that over time all societies are drawn into a process of change which increases wealth, transforms labour and alters how people relate. The arguments are over the direction of change, the drivers, the distribution of benefits and the health impact.

This chapter shows why public health thinking should address the Economic Transition via the categories used in classical political economy, capital, land and labour. Capital is a combination of hidden labour and resources which affect health. Land is the ecological stock and thus hidden as well as visible health. And labour is both energy power and knowledge, both of which have immediate health ramifications. Our argument is that mainstream economics today has corralled economic discourse into a focus primarily around economic capital, while any outstanding issues are merely those of 'forms of capital' – human capital, cultural capital and social capital. The latter concept is often being unthinkingly imported into the public health field, an issue we return to in our discussion of culture (see Chapter 11). Questions of labour and labouring are conceived in modern economics as forms of capital – human capital – which reverse the older political economy. Everything becomes capital, much as all economics is reducible to markets. If it is not in a market, it ought to be. This way of thinking about existence leaves or downplays the fundamental transformative role of work, leaving aside the issue that the 'bearer' of this capital is a living, breathing human being whose existence can be more or less healthy. Thus the connections between labour – the act of work – and health have been severed unnecessarily. In this respect, our conception of the Economic Transition returns to older notions within public health, not least that of the founders of the British National Health Service, who wanted health services based around occupational health, recognising the workplace as a primary setting and shaper of human health and longevity. With modern data on income disparities' impact on life expectancy, we note the return of such attention. This is overdue and central to Ecological Public Health.

The Economic Transition points to a process of change observed by many analysts and historians. With variations, they broadly agree that a transition began from pre-agricultural to agricultural-based economies around 12,000 years ago.[1] This then developed with trade and mercantile operations erratically over the last thousand years, but developed rapidly into fully industrialised economies in the last two centuries or so. Not all societies may become fully industrialised, but none is exempt from its impact, if only by trade and now by media information spread. As much of the West deindustrialised in the late twentieth century, it transferred its 'dirty' work and industries to the East and South.

The contentious element of this Economic Transition, as we discuss, lies in how this process of economic change occurs, who wins and loses (including the loss of ecological 'stock'), what drives it and where economic activity occurs. Some argue that an entire sequence of change has emerged. They have suggested that economies go – perhaps have to go – through set unilinear phases of development. If pre-agricultural economies were characterised by nomadic, hunter-gatherer economics, reliant on the bounty of nature, then agricultural economies are about generating the organised fruits of the land for local consumption and moving into wider exchange, with settled existence being a prerequisite. This was outlined in the Urban Transition (see Chapter 6). Early industrial economies, which follow, are mainly about the reorganisation of human labour to generate efficiencies with limited technological input. They then further develop through non-human energy sources, and the alliance of science and technology. This reshapes work, and enables modern capitalist economies to emerge.[2] Post-industrial economies then emerge, centred on 'services', with the prime focus of wealth generation again being human resources. There is a hidden conventional economy, however, in the form of distant industrial economies which provide goods which were previously made more nationally or regionally. In fact, the so-called post-industrial economy is really a globalising system of supply chain management, with industry and agrarian inputs centrally organised by powerful corporations and chains of command.

The notion of an Economic Transition from agrarian to industrial capitalism remains a constant in much health and economic thinking. Some economic texts go even so far as to portray the relationship through an equation: 'wealth equals health'.[3] Others, however, point out that health improvements are not necessarily directly linked to indices of economic growth.[4] The relationship between economics, as defined by wealth, and health, as defined by mortality, is not simple; it was explored under the Demographic and Epidemiological Transitions.

We appreciate the elegance of this portrayal of the Economic Transition as occurring in phases of development. Intuitively it makes sense, and it runs through many conceptions of progress, but we note that there are varying interpretations of how that evolution occurs and whether it is orderly. A first interpretation sees the transition as a series of stages, unfolding as an almost unilinear and set developmental sequence. The second sees complexity as the core feature of the transition, which has no universal or set pattern. A third approach, today's mainstream, apparently eschews economic history altogether and presents progress as the application of a set of ideas known as 'market rules'. A fourth interpretation, touched upon at the end of the previous chapter, suggests that progress might mean reversal to a new steady state, whose level of development is yet to be determined, some seeing it as today's Western pattern of living, others seeing it as a reversion to a 'lower' state because of the crisis of the diminution of the ecological stock.

To make matters even more difficult, some thinkers weave across these interpretations or shift position over their own lives (not a criticism). We begin this exploration with the classical economists such as Adam Smith, David Ricardo and others, noting that the term 'classical economics' is from Karl Marx, who for obvious reasons was building upon but dissociating himself from them. The classical economists were primarily concerned about the interplay of land, labour and capital, suggesting that economics was political economics, firmly part of public discourse and policy. For them economics had a number of foci. One was political, another was moral, and yet another was the relationship of nature to society itself. Classical political economy ranged across all these foci. This breadth of emphasis was due in part to their witnessing the emerging and altering role of the State within and alongside production and exchange.

Arguments about economic development

The serious debate about the Economic Transition probably begins with Scottish moral philosopher and political economist Adam Smith (1723–90). '[W]hat is properly called moral philosophy', said Smith, is to 'investigate and explain those connecting principles' of 'common life . . . arranged in some methodical order.'[5] By 'moral philosophy' is meant something closer to what now might be called sociology. Smith is lionised as the founding father of modern economics, but he did not see himself as an economist in current terms. In the eighteenth century, still in the merchant phase of capitalist development, there was no common perception of the economy as a separate object of analysis. Discourses on money, trade and commerce treated economic phenomena as properties of physical nature.[6] Smith's thinking ranged seamlessly from the moral to the biological. Smith lived through and observed many social changes: the rationalisation of agriculture, the massive expulsion of peasants from their plots granted by customary law, the displacement of populations, the emergence of cities as centres of commerce, and long-distance trade. Smith, though interested in the past, could see economic events through the filter of his own life and times. He knew nothing of the industrial age, let alone 'post-industrial' consumer capitalism. Remarkably therefore, Smith's ideas are presented as having a contemporary relevance by an economics profession which increasingly eschews history.

The great economist John Maynard Keynes observed in 1936 that society faced the danger that all current events (the Great Depression of the 1930s) were being played out according to the vision of some defunct economist.[7] Smith is a primary point of reference. It is Smith who is cited as coining the expression 'invisible hand of the market', which is today used as a metaphor for the market or price mechanism guiding economic activity and delivering unintended benefits for all. A typical reference to the modern relevance of Smith's expression is that given by the 'complexity economist' Eric Beinhocker, also considered later. According to Beinhocker, Smith thought that self-interest and competitive markets would create a balanced economy, thus bringing eighteenth-century thought into line with a twentieth-century prophet of the unregulated market, Gordon Gekko from the 1987 Hollywood film *Wall Street*. Gekko's credo was 'Greed is good.' This is a 'rather surprising conclusion', Beinhocker thought.[8] However, Smith didn't think this at all. Smith certainly celebrated the invisible hand as a way of breaking up the then dominant medieval practice of guild-led cartels, where prices were fixed by gentlemen's agreements. It was more democratic, he argued, to open such processes up to public scrutiny and open exchange. He saw this as the responsibility of the State. One economic historian who has traced Smith's original thinking has summarised what Smith meant in *The Wealth of Nations* as simply 'the inducement a merchant has to keep his capital at home, thereby increasing the domestic capital stock and enhancing military power'.[9] Another historian, having undertaken a textual analysis of Smith's use of the term in his entire corpus of work, discerns not one type of invisible hand but five, others being less a description of the market mechanism than a human projection on to benevolent intentionality.[10] Adam Smith spoken of in awe and too often actually unread in the twenty-first century by modern economists would be not wholly recognisable to the eighteenth-century man himself.

Smith saw societal development in historical terms, although archaeological texts were then few. He filled historical gaps with conjecture. He offers a four-stage view of human history: hunting, shepherding, farming and then commerce. Humanity began in pre-civilisation and ends with his contemporary period of merchant capitalism, where economic evolution stops. These phases are shaped around the principal means of economic activity. Each stage is presented as a more advanced state of society than the previous.[11] Smith acknowledged that there could be setbacks, such as the collapse of past commercial societies like Classical Greece, for which he provided no explanation. Smith offers, in effect, a materialist and social conception of history, that is to say he gives primacy to technical and societal development in describing the unfolding of economic advance.[12]

Malthus disagreed with Smith, broadly preferring arguments against growth or seeing growth balanced against larger material setbacks and political ends. Writing after Smith, and in his footsteps, Malthus is the first British representative of economics as a professionalising discipline. Malthus's primary objective in writing *An Essay on the Principle of Population* was to counter British utopian thought, as exemplified by William Godwin (1756–1836), but more centrally French utopian thinking spawned by the (dangerous) 1789 Revolution represented by Baron Condorcet. The subtitle of the book refers to both Godwin and Condorcet. Progress in human affairs for Malthus was ultimately a matter of political decisions and aspirations alone, with the economic capacity of society sidelined or even ignored.[13] In other words, transforming the human condition was the purpose of political discourse. The contemporary condition of humanity, however, was dominated by poverty. Malthus was concerned about whether this was inevitable, natural or preventable. Change, he argued, involved far more than aspirations or good intentions. Although Malthus was deeply religious, and typically seen as a conservative, he saw the enduring human challenge more in terms of resolving basic questions of scarcity, a matter more to do with the book of nature than the Bible.[14]

For Malthus the conditions of scarcity were set by the availability of arable land, which, as Adam Smith had earlier observed, could not be made more productive by specialisation alone. In this respect the condition of humankind hardly differed from that of other species. 'Through the animal and vegetable kingdoms, nature has scattered the seeds of life abroad with the most profuse and liberal hand. She has been comparatively sparing in the room and nourishment necessary to rear them.'[15] Lack of land, given population pressure, led to poor nutrition and hence to poor health. Malthus also saw that poor nutrition precipitated a greater vulnerability to epidemic disease, as we have noted in previous chapters. He thus viewed social development, inasmuch as it could occur at all, from the standpoint of a primarily agricultural society – and only later acknowledged the impact of industrialisation.[16] Malthus's theme, written just as the British industrial revolution was emerging, was of the ever-present potential of extreme scarcity. This he expressed mathematically, in effect a bioeconomic law, as 'population, when unchecked, increases in a geometrical ratio . . . [while] subsistence increases only in an arithmetical ratio'. His prognosis was of limited growth potential for agricultural productivity. If population numbers rise, the mismatch of supply and mouths would rapidly expose limits to growth, the so-called Malthusian trap. Other pressures would restrain population with dire and draconian effects. Malthus proposed a notion of economic change based on the fundamental tensions between the fecundity of nature and the fecundity of the human species.

The objections to Malthus's views were immediate and numerous, and continue to this day, as we have noted. His analysis also received many supporters and popularisers, many of whom took a different ethical position from his own. Despite numerous *ad hominem* criticisms, he viewed the processes he described as regrettable. Today, alongside the apparent obsolescence of his views, there are equally mixed views among economists about whether Malthus was actually right about the limiting effects of the agricultural economy prior to the modernisation that took off in the mid- to late nineteenth century.[17] He could be dismissed as plain wrong, or at least it could be argued that the boundaries of what he saw as natural environmental limits have been constantly breached and extended. The modern economist's answer to Malthus's problem of scarcity and resource limitation is given by the notion of input and technical substitution. Productive capacity has been extended by fertilisers (initially guano), pest control, cropping practices and machinery, for example. Above all, in Malthus's time, Britain extended its feeding capacity by food imports, about which Malthus had mixed feelings, and also by raising the productivity of agricultural production and new forms of energy.[18]

The fact that Malthus was 'wrong' for the next two centuries has not dissipated his big thesis. As the economist Fred Hirsch once observed, substitution may not always be adequate to 'counterbalance the constraints resulting from scarce physical factors of production'.[19] Furthermore the limits to growth may be ecological not only in a meaning strictly limited to resources – that is to say nature – but also in the social aspects. What has emerged is the modern notion of 'carrying capacity' (the words themselves come directly from the cargo limits of merchant shipping). This has more recently been defined as the theoretical maximum population that an area can sustain given technological capacities and natural constraints.[20] As we saw in the previous chapter, the Malthusian trap has actually been obviated by the availability of new, far cheaper forms of energy. The Economic Transition was sketched particularly by David Ricardo, interested in the shift from a predominantly agrarian society with capitalist elements to a period of 'capitalism proper', but perhaps the man who most articulately explored this process and where it might lead is Karl Marx, a very different sort of economic theorist.[21]

To Marx (1818–83), often writing with his friend Friedrich Engels (1820–95), political economists like Smith, Malthus or Ricardo offered a welcome alternative to the philosophically idealistic formulations of historical progress found in their German homeland, specifically in the writings of Georg Hegel and Immanuel Kant. Unlike Smith, however, Marx did not think commercial society to be the final stage of history but viewed the social tensions of the current and previous epochs in far starker terms, not only as the subtext of historical change but also its motor. Theirs was a history constructed through a filter of class relationships, models of ownership and power, technical change and the play of world-historical events, such as the rise and fall of empire. The early stage of human civilisation, which Marx called 'primitive communism' (in today's language 'communalism'), roughly coincides with Smith's hunting period. Two other stages, slave society and feudalism, coincided with agriculturally based societies. Agriculture developed with and from the collapse of the slave system managed through the Roman Empire. Marx was completely uninterested in writing history to moulder on library shelves, and his arguments on earlier epochs are merely a rough sketch for a different purpose, which was to understand and theorise the logic of historical change in order to dissect the shape and direction of industrial capitalism.

Smith, it should be remembered, viewed merchant capitalism – towards which he often expressed equivocal thoughts – as the final stage of economic development, but this had already been surpassed by the 1820s.[22] This is not to say that some features of modern 'consumer capitalism' were not already present.[23] Indeed it was famously Smith himself who identified important constituents of the production methods which capitalism would require: task separation, mass production, constant trade. Marx and Engels proposed that the desirable future for society would emerge and had been sketched but badly by utopians. They argued that the main accomplishment of society's capitalist phase, the encouragement and release of technical forces, was already under way and would heighten class tensions and dynamics. Accepting their own strictures on the naivety of utopian speculation, they gave little attention to the economic or even ethical character of this future society, which they termed 'communism'. Instead they focused entirely on observing the unfolding dynamics of socio-economic development.

Marx and Engels sought to expose what is sometimes referred to as the iron laws of history. In this, they were influenced by Hegel in pursuing the logic and order of economic development. Actually, they did not depict the capitalist system as operating on the basis of sealed logic. Its conditions of development were modifiable, they argued. Social reform can soften the brutality of factory systems ('primitive accumulation') and can be introduced to respond to the collective sense of threat to dominant groups. Engels, in particular, observed the health threats to the rich, and Marx, too, recounted that factory legislation, once resisted by factory owners and political leaders as an impediment to the expression of 'personal freedom', could actually be advantageous in the real world of politics. (Even today, voices are raised against health and safety legislation as an infringement of human liberty, usually by those not exposed to dangerous equipment.) It is often said, erroneously, that Marx thought labour the 'ultimate source of value'.[24] In fact, Marx, following earlier political economists, took full regard of the place of nature, and some of those following in his footsteps point out that many of his observations are consistent with contemporary environmental thinking.[25]

What perhaps marks out Marx and Engels from the analysts of the Economic Transition who pre-dated them is the attention and significance they accorded to social classes and movements; in particular, they focused on the organised working class. If the industrial age was uniquely new, so too was the working class as a social movement. As historian Charles Tilly has more recently observed, between 1750 and 1840 ordinary British people abandoned old forms of protest such as collective seizures of grain, the sacking of buildings, or the public humiliation of officials and replaced them by marches, petitions, public meetings, and other new forms of social movement politics. The change created – perhaps for the first time anywhere and despite a limited franchise – mass participation in national politics.[26] Supporters saw the rise of lower-class power as inevitable, but Engels for one observed that the working class was often prepared to accommodate its own oppression; it was prepared to accept reform even though 'objectively' a substitute for real change. The picture painted is of the Economic Transition as creating stark inequalities (which we know to generate health inequalities) but also a tendency to boom and bust cycles within underlying economic growth. This was, Engels charged, capitalism's Achilles heel, its 'tipping point' in modern parlance.

Marx welcomed the political economists' focus on the material world, which gave primacy to the labour process, land, trade and wealth (value) creation. He shared Malthus's criticism of naive utopian thought, but he was also famously withering about Malthus himself. In this, he was not just discourteous in Victorian terms; Malthus was described by almost all as a kindly parson. We wonder if he also had some worries about whether Malthus had a case. If scarcity did indeed have its 'roots in nature', as Malthus had supposed, then the transition to the next phase of society, socialism, would be impossible.[27] Perhaps, too, the spectre of a society limited by scarcity helps explain why the *Communist Manifesto*, Marx and Engels's most famous work, was so full of praise of the technological achievements of capitalism. In this respect, Marx and Engels were more prescient than Malthus. From the nineteenth century, European capitalism unleashed a phase of remarkable economic growth not just of industry but of the land. From 1500 to 1820, world per capita income rose by a mere 0.05 per cent a year. From 1820 to 2001, it averaged 1.23 per cent, nearly 25 times as fast.[28]

The views of Smith, Malthus, Marx, Engels and others of the period remain significant for economics and politics today for different reasons than they might have selected for themselves. Smith's mentions of the invisible hand of the market have become a justifying principle for hypothetical free markets. Malthus is presented as a population theorist bewailing population growth when he was nothing of the kind. Marx and Engels are forever associated with alternative societies established in backward economies, in complete contrast to their notion of the transition from capitalism to socialism on the basis of technological change and the elimination of class divisions. The ironies are many, not least that one country subscribing to Marxism, the USSR, returned officially to capitalism, while another, China, has become a form of state capitalism and the pacemaker of the world economy.

The twentieth-century arguments

From the mid-twentieth century, an important argument emerged about how best to develop underdeveloped economies and therefore improve the social and health circumstances of populations. From the ending of the Second World War, the problems of development were thrust upon economists by the rapid break-up of colonial empires and the instant irrelevancy of colonial economic models. If the term 'economic development' had been rarely used before the 1940s, the ascendancy of nationalist governments in Africa and Asia pushed economic development on to the agenda of the new economic bodies of the United Nations (UN), formed in 1945. The World Bank was but one institution formed by the UN to steer economic development. As Gerald M. Meier from the World Bank reflected, the 'major capitalist countries' now began to recognise the grave danger 'that former colonies might, if there was little social progress, fall under communist domination: investment opportunities and access to markets and sources of raw materials would then be diminished'.[29]

Walter Rostow (1916–2003) was one of those who gave particular thought to this problem. Rostow famously updated the stages model first mapped by the classical and then Marxist economists. He used the term 'transition' in so doing. Rostow was an economic historian who became America's dominant academic commentator on economic development. For him, transition described the passage from traditional society to advanced capitalist economy. In 1960 Rostow suggested that countries passed through five stages of economic development.[30] He updated Smith's formula on the direction of economic advance by adding a new 'end point' in the form of advanced capitalism (rather than merchant capitalism). Rostow's stages went through, firstly, traditional society, then a transitional stage (the preconditions for take-off), take-off, drive to maturity, and finally high mass consumption. If Smith's discourse on historical change had been constructed merely to delight his students in Glasgow University lecture theatres, Rostow's appeal was to a wider audience, not least a USA locked in ideological combat with the Soviet Union in the Cold War. He helped contrast US material progress with the reality of USSR command economics. Although Rostow constructed his stages from European economic development, his theory was aimed at the developing world, where increasingly Marxist – more often Maoist – ideas had some attraction. For Rostow the key to tackling underdevelopment was investment, economic aid, training and education, all of which the USA had and could offer in abundance. It was an approach which had worked for Western Europe through the form of the post-Second World War Marshall Plan for European reconstruction, on which Rostow had advised.[31]

Rostow's thesis undermined the walls of socialist thought. No longer did capitalism need to be weighed down by Malthusian or Marxian doubts or crises; it offered the promise of wealth for all, which would bring health. That said, the wounding criticism of his theory largely came from fellow mainstream economists, who charged that Rostow's analysis lacked much correspondence to actual historical process. There was no common path to economic development or sudden take-offs.[32] Rather there was a general expansion of economic growth, with Britain setting the lead until the 1880s and the USA thereafter.[33] Despite their rejection by other economists, Rostow's views formed an especially attractive and coherent justification for the politically expedient message to developing countries: 'Follow our path and you will become as rich as us.' Economic Transition in Rostow's terms is essentially a modernisation story with a specifically (and post-European colonial) American twist. And for the poor of many societies, for example in Central and South America, the distant attraction of the American Dream has continued to draw immigration northwards.

The debate around Rostow's economics have since focused on the successes and failures of economic development. His historical and implicitly optimistic picture of economic growth now occupies a quiet backwater in the history of development studies, displaced by a decidedly non-historical perspective, what became known as the Washington Consensus. This was a term coined by economist John Williamson in the late 1980s to refer to a package of ten policy instruments which were believed to 'reform' economic development.[34] These become synonymous with neoliberal economics as represented in public policy, although Williamson has dissociated himself from that, arguing that the neoliberal experiment exemplified by President Reagan in the USA and Mrs Thatcher in the UK had mostly been 'discarded as unpractical or undesirable fads', with the exception of privatisation.[35] Despite such disagreement, the word 'Consensus' has stuck to Washington Consensus, much as its critics might have preferred 'Dissensus'. Much of the criticism stemmed from how policies were imposed. In his own retrospective analysis of how the term was used by his critics, Williamson paradoxically accepted that it was correct if describing the policies applied by the Bretton Woods institutions – the World Bank, the International Monetary Fund (IMF) and other bodies – on 'client countries'. Among Williamson's ten original policy instruments in the package were: fiscal policy discipline; redirection of public subsidies; tax reform; trade liberalisation; privatisation of state enterprises; deregulation; and legal security for property rights. Thus, if the Rostow-style model of economic and social modernisation provided a place for the State to unfold and direct historical processes, the new approach substituted market mechanisms in its place. In this picture, economic history is irrelevant; what matters is the application of market processes in any national or international economic transaction.[36] This includes health. Healthcare reform became a key test for how extensively the privatisation process had been enshrined. Health services have to be market-driven and interpreted.

An alternative Economic Transition model to Rostow's had been offered by Kenneth Boulding before the ascendancy of the Washington Consensus. Boulding returned the term closer to Malthus's interpretation. Whereas Rostow had offered a cornucopia for all, the aspiration of walk-in refrigerators and gas-guzzling town cars, Boulding offered the prospect of a far more sombre future. In his 1959 introduction to Malthus's *Population: The First Essay*, Boulding suggested that 'the Malthusian system, given the premises, is as irrefutable as a syllogism, and no amount of experience can stand up against watertight logic'.[37]

Boulding was proffering a bioeconomic model. He agreed with Malthus's strictures on scarcity and considered it the first duty of the economist to be 'dismal' – the epithet first applied to Malthus but which stuck more broadly, and inaccurately, to the field of economics itself. Economics ought not to be studying only a narrow slice of the human experience, financial exchange, but a wider version of the economy as part of natural–human systems. For Boulding, war, overpopulation and the exhaustion of natural resources were the new 'Malthusian traps' threatening the economy and society, although they could, with ingenuity, be avoided. Boulding was stating that economics has no option but to align itself with ecological thinking. Modern economists might joke about their discipline being the dismal science, but Boulding was highlighting their naive optimism if they continued to deny the connection between economics and nature.

Boulding (1910–93) was born in Liverpool, UK, but lived and worked in the USA. A one-time president of the American Economic Association, with honorary doctorates from a total of 33 universities(!), he set out his own genealogy of human economic development with a theoretical schema to explain it. He portrayed three periods of 'rapid growth'. These were: firstly, the transition from Palaeolithic to Neolithic society; secondly, from Neolithic to 'civilised society'; and, finally, from civilisation to 'post-civilised society', the latter phase being applied to the twentieth century, which he saw as shattering any ecological pretence at viability.[38] This damning account was based on his evolutionary perspective. Like another economist before him, Thorstein Veblen (1857–1929), Boulding saw economic development as a process analogous to biological evolution, that is to say a process which began with simple organisms or structures and built by adding complexity. Veblen, in contrast, had attempted a formulation much closer to Darwin's own conceptions of evolution.[39]

Veblen's thinking was based on the perception that human development was judged only partly by the state of wealth but in particular by its acquisition of technical knowledge or know-how. He discerned four stages in the evolution of mankind: the peaceable savagery era, the barbarian era, the handicraft (and petty trade) era, and the machine age. Although he accepted Marx's critique of capitalism, he took from Darwin the thought that evolution was continuous, and followed no predetermined course or unique pattern of development.[40] While viewing society in similarly evolutionary terms, Boulding considered the behavioural zone to be only partially determined by practical limits and intrinsic demand properties. He thus rejected for example the then fashionable US psychologist B.F. Skinner's behaviourist analysis for its poor understanding of human behaviours as solely animal responses, not least because he conceived of 'animal' behaviour outside their ecological niches.[41]

Both Boulding and Rostow were politically engaged, but not in the directions that might be expected. Boulding found his political home in the American Republican Party for more than a decade, while Rostow, conversely, was an ardent Democrat. Rostow moreover became US Democratic President Lyndon Johnson's national security adviser and was a staunch advocate of 'domino theory', used to inform the unsuccessful US military strategy in South-East Asia in the 1960s.[42] Boulding meanwhile (like President Richard Nixon, a Quaker) was an active peace campaigner. While these political differences were considerable, both maintained that economic development should follow a capitalist course.

As with Veblen, writing more than a half-century before him, Rostow's central analytic framework was consumption. In this, he merely enshrined what could be observed in US capitalism: extraordinary use of resources fuelling purchase of goods. For Boulding, by contrast, consumption meant the destruction of a stock – as in the depletion of fossil fuels and minerals. What the mainstream economist therefore calls 'capital' was to him nothing more than human knowledge imposed on and extracting the material world.[43] Knowledge and the growth of knowledge were therefore essential keys to economic development. The other parts of the process – investment, financial systems, economic organisations and institutions – he characterised as only the mechanisms by which a knowledge process was created and expressed.

In his attempts to generate a popular audience for these views – his public appearances in the USA being stymied by a British accent and stammer – Boulding sought to package his ideas in popular metaphor. He proposed that the USA operated a 'cowboy' economy, defined by the wasteful use of non-renewable resources, which ought to be replaced by a 'spaceship' economy – a place which by definition requires for its survival the ending of waste and the use of renewable energy sources. Together with the lesser-known work of fellow economist Nicholas Georgescu-Roegen (see Chapter 7), his work helped generate the new branch of environmental economics in the late 1960s, and hence ecological economics today, and raised the political level of concern about the finitude of planetary resources. An illustration was the 1972 Club of Rome report *The Limits to Growth*.[44] Based on calculations of known energy resources, the report projected a global economic collapse some time before AD 2100 as a result of limits to energy and natural resources needed to meet rising global levels of consumption and the resulting waste of ever-expanding production. Although committed to market-based perspectives, the Club of Rome recognised the challenges industrial capitalism presents to maintaining the eco-systems on which all life on the planet depends. At the time, the report attracted considerable attention and was influential in the establishment of the World Commission on Environment and Development by the United Nations General Assembly in 1983. Despite its dire warnings, *The Limits to Growth* had limited effect on Western production and consumption, which continued to grow.[45] Twenty years later, the Club of Rome released a follow-up study entitled *Beyond the Limits: Global Collapse or a Sustainable Future*.[46] Using new data, the book sombrely affirmed the grim conclusions of the Club's initial report. Again, it had limited traction within the political framework.

The current fault-line: market economics versus ecological economics

This account of the emergence of thinking about the Economic Transition has suggested differing approaches, not least in formulating the nature and desirability of economic growth. Surprising alliances have emerged across history and ideological boundaries. Rostow and Marx, for example, agree on the nigh inevitability of advance into and beyond industrial capitalism. Some questions arise which now need to be noted and which already feature in twenty-first-century political economy. What is development? Can economic growth be decoupled from environmental or health damage? Is there a limit to the advance of general well-being from endless economic development? Can health and the environment be costed and internalised into dominant market economics? How can the twenty-first century shape policies which respond to the stark evidence about inequalities in quality of life? What are the economic institutions through which human activity is conducted: if not the market, what? All these questions emerge from previous thinkers recognising the immensity of the legacy of the Economic Transition.

Running through all these questions is the shocking possibility that markets might not be everything, that markets are human creations which carry human frailties, a weakness Adam Smith recognised and which newly fashionable 'behavioural economics' presents as a new and distinctive paradigm.[47] 'Neoclassical economics is based on the premise that models that characterise rational, optimising behavior also characterise human behavior', says the Chicago economist Richard Thaler.[48] Smith would have agreed, but then he would have thought any suggestion that markets could operate through such terms absurd. People may make calculations, but their interpretations of risk are often in error. In his discussion of gambling, for instance, then as now employed as a mechanism for funding the State, Smith marvelled at the people's capacity to believe they might win when evidence suggested otherwise. People gambled on lotteries when 'the world neither ever saw, nor will ever see, a perfectly fair lottery', he wrote.[49] If a lottery was truly fair, he reasoned, the people running it would never make anything from it. There was no man living, he reasoned, who didn't share part of an 'over-weening conceit' in overestimating their likely good fortune. Younger people, he observed, operated their lives with a 'contempt of risk'. Smith saw this feature as a deeply embedded human trait but also a failing. In more psychological language, such false expectations promote wishful thinking, denial, and a maladaptive delay in confronting reality. In social anthropologist Lionel Tiger's view, however, 'making optimistic symbols and anticipating optimistic outcomes of undecided situations is as much part of human nature' as any other human biological feature.[50]

Optimism can be presented as both adaptive and maladaptive, according to viewpoint. For some it might offer a positive illusion, for example leading the sick person to get better, while in others it might only result in wasting time on non-beneficial pursuits, gambling being Adam Smith's prime example. Whatever the unlikely resolution of this conundrum, two and a quarter centuries on, Smith's observations are now writ large. With evidence that current economies (not to say economics) are mis-serving the future of humanity by overestimating fortunate outcomes in financial markets or continuing the mining of the infrastructure of existence or presenting a world in which people's well-being endlessly rises, how can anyone argue that general economic welfare is advanced by the optimistic values associated with greater consumption? While agreeing with Smith's patently true observation that young people are more likely to be risk-takers, it is equally true that they may be more aware of the environmental consequences of their actions since they live in an era in which the language of ecological limits is being forced into the public narrative. That said, young people are more reliant on resource-hungry technology and less tied to historical phases of social rationing. What this discussion primarily shows is that, like Malthus, Smith was really a bioeconomist in that he, like others since, saw the interconnections of the environment, bodies, mind, culture and society. He saw how psychologically complex these relationships were, an understanding which modern economists are now just rediscovering.

This fault-line between dominant market economics (or neoclassical or neoliberal economics) and what is called in the literature ecological economics is now of paramount importance for any twenty-first-century approach to public health and other civilising functions.[51] On the one hand there is an approach to economics which over time has narrowed political economy from the broad interdisciplinary vision of the classical thinkers to the operation of the price mechanism almost alone. Economics has been reduced to its subjectivist or 'hedonistic' aspects – what the customer desires. Faced by rising evidence of environmental and health harm, this conventional school has taken to valuing 'externalities' such as the costs of ill-health or impact on eco-systems services. And on the other hand there is a tradition of ecological economics which derives its logic also from the classical thinkers but incorporates the notion of ecological space as the paramount framework within which human labour and exchange occur. At the margins to both is a discussion of whether the quality of human existence and for that matter advances in public health are best served by either set of approaches.

Nicholas Georgescu-Roegen described himself explicitly as a 'bioeconomist'.[52] He became notable for his analysis of the material, particularly physical, basis of economic activity, insisting that descriptions of economic phenomena, especially mathematical descriptions, must go beyond relative market prices to take into account the basic physics of nature itself, in particular in the conversion from low- to high-entropy states.[53] Such a viewpoint, as we have seen earlier, offers a strong contrast with the economics of his time in which short time scales were all that apparently mattered. It earned him an implicit rebuke from Paul Samuelson, the then leading representative of US mainstream economics, who dismissed any discussion of entropy in the social sciences as the sign of a 'crank'.[54] For Georgescu-Roegen, who in childhood in his native Romania observed how the scope of human lives was limited by subsistence agriculture, economic analysis must be grounded in the reality of the physical and social universe in which humans are embedded. For him human choices always occur in a social context, which therefore placed strict qualitative limits on what economists often refer to as the laws of supply and demand. The mathematical formulae on which economics was increasingly based only helped to conceal the falsity of the view that all commodities were comparable and substitutable, he thought. As he trenchantly put it, '[h]e who does not have enough to eat cannot satisfy his hunger by wearing more shirts'.[55] This approach underscored his perspective on nature.

Georgescu-Roegen's work informed the thinking of explicitly ecological economists such as Herman Daly. The twentieth-century economic crisis, according to Daly, echoing Kenneth Boulding, was its incapacity to recognise that economic markets are merely a sub-set of the ecological system. Figure 8.1 is his depiction of how economic activity fills and possibly exceeds ecological space; he describes the shift in human history as from 'empty world' to 'full world', with economic activity as a process of transforming material coming to fill previously ample space. This was a metaphor of course. But Rockstrom and colleagues estimated exactly that process happening in a much cited paper in *Nature* in 2009.[56] They calculated that the nitrogen cycle and rate of biodiversity loss had already gone through long-term ecological limits.

What is not fully known, and possibly never will be, is the limits of this ecological space, captured by the concept of 'carrying capacity'. This notion is drawn

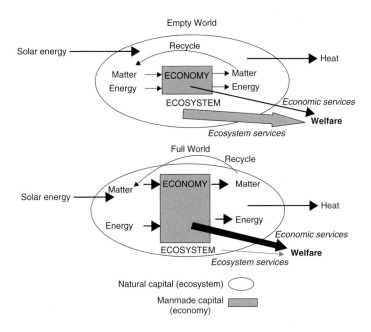

FIGURE 8.1   Herman Daly's 'empty-world versus full-world economics'

from the image of a boat gradually filled to the brim with cargo, thus placing cargo and crew in danger, with clear Malthusian echoes. It is for this reason that a group of economists, led by economics Nobel laureate Kenneth Arrow, have recommended focusing not on the measurement of carrying capacity – which they worry might be no more than inspired guesswork – but on the complex nature of ecological resilience.[57] The implication here is that estimating the linear impact of economic growth on ecology may be an illusionary exercise. By the time economists have established a methodology for doing so, it may no longer be relevant.

Arrow and colleagues suggested that a critical factor for deciding how well humanity addresses the crisis of ecological versus market economics might be the institutions within which economic activity occurs and by which it is shaped. Institutions need to be designed to fit the purpose; currently economic rules and terms of reference, by implication, are not fit for purpose. In Herman Daly's case what is implied is a return to first principles, the advocacy of a 'steady-state' or 'no-growth' society, thus invoking John Stuart Mill's 'stationary state society', introduced in Chapter 3, and proposed at the very outset of modern market economics.[58] Other expressions offered include 'prosperity without growth' and 'sustainable de-growth', terms used both for analysis and as banners for social movements.[59] What also has to be clarified is how far this new version of economics is compatible with capitalism, acknowledging that capitalism can be manifest in many forms. Just as John Maynard Keynes's critique of 1930s capitalism for ignoring the social costs of its development helped redesign the post-Second World War economic architecture, might ecological economics help rescue today's architecture from three decades of neoliberal domination and denial of environmental harm? Some think this a distinct possibility.[60] A possible ideological battle is being sketched of market economics as a latter-day Goliath versus ecological economics as the modern David. If this metaphor holds then it might also be added that Goliath has continued to grow in size, win plaudits for his victories and attract and maintain powerful friends, while the David of ecological economics has remained puny. His stones only bounce off.

Certainly, neoliberal market economics became the dominant paradigm from the late 1970s, and it remains so today. Chicago economist Theodore Schultz, in his speech on receipt of the Nobel Prize in economics in 1979, claimed that 'standard economic theory' was an entirely adequate means for understanding economic development and pressures of resource scarcity. Land (as a source of limits), said Schultz, was 'overrated': hence 'Mankind's future is not foreordained by space, energy and cropland. It will be determined by the intelligent evolution of humanity.'[61] In effect, therefore, nature posed few or no limits. The notion of a contestable Economic Transition based upon rival assessments of broadly based 'political economic' perspectives is further sidelined by the bold notion that human behaviour, in its very essence, is constructed through rational economic choices, the notion that while psychology was present in all decision making it relied on strict consistency of preferences. The most remarkable feature of this new orthodoxy, whether presented as the open-ended, unconstrained vision of economic development offered by Schultz or the rational economic choice model of Gary Becker, his colleague at the University of Chicago (also a Nobel Prize winner), or in the updated form of behavioural economics (which substitutes psychological complexity for economic rationality but otherwise disdains any attempt to reduce the scope of markets), is the breadth of its ambition. Other social scientists, marginalised or simply ignored, can only look on in wonder. For sociologists the reduction of human existence down to economic factors (even including the incipiently individualistic contribution of psychology) was a 'takeover bid' for the explanation of all of human behaviour.[62] For economists still steeped in the political economy tradition, it represented nothing less than 'economic imperialism', as Ben Fine has put it.[63]

The most remarkable aspect of neoliberal market economics has been its resilience in the face of its own stunning failure. In 2008, the orthodoxy of the self-regulating market imploded with the collapse of the Western credit bubble, after years of speculation and rule-fixing to suit a particular version of the role of debt-inducing banking and lending.[64] According to political scientists Francis Fukuyama and Seth Colby, the former an adviser of the Bush administration, the liberalisation measures implemented by professional economists had 'contributed to a massive global recession that, from peak to trough, wiped out $40 trillion in savings' and caused 'U.S. public debt as a percentage of GDP to increase from 42 percent to somewhere between 60 and 80 percent, according to estimates'.[65] The picture they offer of the profession is something of an ungovernable, introspective cult. Alas, it has power over the conditions for public health.

Given that economics had started out, as we saw, with an explicitly moral frame of reference, how and why can this situation – if the accusation be true – have occurred? There are several explanations offered. For Fukuyama and Colby the conclusion is hardly economics-profession-friendly: it results from the pervasiveness of questionable premises, oversimplified models and ideological bias. A much softer variant of this explanation is offered by another Nobel laureate, Paul Krugman, himself an economist and advocate of what is called the 'neoclassical synthesis'. He feels that his colleagues were blinded by their own mathematical science.[66] Indeed, as the Swedish ecological theorist Peter Söderbaum has remarked, the Bank of Sweden (Riksbanken) Prize in Economic Sciences in Memory of Alfred Nobel, may be part of the problem, since it is based on positivism as a theory of science and therefore tends to support neoclassical (market) economics.[67] Whatever the lure of numbers, and certainly the presence of equations in most modern economics papers today acts to emulate the appeal and rigour of the physical sciences, a career in economics would certainly be uninviting without considerable mathematical dexterity. The consequence is that almost all academic resources in economics have, in recent years, been devoted to mathematical economics, in particular the establishment of deductive models based upon the presumption of event regularities or correlations, an outcome that economic philosopher Tony Lawson characterises as 'erroneous thinking'.[68]

For others, the explanation is more social in form. Former IMF chief economist Simon Johnson and his colleague James Kwak suggest that the economics profession became, in so many words, highly influenced if not actually corrupted via the strong mutual relationships with avaricious banks.[69] Perhaps one of the kinder explanations for the mismatch between the claims of economic prediction and real events is that of 'cognitive dissonance'. This is the psychological incapacity of economists to consider information sources other than in terms acceptable to themselves. This criticism turns the psychological pretensions of market economics on their head.[70] In any case, among the copious diagnoses of the financial wreckage of Western economies from 2008, there are now calls for the economics profession to address its own ethical standards. This would doubtless have amused Adam Smith.[71]

Against this apparent failure of market economics, ecological economics has established a critique but not much further. For example, while it is often claimed that competitive energy markets produce energy efficiency improvements, these are shown to be overtaken by 'rebound effects' which actually increase energy consumption.[72] The problem is, as Spash and Ryan have identified, much of what is called ecological economics takes its cue from market economics, for example by devising schemes like carbon pricing. In contrast the original promise of ecological economics was to offer an alternative to the mainstream.[73] Its weakness in this regard might be explained by the same factors which have undergirded the resilience of market economics even while it singularly failed to predict or afterwards explain the world financial crisis. As noted, money, recognition, publication and awards (including the Nobel!) go to those who work within, or amend, the existing market assumptions rather than those who provide a fundamental critique. As yet no new John Maynard Keynes (who personally eschewed mathematical modelling and raged against banks) has emerged from the centre of the establishment who is able to command a broader rescue vision. The nearest possible equivalent, the economist Lord (Nicholas) Stern, has tended to restrict himself to climate change.[74] Nor are there any sightings of a reborn Karl Marx able to provide what the Frankfurt school of social scientists have called an 'immanent critique' of economics and construct an alternative. But even if he or she did, would the economics field notice?

Nevertheless there have been attempts to offer fresh thinking. The tradition of evolutionary economics thinking, as we noted earlier, began with Veblen. It has taken on a new idiom, however, with the term 'complexity economics'. Eric Beinhocker, an economist with McKinsey, the management consultants, has presented an updated account. He presents the economy as a 'complex adaptive system' in which general evolutionary laws operate and where market advantage is gained by the mastery of two of its properties: technology (separated into physical technology and social technology) and business design.[75] By good fortune these are precisely the business services offered by McKinsey! Beinhocker's approach is more subtle than this apparent slight suggests. Complexity economics imports its concepts from beyond the business world. Against neoclassical economics, the economic world is seen as a historical creation with dynamic properties. Transition is implicit. Where conventional economics understands economies only through ahistorical and diachronic terms, for Beinhocker and others the economic system is understood synchronically. An economy is thought to evolve, to be thermodynamic (and therefore also entropic), emergent (having different properties at different levels of scale), open and non-linear, and to provide limited or 'fuzzy' information. Conventional economics, according to this view, has its successes. It is able to map and model non-complex, non-adaptive characteristics of systems, but this applies the modelling assumptions of mathematical physics, a reason why so many physicists are employed in economic modelling. The picture is of economies as evolutionary systems which are adaptive. Thus the evolution of an economy moves beyond being a mere metaphor drawn from biology into becoming a 'reality'.

In the neoclassical version of the economy, in contrast, the properties of both the physical world and the social world are more or less static and unchanging, opening the possibility of a reductionist understanding of economic processes. The difference between the two perspectives is important. Either the economy is adaptive or evolutionary, in which case complexity analysis applies, or it is operated according to simpler, unchanging physical laws. Even in Adam Smith, economies were said to evolve through stages; in Malthus there is a constant tension between agriculture and human population growth; in Marx the surface appearance of financial systems conceals dialectical processes. For these political economy theorists there was a dynamic, historical interplay of human and natural worlds. They painted a bioeconomic system. Indeed the fact that the world economies have changed dramatically since, from merchant to advanced capitalism, underlines the point. Economies are historically formed, organic, self-constructing, imperfect, volatile and disruptive. While the assumptions that economic rules operate like mathematical physics may be extremely effective in certain environments, for example those with electrical, chemical or mechanical properties, they are entirely ineffective in circumstances which have evolutionary properties. This is not therefore just a collision of ideas; it is a variance of perceived realities.

Another account builds on the thinking mapped by the Club of Rome. This suggests the need for 'natural capitalism', which can better satisfy customers' long-term interests yet deliver profits by solving environmental problems.[76] There are many more offerings of this type. Perhaps the most optimistic of all has been sketched by someone who experienced at first hand the creative destruction – to use Schumpeter's expression – of modern capitalism. Matt Ridley, former board chair of the failed British bank Northern Rock, which was rescued by huge borrowings from the British taxpayer and de facto nationalised, presents a notion of human evolution as one with a pure vision of market dynamics. For him, mainstream economics ought to remain supreme because markets and trade have driven human prosperity from early times. The natural order, Darwinian evolution and twenty-first-century markets need to be better aligned.[77] As Spash and Ryan have commented, such neoliberal economics is 'pro-growth, pro-development technological optimism'.[78]

Work, labour and health

John Maynard Keynes (1883–1946), the British economist, is associated with the redesign of post-Second World War economic financial architecture. His ideas helped shape the mid-twentieth century. In some respects he was a conservative figure who by upbringing had little experience or understanding of the lives of people beyond his own class and elite social group. If, as an economist and civil servant, he had much to say about work, he therefore had less to say about labouring (in the sense of physical energy expenditure such as bothers public health) or the immediate circumstances of work (such as bothers occupational health). Unemployment had peaked in 1932, but the dramatic fall in Western unemployment had to wait for the outbreak of the Second World War, which rebuilt full employment in pursuit of war. Keynes knew that stability of the economic system meant dealing with its major flaws. In his 1936 seminal work *The General Theory of Employment, Interest, and Money*, Keynes observed that the 'outstanding faults' of the economic system were 'its failure to provide for full employment and its arbitrary and inequitable distribution of wealth and incomes'.[79] These were matters, he argued, with which the mainstream economics of the day was largely unconcerned. That severe inequality was present in Britain was hardly unknown, but the situation in other 'Anglo-Saxon' countries was thought to be better. It was not. In the USA, which by then had economically overtaken Britain, the share of wealth owned by the top 1 per cent of income earners was close to 40 per cent in the early decades of the twentieth century.[80]

Over the following decades, wartime command economies which boosted employment, the new economic system Keynes designed and more progressive taxation meant that British and US disparities declined. After narrowing in the post-war reconstruction, gross intra-national inequalities of wealth returned from the 1980s. By 2007, according to Emmanuel Saez of the University of California at Berkeley, the income share of the top 10 per cent of the US population was equal to 49.7 per cent of total incomes, a level higher than in any other year since 1917. Figure 8.2 plots the percentage of national wealth given to the top 5 per cent of the population in the USA, the UK and Sweden across the twentieth century to today. The trend appears the same whether it is the top 1, 5 or 10 per cent. It shows how inequalities declined from a high point in the 1920s to a low point in the 1950s for all three countries. By the 1980s, despite steady economic growth, Sweden was a less unequal society, but from the late 1980s on even Sweden succumbed to mounting inequality. Factors which explain this rise in inequality include not just technological change but also the progressive abandonment of redistributive and employment policies which had reduced inequality from the 1940s. Data on inequalities in the developing world is far less available than in the rich world. What is known is that while the economies of China and India have been expanding at a rapid rate, the former at around 10 per cent per annum, inequality has been rising also, particularly between the very rich – the top 1 per cent – and the rest of society. In South Africa the wealth gap has actually increased during the post-apartheid era. Keynesian economics had fallen from favour with the rise of a neoliberal approach,[81] discussed earlier, in the form of Chicago economics (exemplified by Theodore Schultz and Milton Friedman) and the

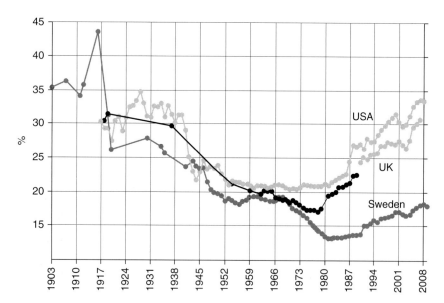

FIGURE 8.2   Income shares of the top 5 per cent in the USA, the UK and Sweden, 1900–2010

policy injection of structural adjustment policies and the Washington Consensus at the international level.

The majority of the member countries of the OECD, the 34 richest countries in the world, have experienced a rise in inequality since the mid-1980s, as shown in Figure 8.3. In OECD countries today, the average income of the richest 10 per cent of the population is about nine times that of the poorest 10 per cent – a ratio of 9 to 1. However, the ratio varies widely from one country to another. It is much lower than the OECD average in the Nordic and many continental European countries, but reaches 10 to 1 in Italy, Japan, Korea and the United Kingdom, around 14 to 1 in Israel, Turkey and the United States, and 27 to 1 in Mexico and Chile. Only two countries, Turkey and Greece, witnessed decreasing inequality, but the latter became engulfed in economic crisis in 2011.

From the 1980s in the Anglo-Saxon world of US and UK capitalism, a package of policies was gradually injected designed to reshape expectations of work. These included the undermining of trade unions, a shift from state to individual corporate provision of health and retirement benefits, and a general lowering of social norms on pay inequality. This package succeeded politically, as is evidenced by the general acceptance of huge disparities in disposable wealth. Indeed, modern 'celebrity culture' almost glorifies the acceptance of flaunted wealth and conspicuous consumption. One reaction to evidence on the widening wealth gaps is to argue that it is deserved, and that some labour (such as that of bankers, rock stars and sportspeople) warrants vast pay rates, while most does not.[82] Another response is to deny the inequality data altogether.[83] Back in the 1930s Keynes had accepted that inequality was

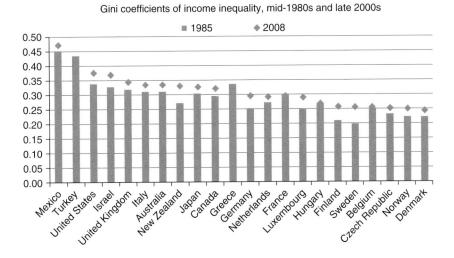

FIGURE 8.3   Income inequality increased in most, but not all, OECD countries

inevitable but proposed that society could prevent excessive inequality. In doing so, he aligned economics with social justice, an argument resurrected by John Rawles and Amartya Sen later in the twentieth century.[84]

As we noted at the end of our discussion of the Epidemiological Transition (see Chapter 5), there has been a long-running concern that economic inequality has a direct impact on health inequalities. After many years of academics 'rediscovering' poverty and inequality, it is perplexing that there is still debate and uncertainty over the precise mechanisms at play. Does income or status explain the poor health of low-income groups? Or is it explained by deindustrialisation and the loss of work and jobs on offer? Is it the changing nature of work or changed behaviour which follows from worklessness, the shift towards poor diet and alcohol and tobacco use? Studies suggest all of these. The facts remain that work and worklessness both frame health. Oscar Wilde, if alive today, could no longer ironically remark that 'Work is the curse of the drinking classes.'

Work is central to life. It gives meaning, accords status and provides a focus to the day. Meaning might not be given by the labour process itself – the dream of utopian socialists such as the artisan, artist and designer William Morris (1834–96), who argued for a craft economy to give dignity to labour[85] – but it can be given through the everyday associations and social contact that people make through their work. The academic literature agrees with common sense. In subsistence societies, where work is shaped by the necessity of provision, work is frequently physical and energy-demanding. In post-industrial societies, work uses the human body less for physically demanding labour. Yet, in all sorts of societies, social esteem is indicated by one's place in the division of labour. How we are valued by others matters enormously. Unequal valuation of work results in unequal valuation of self. If people find out that they are paid less than others doing what they feel are equivalent jobs their sense of fairness is disturbed.[86]

These apparently sociological and psychological dimensions are only part of the picture. Work is the linkage between the Energy Transition (see Chapter 7) and the Economic Transition. Economic progress is deemed to have occurred when non-human energy through sources such as coal and electricity replaces direct human labour. Yet this shift is now known to be a contribution to the rise of overweight and obesity, and climate change. People in rich societies have difficulties in fully using the calorific energy they eat or drink: hence the mismatch analyses of the epidemiologist Ian Roberts or of physicians Peter Gluckman and Mark Hanson.[87] Indeed, supposedly modern economies often devalue human physical labour, viewing it as the past, yet now encourage the overfed to go to gyms to walk or run on stationary runways as a response to the obesity pandemic. One can laugh at the absurdity, yet to have a machine capable of digging a ditch or to help build things in a short time can be miraculous, and does reduce an older historical problem of bodies being literally worn out by hard physical labour.

Another strand of health thinking about work has stressed how human physical and mental potential can be undermined by poor health. Undernourishment due to poor income can reduce the capacity to work. From the nineteenth century to today, many studies, reports and campaigns have reiterated this point, with public health representatives championing the case for minimum standards of living, and arguably turning it from a radical demand to a question of scientific adjudication.[88] The core arguments here are simple, and so is the question that follows it: what is the level of income (derived from work) required to enable humans with varied physiological needs to perform different tasks? In the USA in the early twentieth century, W.O. Atwater (1844–1907), an early nutrition scientist, pioneered the calculation of how much food, and therefore income, different workforces required to live and work adequately.[89] In the UK, this thinking was adopted and refined by B. Seebohm Rowntree (1871–1954), scion of the chocolate manufacturing family, to research and consider the living standards and the requirements of labour, with much of his research conducted in his home city of York, England and on his own workforce in a series of studies over half a century.[90] His findings helped formulate thinking for post-Second World War welfare reforms. It enshrined a complex understanding of the relationship between physical labour and the inputs necessary to maintain it, particularly diet. Rowntree, like Keynes, focused less on the actual process of work and more on the sensitive issue of how to value work in economic terms: what is a fair rate of pay for the labour sufficient to purchase the means for a healthy existence? By the end of his studies, Rowntree concluded that minimum health standards providing physiological adequacy should be raised to include sufficient income for people to have pleasure and dignity through their diets too.[91]

The conditions of work, not just the labour process itself, have a fundamental impact on health. As we have noted, Britain was to be the first country to industrialise and among the first to experiment with deindustrialisation, in a long wind-down of its early manufacturing base. The shift from primary production to industrialisation to post-industrial society has brought a parallel shift in work and forms of health-related occupational risks. Many large manufacturing industrial sectors such as shipbuilding and mining, growth areas in the nineteenth century, went into decline. Trade unions rose and then fell in influence. It has been suggested that the century following 1900 brought better working conditions generally, falling hours, increased real wages, greater flexibility in work and increased female participation in the workforce.[92] This generalisation is undoubtedly true for the West, but not the whole picture. The direct physical risks associated with work processes have certainly declined in the West. Accident prevention became a more systematic feature of the workplace management, with particular emphases in risky workplaces such as armaments factories emerging in the First World War.

Jürgen Kuczynski (1904–97), the German Jewish economic statistician, undertook a review of accidents at work in Britain in 1942 (to which he had escaped), part of an enormous study of labour relations under industrial capitalism covering Germany, the USA, France and other countries.[93] He observed that during the First World War only fatal accidents at work were recorded, with 1,579 occurring in factories and workshops in 1918. Mines and quarries were separately collated, and non-fatal accidents were not recorded. By the Second World War, reporting of accidents had improved in Britain. In 1941, there were 1,646 fatal accidents in all work settings and 269,652 non-fatal accidents. Kuczynski also noted that accidents were by then being reported by gender. In 1941, 42,857 accidents were reported for women but, as women replaced men on the factory floor in the war effort, this figure jumped to 71,244 in 1942. A decade before, in the dawn of the scientific management era, American safety engineer Herbert Heinrich, whose work is considered more fully below, suggested that in the analysis of industrial accidents there was a strong statistical relationship between frequencies in major injuries and minor injuries,[94] although this idea is discredited today.[95]

In 1974, the year when the UK Health and Safety at Work Act was introduced, the number of fatal injuries to employees was down to 651. The data for 2009–10, nearly four decades later, showed a further fall, with 152 workers killed at work.[96] The construction industry and agriculture accounted for half of all these deaths. This is an undoubted improvement, yet the headline picture is more complex than it first appears. In 2009–10, 2,249 deaths were attributed to mesothelioma, a previously rare cancer caused in almost all cases by exposure to asbestos dust, with victims primarily being trade-associated from asbestos use at work. The trades most at risk were carpenters and plumbers, but the disease emerged decades after exposure. UK mesothelioma mortality is the highest total worldwide.[97]

European work conditions have enormously improved in the twentieth century, but some of the riskiest, dirtiest or most intensive work conditions have been shifted to countries with poor work conditions and regulations and where workers have limited representation and, owing to past historical factors, only limited worker rights and sense of entitlement. Many of the largest world brands have their products manufactured in China, which as we saw earlier (see Chapter 7) became the world's largest user of energy and largest industrial employer. Apple Corporation, the electronic goods brand, does not actually make the iPad and iPhone, but they are made by Foxconn (Hon Hai Precision Industry) headquartered in Taipei, Taiwan. It has 611,000 employees worldwide and is the largest exporter from Greater China and also a major manufacturer in the Czech Republic, where it is the second largest exporter. The company makes products for many of the major Western high street electronics brands. Bloomberg News sought explanations from the company as to why there were reports of ten Foxconn staff committing suicide at its Chinese plants in the first half of 2010.[98] One worker interviewed said, 'Life is meaningless. Every day, I repeat the same thing I did yesterday.' Bloomberg reported that 86 per cent of the workers in its Shenzhen, China, plant were under 25 years old and lived in white dormitories with eight to ten people sleeping in a room. It also reported that the living quarters, with stairs running up the outside walls, were covered with nets to prevent people from jumping to their deaths. Bloomberg reported that the pressure on workers came from the business model. Unlike Apple, which sold its Foxconn-made products for high financial margins, Foxconn itself made tiny margins, resulting in intense pressure to lower production costs. Reviewing the whole Chinese-based brand assembly manufacturing sector, China Labor Watch, a tiny NGO with offices in Mainland China and in New York, reported that workers had few rights to complain about conditions. It found that workers' ability to organise and express their grievances was extremely limited, and daily overtime work was obligatory, with in excess of 100 hours being the working week norm. The majority of the factories surveyed failed to pay wages in accordance with Chinese labour laws or in accordance with the minimum wage.[99] These are almost Dickensian work conditions, hidden from Western consumer sight, but the reality of a globalised supply chain system.

Work can be risky in ways that at first seem unconnected with the labour process. Cars and trucks are now a work site, much as factories are in industrial systems. The UK House of Commons Transport Committee estimated that in 2007 between 750 and 1,000 drivers died in accidents related to their work each year.[100] Given EU-legislated restrictions on the hours of commercial transport driving, the UK situation is probably better than in many countries worldwide. A 2005 study argued that deaths related to motor vehicle traffic accounted for 16 per cent of all fatalities in New Zealand, 22 per cent in the USA and 31 per cent in Australia of all work-related deaths.[101] Such a situation – injury to drivers on work assignments – might be thought to be primarily an issue for economically advanced societies. This would miss the fact that low-income countries typically use cheaper, riskier forms of transport, have poor road design, and often have poorly maintained vehicles which are inherently less safe. Their systems of accident surveillance and legal systems of compensation are ineffective or limited. The poorer the country the more the pattern of risk shifts to pedestrians. Although any figures should be taken as only a rough guide, it has been suggested that around 45 per cent of road traffic fatalities in low-income countries are among pedestrians, whereas an estimated 29 per cent in middle-income and 18 per cent in high-income countries are among pedestrians.[102]

Many of these fatalities are work-related. In Tanzania, one study suggested that 62 per cent of work-related injuries occurred on roads; walking along the roadside to or from work was the most common category of risk.[103] Traumatic injuries at fixed work sites such as a factory are more likely to get attention, but because these accidents occur on or beside roads means that the responsibility is either dissipated or shouldered by the victim. The International Labour Organization (ILO), part of the United Nations, collects occupational accident data from all the countries in the world. The ILO includes road traffic accidents as a part of work-related injuries and also, as one might expect, occupational or work-related disease. It also admits that reasonably reliable data is obtained only from a rather limited number of countries, around one-third of the 174 ILO member states.[104] The total world picture it assembles, a fatal occupational accident rate of 14 per 100,000 workers, or 335,000 fatalities a year worldwide, is a rough estimate when better data is needed.

Today in Western countries there is far more information about work-related injury, including self-assessed conditions. In the UK, for example, an estimated 1.3 million people who had worked in the last 12 months, and a further 0.8 million former workers, suffered from ill-health which they judged work-related. Musculoskeletal disorders were the most common type of work-related illness, but mental ill-health gives rise to more working days lost. Such information is self-reported, as are accidents outside the workplace, a source of data which raises questions about boundaries between work and non-work, what is body and what is mind. In human relations management this is often presented as the 'work–life balance' problem, as if work was something one was meant to suffer and pleasure is only possible in one's own free non-working time. In the name of neoliberal economics, not Keynesianism, right-wing thinkers maintain a constant attack on health and safety legislation as unwarranted intervention in the name of health nannies. The reality of work–health links is rarely discussed.

The serious analysis of work and health centres on better understanding the interaction of people, machines and the work environment. Even for light labour such as office work, new technologies such as computers led to new forms of ill-health such as strains to hands, eyes and backs. A so-called 'systems approach' to occupational health has advanced the understanding of effective prevention. Some of the roots of this perspective lie in the analyses of safety engineer H.W. Heinrich in the early 1930s. For Heinrich (1886–1962) it was not enough to analyse a single person or machine in isolation but to examine overall processes. He stated that every incident results from a series of events, the last one being the accident itself. What he called the domino theory presented an accident sequence likened to a row of dominoes knocking each other down in a row. Later researchers introduced the role of managerial error and property loss and the view that the causes of accidents are complex and interactive and far less behaviourally based than in Heinrich's model. Whereas Heinrich attempted to systematise work risks – raising the question of whether an accident was truly accidental – the production management focus promoted by W. Edwards Deming (1990–93) implicitly shifted the understanding of accidents to the inherent quality dimensions of the production process. He used statistics to establish knowledge, not just information, on the performance of the work system. Deming's ideas gave birth to the total quality movement and a particular boost to Japanese industrial production following the Second World War. It is now associated with Toyota's just-in-time management, also used by food retailers. This emphasises logistics and minute management of the workforce to deliver all parts at the right moment, with minimal delay. Underlying these ideas were a set of important, even philosophical, principles linking production, product quality and work-related risk. Deming's objective was not merely an exhortation to workers to produce more and to management to generate higher profit. In one of his last books he observed that 'We have been taught by economists that competition will solve our problems. Actually competition, we now see, is destructive.'[105] Deming argued that the resources used in production were 'temporary blessings', thus resurrecting the discussion of energy and material constraints that we outlined earlier in the work of Boulding and Georgescu-Roegen.

Factory production, as we have seen, is merely one work setting, and in some societies a declining one. The world's largest workforce is still agriculture, which has 1.1 billion, of whom only 450 million are waged.[106] Even with attention to accident prevention, some industries remain highly risky, particularly agriculture, which even in the rich UK has the highest rate of fatalities of any occupation.[107] In the developing world, agriculture is a risky business from poor handling of agrichemicals and poisonings.[108] In lower-income countries work risks are treated more lightly: poor or no provision of protective clothing, poor training in risk assessment, differentiation of the workforce according to work status and gender, little scope for employee redress, and lack of trade union rights.

In focusing on the differential health risks between grades of employees, health researchers have emphasised organisational, income and cultural factors and how they interact in the workplace. The British Whitehall studies, begun by Geoffrey Rose and colleagues in 1967, provide another dimension to ostensibly work-related health risk. It examined the health of male civil servants in England between the ages of 20 and 64. It found that men in the lowest grade (messengers) had 3.6 times the coronary heart mortality of men in the highest employment grade (adminis-trators). Men in the lower employment grades were shorter and heavier for their height, had higher blood pressure and higher plasma glucose, smoked more, and reported less leisure-time physical activity than men in the higher grades.[109] Most of the men in this study had physically undemanding occupations. Decades later, the study was rerun. Risk factors had changed in the meantime. Nevertheless, the pro-file of vulnerability, what the researchers now called the 'social gradient', remained. Compared with men in the lowest 5 per cent of a risk score based on smoking, diabetes, employment grade, and continuous levels of blood pressure, cholesterol concentration, and body mass index (BMI), men in the highest 5 per cent had a 15-year shorter life expectancy from the age of 50.[110] Work stress was one factor and was associated with weight gain among obese men but weight loss among lean men.[111] The converse may also be true. If workers find their life satisfying, their health improves and the mortality risk from coronary heart disease lessens.[112]

The Whitehall studies offer a picture of incrementally graded patterns of inequal-ity linked to but not fully explained by a worker's position in large-scale organisa-tions. It leads to many difficult questions. How much are health inequalities due to work processes and how much due to generally prevailing social inequalities? How much can be attributed to bodies and how much to minds? Indeed, is such dualistic thinking worthwhile? What began as a study of differential health patterns among civil servants broadened into what became the 'social determinants of health' perspective, adopted by the WHO. The notion of 'social' determinants of health is really 'societal' and systemic. As the Whitehall authors note: 'These circumstances are shaped by the distribution of money, power, and resources at global, national, and local levels, which are themselves influenced by policy choices. The social determinants of health are mostly responsible for health inequities – the unfair and avoidable differences in health status seen within and between countries.'[113]

One of the consequences of deindustrialisation has been the shift in employment to the services sector. As we have noted above, this actually often means less than it sounds, being a downward shift into a new division of labour and the breaking of labour forces into smaller units and their internationalisation.[114] Deindustrialisa-tion can produce an entire culture of worklessness in formerly industrial areas. As a consequence of the decline in working-class jobs, a new workless category has been created: the discouraged jobless, people designated too ill to work but also adminis-tratively inconvenient to categorise as unemployed or job-seekers. The connection between unemployment and health is clear. Worrying about being unemployed, especially among older workers, may precipitate depression.[115] Unemployment itself may lead to declines in psychological and physical health and an increased incidence of suicide.[116] Suicide rates are linked to movements in the business cycle: economic depression leads to mental depression.[117] The longer people are out of work but seeking it, the greater the risk of mental health problems.[118]

The principal underlying question is that of class in modern societies. In previous decades social class was an accepted national analytic category. Today, as Klaus Eder has remarked, classes have been 'culturally dissolved'.[119] The result is that class structure is itself defined by patterns of inequality and the mode of understanding such inequality. As the sociologist Zygmunt Bauman has noted, being poor today in Western societies derives its meaning not just from being unemployed but from being a flawed consumer.[120]

How much is the persistence of poor health due to past deindustrialisation? Can any one factor, even from the past, be isolated as an explanation? This was asked about a part of Scotland, a country which has the highest mortality rates and lowest life expectancy of any Western European nation. Its western central area, the region radiating out from Glasgow, presents the worst health trends in Scotland, which makes Glasgow the unhealthiest urban area in the whole of Western Europe.[121] Glasgow was once one of the shipbuilding and engineering centres of the world, progressively losing this role from the 1950s. Comparing this area with ten other post-industrial regions across Europe, public health researchers were perplexed. Some facts are obvious: poverty underpins post-industrial decline. It manifests itself in health terms through interactions with other structural, behavioural, psychosocial and cultural factors. While it was therefore tempting, said the Glasgow University researchers, to explain this area's poor health with deindustrialisation, they found only limited support for it within the data they examined. The data raised more questions than can be answered. This picture of poor health and health inequality is not just a matter of economic phases of boom and slump, nor is it likely to be some mysterious 'factor X'. Rather it would seem that it is the entire aspect of place, people, economy and culture – into which are mixed many unknowns or qualitative 'hard-to-describes'. Public health thinking has tended to focus on some certainties, such as smoking, low fruit and vegetable consumption, or alcohol, all manifest in Scotland,[122] but the complexity of factors involved – material, biological, cultural and social – suggests the need for a systemic or Ecological Public Health analysis.

The Economic Transition and public health

The classical economists recognised economics as occurring in natural settings. Yet, to read many modern economists, the reliance of human endeavour on the planet seems to have been lost. We are not alone in suggesting that the future of public health thinking about economics will also have to recover more complex and complete understanding, not least of work and the structural nature of inequalities discussed in this chapter. Our analysis questions the reduction of public health's engagement with economics to 'market' thinking. More complex, ecological thinking is required. Notions of State, corporate and civil society responsibility need to be on a more equal footing. The outcome of the discussion of the Economic Transition for public health, we suggest, is a stronger acquaintance between public health and economics, as long as the latter is reformulated to encompass questions of Nature and human relations which were once part of a seamless discussion of political economy. We have highlighted thinkers in this chapter who pioneered such integration. Their argument is for de-compartmentalisation and for the repositioning of economics within the full range of social sciences. The more mathematical tendencies in modern economics have lost sight of people, their health and the circumstances, social and environmental, which define progress.

We have seen that the assumption of economic growth translating into better health is problematic. The argument from the stages of growth and market theorists that there is an inevitable line of health improvement cannot be supported. The rise of non-communicable diseases (NCDs) seen in previous chapters is another illustration of the fact that there is no direct correspondence between improved wealth and improved well-being. We have seen, too, that the Economic Transition draws primarily on the Techno-Economic model of health but is constantly drawn into other domains and dimensions of existence. In that sense, if modern economics is to help address Ecological Public Health challenges, it will celebrate more the broad and interdisciplinary, in modern terms, approach of the classical political economy thinkers from the Enlightenment to today. Table 8.1 summarises some of what has been learnt by the account here and is presented as an aide-memoire before we turn to the notion of a Nutrition Transition in the next chapter, and after that into more overtly social and cultural issues which shape the conditions for twenty-first-century public health.

TABLE 8.1 Four approaches to the Economic Transition

Approach to Economic Transition	Approach			
	Stages of growth	Complexity	Market	Steady state
Core idea	Economic Transitions go through an orderly sequence en route to prosperity.	The economic system is a full evolutionary system.	Order follows from applying market or money values to everything.	Economic activity has to fit into ecological realities, i.e. nature.
Key thinkers	A. Smith, K. Marx, W.W. Rostow.	T. Veblen, E. Beinhocker, N.N. Taleb.	M. Friedman, F. Hayek, T. Shultz.	J.S. Mill, R. Malthus, K. Boulding, Club of Rome, H. Daly, T. Jackson.
Policy approach	Investing people at lower stages of growth will speed up their transition.	Pragmatism rules.	Social, health, environment, culture: all have to be tailored to fit economic 'rules'.	Economics is no longer the key policy tool; sustainability becomes the key principle.

TABLE 8.1 Continued

Approach to Economic Transition	Approach			
	Stages of growth	*Complexity*	*Market*	*Steady state*
Main criticisms made of the approach	Too mechanistic.	Implications for policy unclear, since everything is in motion.	Reductionist.	Turns dominant economics on its head; requires a different world order.
Implications for public health	Better health follows each stage.	Quality of public health important for evolutionary success.	It is part of human and social capital, to be costed.	A key indicator of sustainability.
Approach to nature and resources	Resources are linked to economic expansion.	Economics draws natural and thermo-dynamic law.	Resources are endless and therefore resource limits are irrelevant for economics.	Ecological resources have to be maintained as the bedrock of existence.
Approach to capital	Capital is required for economic expansion.	Knowledge is critical component of capital in an evolutionary system.	Everything is a form of capital.	Ecological capital is more important than financial capital.
Approach to work and labour	Progress is to replace human labour with technological knowledge.	Technical labour is key. Knowledge of evolutionary system is key to economic advantage.	Flexible labour markets need to be encouraged and restrictions removed.	For J.S. Mill, labour ultimately needs to be organised and used in co-operative functions for the general good. In modern forms this becomes 'for sustainability'.
Current political impact in the West	Renewed interest as a way of looking at capitalism as a dynamic system.	Renewed interest, particularly by some management consultancies.	Dominant perspective for economic co-ordination, but under stress.	Marginal, but seen as possible new paradigm owing to world recession in the early twenty-first century.
Where operating?	Some leverage in some nominally planned economies, e.g. China.	Information technology, informatics, management theory.	Globally.	No economy yet, but some support in particular commodities and companies, e.g. energy inputs, food.

9

NUTRITION TRANSITION

The 'Nutrition Transition', as was true for the Demographic and Epidemiological Transitions, was a term coined by an individual researcher, who then proceeded to refine and extend the concept. The Nutrition Transition is a concept mapped by Barry Popkin, an American economist and epidemiologist, and current from the 1990s. It describes a historical pattern of change in diet and physical activity witnessed particularly in the twentieth century across the world, as people became richer.[1] In over two decades of work, studying about half the planet's populations, Popkin and colleagues have suggested that as societies modernise they converge towards a particular dietary configuration, one which is high in saturated fats, sugar and refined foods but low in fibre, often termed the 'Western diet'.

The word 'nutrition' is derived from Latin via Old French. The meaning is simple: to be nourished. The shift in nutrition accompanies the emergence of lifestyles characterised by lower levels of activity. These changes are reflected in 'nutritional outcomes, such as changes in average stature, body composition, and morbidity'.[2] These latter indicators are why this is such an important transition for public health; height, weight, girth and the relative (in)appropriateness of intake and output from the body directly affect population and individual disease profiles and social consequences. Repeatedly, Popkin has explicitly related the Nutrition Transition to the predecessor Demographic and Epidemiological Transitions (see Figure 9.1). That relationship has been summarised thus:[3]

> Two historic processes of change occur simultaneously with, or precede, the 'Nutrition Transition'. One is the Demographic Transition – the shift from a pattern of high fertility and mortality to one of low fertility and mortality (typical of modern industrialised countries). The second is the Epidemiological Transition, first described by Omran; the shift from a pattern of high prevalence of infectious disease associated with malnutrition,

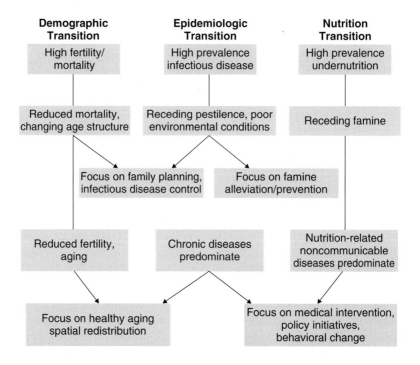

FIGURE 9.1 Popkin's schema of how the Demographic, Epidemiological and Nutrition Transitions interrelate

periodic famine, and poor environmental sanitation to one of high prevalence of chronic and degenerative disease associated with urban–industrial lifestyles.

In effect we see that the Nutrition Transition, as described by Popkin, is the outcome of the fusion of two processes: dietary change and physical activity change. By implication, given the impact of the Demographic and Epidemiological Transitions, other shifts in background circumstances are implicated. The Demographic Transition implies changes in family size and therefore possible changes in dietary circumstances of households. The Epidemiological Transition refers to the changing disease conditions, including the microbial context, which may have a bearing on physiological nutritional processes, a point made by Thomas Malthus two centuries earlier. Both Popkin and Malthus depict long societal processes, Malthus at the end of the eighteenth century and Popkin at the end of the twentieth century and beyond. For Popkin, the archetype Nutrition Transition is that experienced by the USA, a society which is by degrees becoming physically heavier and, with the likely growth of non-communicable and chronic diseases, associated with this apparently new mix of dietary and physical activity change.

The concept of the Nutrition Transition has rightly been lauded, but in this chapter we suggest that some modification and amplification emerge through taking a longer perspective on the patterns of nutrition change and the drivers which shape them. In particular, we propose that what is referred to as the Nutrition Transition, offered as only one process, is in fact the weaving together of many.[4] The Nutrition Transition, as conventionally depicted, can be criticised for underplaying the importance of cultural change as a driver. We outline our thinking on the Cultural Transition later (see Chapter 11). To be fair, culture is acknowledged by Popkin and colleagues, for example in studies of the explosion of soft drink consumption and when noting that assimilation to American cultural norms places immigrant children at particular risk.[5] Yet in our view the variability in food cultures, and the potential shift towards a post-transition food culture, warrants more attention than the nutritionists have thus far given it. Indeed, the cultural element within the Nutrition Transition may even be key to resolving the problem. The alternative is to accept the inevitability of current trends and their accompanying economic and health costs. We have elsewhere argued for the unbundling of the Nutrition Transition.[6]

Popkin's work has focused on recent dietary shifts in China, Asia and Latin America. The phenomenon is now beyond doubt. In studies collating data from 100 countries, he and colleagues have shown the remarkable acceleration of the Nutrition Transition.[7] But are such shifts malleable? The Nutrition Transition is a schema, not necessarily an inevitable truth. The question is why and how is this happening? Given the impact of the Urban Transition (see Chapter 6), one could even posit that the Nutrition Transition is influenced by urbanisation as that social form has come to dominate human life. The overarching theme of the Nutrition Transition is that there is a mismatch between food supply, environment, bodies and culture or minds, i.e. how humans live in modernity. On that, many analysts could agree, but immediately they then diverge over the explanation. Is the Nutrition Transition due to inappropriate genes (i.e. an evolutionary mismatch) or the wrong mindsets (i.e. a cognitive mismatch) or the wrong food availability (i.e. food supply mismatch) or other circumstances or even, to stretch a point, an 'obesity virus'? Different disciplines each approach this historical shift with their own predilections. Popular journalism feeds easily on speculation.

Another perspective on the Nutrition Transition, or at least on the changes in the volume of nutrition in shifting environmental conditions, is found in the writing of Nobel laureate Robert Fogel and Dora Costa. They describe what they have termed the process of 'technophysio evolution'.[8] This proposed a link between technological change and physiological change, and they invoke Darwinian evolution as the underlying biological explanation. They suggest that human physiology is the repository of massively changed inputs and environment. A new pattern is emerging of increased energy availability, improved resistance to infection, improved food production and higher incomes enabling better living conditions. Fogel and Costa propose that this mix is subject to potential change, all except genetic pre-potential. The result is a qualitatively new mix which is now setting humans apart from animals and 'from all previous generations of homo sapiens'.[9] The result of these changes in nutritional status is a dramatic improvement in the physiological stock of human beings.

While the two concepts, Nutrition Transition and 'technophysio evolution', might not be rivals, they do appear to offer different interpretations of the same broad transition. For Popkin and associates, the outcome of the Nutrition Transition is a world in which health outcomes progressively worsen as dietary choice expands. In their account of the technophysio evolution, Fogel and Costa depict a world in a process of physiological improvement. In their view the prevalence of chronic disease is falling, whereas the impression of the public health field is the reverse. The Epidemiological Transition as we saw speaks of the age of degenerative diseases, but Omran did not say that degenerative diseases have risen; he said that they appear because people are living longer. What further troubles Fogel and colleagues is the steady rise in US healthcare costs, which Fogel elsewhere notes are set to rise to 29 per cent of US GDP by 2040.[10] Latterly, Fogel and others have acknowledged how obesity does present a new set of problems. However, they downplay its importance by stating that the predictions of its effects are 'speculative', while the overall rises in expectation of life 'show no signs of stopping'.[11] There is some uncertainty in this analysis, since they acknowledge the environmentally driven potential for famines today.

The importance of nutrition: bodies and environments

Why is nutrition important? This question may be self-evident to nutritionists but not so to everyone else. After all, Western societies have plenty of food. Some have a glut and, over the last half-century, food choices and food availability have grown to a remarkable extent even for relatively low-income households. But the story of human nutrition cannot be reduced to choice, availability or even price, although all remain important.

In the twentieth century, nutrition science has grown increasingly sophisticated in how it measures and judges dietary adequacy and dietary consequences for health. By the middle of the twentieth century, a fairly consistent picture had emerged from nutrition science, sufficient for its advice to become a key element in public policy and public health practice, and for it to be adopted as a key source of health advice to governments through the fledgling International Health Organization (forerunner to the WHO) in the 1930s.[12] In the post-Second World War period, nutrition science consolidated and became ever more sophisticated with the incorporation of genetics, biochemistry and the lessons of food technology. But, almost as soon as this acceptance into mainstream public policy and scientific respectability occurred, a new radical critique emerged from epidemiology. In his now celebrated Seven Nations study, the US epidemiologist Ancel Keys (1904–2004) showed that when countries became richer this fact did not automatically translate into their eating a better diet or longer life expectancy.[13] In fact, Keys's research showed the relatively poor Greeks (on the island of Crete) and the Japanese had better diets and health-related profiles than the US, the UK or the Finns. The possibility that the Western diet might have consequences had been raised. Today, the pursuit of the ideal diet – be this based on the US food pyramid, the UK's healthy plate, or the more popular versions of the Mediterranean or Japanese diet – is the stuff of newspaper columns as well as public health policy.

Again, a mismatch analysis is being offered, this time as an inappropriate mix of human physiology, food supply, consumer choice and lifestyles. Some analysts have suggested that the ideal diet for humankind might be that of human Palaeolithic ancestors, but this is contested by others as inappropriate for today.[14] That humans were hunter-gatherers for the vast majority of their evolutionary history is not disputed; that case was summarised by Hugh Trowell (1904–89) and Denis Burkitt (1911–93) in their 1981 observations on the differences between patterns of disease in advanced societies and African nomadic groups. They observed that six common medical diseases – blood pressure rising with age and essential hypertension, obesity, diabetes mellitus, coronary heart diseases, gall stones and renal stones – had never been reported 'in any hunter-gatherer nomad group until after some degree of acculturation'. They made an exception of the women of pastoral tribes who may take a lot of milk and become obese.[15]

This verdict implied that the 'modern' diet is not just associated with a range of diseases but mismatched to the genetic and physiological make-up of human bodies. One articulate account of this evolutionary analysis is presented by the work of Michael Crawford, a brain biochemist and nutritionist. He has argued that human intellectual capacity is a legacy of evolution and that part of the reason for the emergence of non-communicable diseases is the inappropriateness and changes in the nature of diet, particularly the importance of essential fatty acids, which constitute such a significant element in human brain size and functioning.[16] He notes that between 60 and 70 per cent of a new-born baby's energy from food and reserves is used by the brain for growth and maintenance. Modern diets, he argues, have altered the nutritional composition of foods. In the case of meat, humankind has moved from consuming meat raised in natural circumstances which has high muscle mass but slight fatty mass to meat which is high in fat and the 'worst' sorts of fats. This shift is due to changes in agricultural systems.

The public health case against this argument is that, while those with a pre-Western diet did not exhibit modern disease patterns, they lived much shorter lives, probably because they lacked the advantage of medical treatment or clean environments free of hazards. Until the later stages of the Epidemiological Transition, as we have already seen, infection was the main cause of mortality. Pre-industrial people suffered greater risk of traumas and parasitic and respiratory infections. The same point remains true both for fairly close genetic relatives, the wild chimpanzee, and for twentieth-century hunter-gatherers.[17] Moreover, even if primitive diets were desirable, they are simply unavailable to the urbanised mass population today. Indeed, anthropologists have documented the decline of existing hunter-gatherers and the traumas of their incorporation into modernity.[18] Trowell and Burkitt, with their African experience, were more than alive to the clash between 'civilisation', bodies and ancient lifestyles. They, like many authors exploring the Nutrition Transition, noted how rapid the change in diet can be when people move continents or ways of life and change dietary intake as a result. When the Kenyan Samburu, for example, who previously ate a traditional diet, were drafted into the army, their salt intake increased five times and blood pressure levels rose significantly. 'Like many Western men they were eating 24 times the sodium requirement of man.'[19]

There is a consensus among researchers from Trowell and Burkitt to Popkin and Crawford that something remarkable in human history was emerging. Popkin's contribution was to conceptualise this process as the Nutrition Transition and to chart its spread in studies of unprecedented global reach.[20] In country after developing country, Popkin and colleagues have shown the rapid shift in diets. The pattern described is of an overall rise in calorific intake, an increase in the range and types of foods consumed, a switch from water to soft drinks, accelerated intake of meat and dairy products, and a shift in the nature and source of foods, from home to international types of eating, and the arrival and influence of global food companies and their products.[21]

Significant changes like these have been noted before, albeit on a smaller geographical scale. In the mid-eighteenth century, as noted before, Adam Smith had commented on the prosperity of the North American colonies (see Chapter 2). At the time, epidemic diseases – smallpox, plague, yellow fever – were virulent,[22] and parasitic diseases were also present. Smith noted that the colonial population had far better access to food than their British contemporaries. John Komlos has established that by the 1780s North American colonist adults were as much as 6.6 centimetres taller than Englishmen, and at 16 years of age American apprentices were some 12 centimetres taller than the poor children of London.[23] The North Americans were taller than all contemporary Europeans, even the well-fed aristocracy. This is retrospectively explained by Komlos by low population densities, a relatively healthier disease environment, and the seemingly endless supply of highly productive arable land in the colonies. In short, he suggests a broader picture of the Nutrition Transition in which it is not a transition in and of itself but a reflection of wider ecological changes (both natural and societal) which do, however, alter the intake of food. This picture was soon set to change, however. Fogel and Costa showed that, in the USA, height fell below late-eighteenth-century levels for much of the nineteenth century. This was accompanied by falling life expectancy.[24] Certainly, there appears to be no iron law about nutritional advance; nutritional status (not just height) can fall just as easily as it can be made to rise, depending on circumstances. As Tocqueville had predicted in the late eighteenth century, American society was moving away from rural pastoralism (which delivered Adam Smith's observed population benefits) and becoming more unequal, not least because of population concentration in towns which brought disease.[25]

There can be little doubt that nutrition has played a leading role in altering public health, but there remain tricky issues in clarifying the interaction of nutrition and environment or circumstances, not least in the choice of indicators. As the nutritionist Nevin Scrimshaw (1918–) has pointed out, malnutrition also increased susceptibility to infectious diseases, yet this fact was completely missing from textbooks dealing with either nutrition or infectious disease up until the 1950s.[26] In fact, lack of hygiene meant that many foodstuffs, particularly milk products, were the actual route for pathogens and a host of other infections.[27] Thus while public health professionals focused on measures of height in the physiological development process, these were actually less an indicator of nutritional status and more a comment on the nutrition–environment interaction. It is only fairly recently accepted, therefore, that the height adult humans achieve is the result of a complex interplay between genetic endowment and environmental exposures during development.[28] Crimmins and Finch have shown how height gain might fall during periods of improving income in newly urban centres, and at the same time a decrease in infections and ensuing inflammation has the potential to increase height independently of improved food intake.[29] Changes in body size could be explained as indicating the complex interactions between the Epidemiological Transition and the Nutrition Transition. Timothy Hatton has suggested that improvements in the disease environment in Britain increased average height by about half a centimetre per decade in the first half of the twentieth century.[30] Increases in height, therefore, might not always follow as a direct consequence of increases in income and nutritional improvement.

Komlos and colleagues have explored these changes through the concept of the biological standard of living.[31] The core idea here is that environment, incomes and food availability shape the body literally. The body's height and girth, together with morbidity and longevity, are indices of general prosperity and well-being. In effect this presents the biological standard of living as a composite explanation which subsumes the Nutrition Transition. It provides a measure of social differences between and within countries. It paints a picture of health and well-being as an interaction of socio-economic levels, health and bodily potential. The power of this perspective is that, whereas Popkin examines the shift from underweight to overweight within a short and recent time frame, depending on availability of data it is possible to take a much longer perspective – connecting with the evolutionary views of writers such as Crawford. When contrasting the USA and Europe, Komlos and colleagues have pointed out how colonial America began its Economic Transition with the highest biological standard of living, as noted above, yet by the twenty-first century the USA was comparing unfavourably with Europe. Not only were Europeans healthier but also taller, reversing the situation of two centuries earlier.[32]

The situation today can be dramatised by the shift from height differentials to weight differentials, but each coexisting with sustained patterns of nutritional deficiency and nutrition-related diseases. In the urbanising US in the nineteenth and early twentieth centuries the fall in height affected both blacks and whites.[33] In the 1930s, Hungarian-born US epidemiologist Joseph Goldberger (1874–1929) from the US Public Health Service examined the patterns of disease among poor, mainly rural communities, in particular the disease pellagra, then thought to be an infectious disease, now known to be due to vitamin B3 (niacin) deficiency. It affected the poor and particularly black communities of the American South.[34] Goldberger, against the prevailing scientific wisdom, was convinced that it was a diet-related disease and conducted experiments and surveys to explore his hypothesis. His results were convincing, but it was left to others to identify niacin as the missing ingredient from the narrow diet of affected communities which lived on a maize- or corn-centred diet. Today, narrow dietary regimes still disfigure the US public health nutritional status and still affect those same groups which concerned Goldberger. The most visible health problem in the USA today is obesity,[35] a precursor to other diseases, notably diabetes type 2. On 2008 projections, all American adults will be obese by 2048, all black women will be obese by 2034, and the number of obese American children will double by 2030.[36]

Another issue which has been much researched and debated and which informs the Nutrition Transition analysis is whether dietary change is due to people becoming richer. Is it because they eat more or because food supply improves or price signals alter between food categories? Engel's law – articulated by Ernst Engel (1821–96), head of the German statistical department in Berlin from 1860 – states that, when household incomes increase, the proportion spent on food and other necessities declines as a proportion of disposable income. Engel was observing the emergence of mass middle-class expenditure, with a differentiation between necessities and luxury (which was measured by his Engel's curve). The implications are considerable, not least for food suppliers, who are forced to chase declining proportional expenditure. This motivates in part the pursuit of value-adding in food products. It also creates ground for the vast expansion of the restaurant and eating-out trade. Nutrition is no longer functional but part of the leisure industry. Food shifts from bodily maintenance to disposable pleasure. Long-term data from the US Department of Agriculture illustrates this general picture across the twentieth century. It shows the steady drop in the percentage of US income being expended on food, while the absolute expenditure rises (see Figures 9.2 and 9.3). This

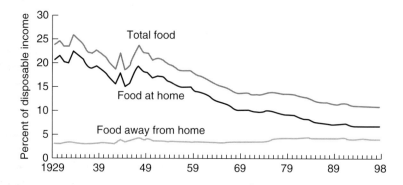

FIGURE 9.2 US spending on food: average disposable income on total, at-home, and away-from-home food, 1929–98

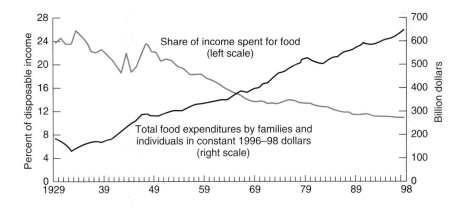

FIGURE 9.3   US food expenditure, 1929–98

picture has been compounded by changes in output from Western agriculture. Long-term data from the US Department of Agriculture shows that the US food supply provided 300 calories more a day per person in 1994 than in 1909. Calories from the US food supply, adjusted for spoilage and waste, increased from 2,220 per person per day in 1970 to 2,680 in 1997. This occurred at a time when people's physical activity was declining, and when health educators were urging behaviour change to eat more wisely.

World data on food also suggests there has been a steady rise in food output and availability over decades (see Table 9.1). In the period given by these Food and Agriculture Organization (FAO) figures, low-income countries increased their calorific intake from meat by 119 per cent, sugar by 127 per cent and vegetable oils by 199 per cent. In China, consumption rose by 305 per cent for sugar, 349 per cent for meat, and 680 per cent for vegetable oils. Meanwhile consumption of pulses and roots declined.[37] Apart from a peak in the early 1970s, linked to the oil crisis of that era, the cost of food declined worldwide until 2002, after which it started an upward trend.

Until the 2008 global financial crisis there was slow general progress in tackling undernutrition and malnutrition. According to the FAO, small import-dependent countries, especially in Africa, were deeply affected by the economic crises and by a parallel food crisis.[38] The latter was stimulated by poor harvests, the diversion of food to other uses, particularly energy generation, and rising prices. The main impact was regional, however. Between 2007 and 2008, the number of undernourished people was essentially constant in economically buoyant Asia (an increase of 0.1 per cent), while it increased by 8 per cent in Africa. The FAO observed that demand from growing economies in Asia was set to grow, but that biofuel production, in North America, South America and Europe, placed additional demands on the food system. Linkages between agricultural and energy markets, as well as an increased frequency of weather shocks, posed additional problems. On the supply

TABLE 9.1 World trends in per capita food consumption (kcal/person/day), 1969–2005

	1969–71 (kcal/person/day)	1979–81 (kcal/person/day)	1989–91 (kcal/person/day)	1999–2001 (kcal/person/day)	2003–05 (kcal/person/day)
World	2,411	2,549	2,704	2,725	2,771
Low-income countries	2,111	2,308	2,520	2,579	2,622
Sub-Saharan Africa	2,100	2,078	2,106	2,128	2,167
Near East/North Africa	2,382	2,834	3,011	2,991	2,995
Latin America and Caribbean	2,465	2,698	2,689	2,798	2,899
South Asia	2,066	2,084	2,329	2,334	2,344
East Asia	2,012	2,317	2,625	2,764	2,839
High-income countries	3,046	3,133	3,292	3,429	3,462
Transition countries	3,323	3,389	3,280	2,884	3,045

side, they observed, there were declining rates of yield growth for some commodities. One major consequence for poor countries and communities is likely to be continuing food price volatility, they observe. In Chapter 5, on the Epidemiological Transition, we considered analyses of the double and sometimes triple burden of disease. The Nutrition Transition certainly adds new disease burdens to older disease burdens, linked to the traditional problems of hunger and malnutrition. It is possible to have rising population weight in urban areas but acute food poverty in the countryside.

The picture elsewhere is quite different. The oft-celebrated Mediterranean diet, the original 'peasant' diet identified as nutritionally beneficial by Keys in Crete and many since,[39] is also in transformation with altered supply. Nikos Alexandratos, former head of the FAO's Global Perspective Studies Unit, has shown how in three Mediterranean countries, Greece, Spain and Italy, a mismatch has also occurred through rising total fat intake, from meats particularly (see Figure 9.4).[40]

Yet another perspective on the Nutrition Transition emerges from the argument that technical changes in food – how it is grown, processed and distributed – might be a significant shaping factor in the Nutrition Transition. Few nutritionists have any romance about primitive diets. Progress is agreed to have occurred when settled agriculture, the spread of techniques and early trade enabled diets to move from being wholly seasonal, based on staple foods (which vary according

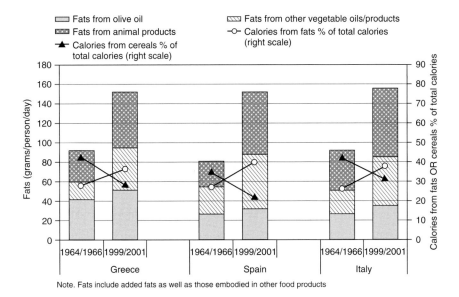

Note. Fats include added fats as well as those embodied in other food products

FIGURE 9.4   Greece, Spain and Italy's diet transition: the rise of fat consumption, 1964–2001

to location and plant availability) and narrow in choice, to diets characterised by greater variety and better storage.

One variant of this technological analysis has offered a pessimistic account of nutritional adulteration. Technologists, this has argued, have denatured some foods and created 'fake' food designed, processed or bred to maximise appeal at point of sale and in the mouth.[41] Particular recent attention has centred on the role of trans-fatty acids – artificially hardened fats favoured in processing. Here there is now strong evidence of a role in coronary heart disease.[42] Another variant of this technological perspective stresses the impact of the emergence of monoculture on the land and, for example, the decline in seed varieties for basic foods, with the industrialisation of agriculture.[43] Against this sober line of assessment, more optimistic arguments stress the value of technical change through nutritional fortification. Examples include fortifying flour with folic acid to prevent spina bifida and the addition of iron and other minerals to ensure at-risk groups achieve the requisite nutritional intake of missing or low nutrients. There have been arguments, however, about how to achieve the correct level and source of fortification.[44] During the Second World War, there was an intense argument within the UK Ministry of Food about whether to fortify white flour or to favour eating non-enriched wholemeal flour.[45] Today the WHO stresses that action to deal with 'micronutrient malnutrition' has advantages which are 'potentially huge', especially in relation to the prevention and control of infectious diseases such as HIV/AIDS, malaria and tuberculosis as well as diet-related chronic diseases.[46] Such policy directions are not merely offered for developing countries and disadvantaged populations. The WHO notes that 'the increased consumption in industrialised countries (and increasingly those in social and economic change) of highly-processed energy-dense but micronutrient-poor foods, is likely adversely to affect micronutrient intake and status'.[47] The WHO estimates that more than 2 billion people, over a quarter of humanity, are affected. Iodising salt, for example, is simple, cheap and health-effective. On the other hand, the ubiquity of trans-fats or the sweetening of foods is driven not by health but by industrial requirements and the price of raw commodities, and by pandering to taste and texture (themselves both desires which are evolutionary residues). What emerges for public health is the need to address who controls the nature of food and food products. In our discussion of the Cultural Transition, we explore how advertising, marketing and cultural pressures are now major features for Ecological Public Health (see Chapter 11). These are clearly on the agenda of nutrition policy worldwide, with increasing concern about the powerful effect of advertising and marketing on driving the uptake of nutritionally inappropriate dietary ingredients.[48]

Environment and physiological growth

How do environmental circumstances affect physiological growth, resistance to infectious disease and vulnerability to chronic ailments? Nutritional intake occurs with certain environmental conditions. The risk of developing chronic diseases in adulthood is influenced not only by genetic and adult lifestyle factors but also by environmental factors acting in early life.[49] One of the classic examples has been rickets, as shown in the stark black-and-white photographs of hospitalised children at the end of the nineteenth century, a time when photography was becoming far more widely used as a hospital teaching tool. Rickets is one of any number of dietary-related chronic diseases, ranging from pellagra, a disease caused by vitamin deficiency, common in the American South, to obesity today. In the case of rickets, this bone development disease was mostly found in northern countries of Europe and notably in England (on the European Continent it was known as the English disease), as well as northern industrial towns of the USA. The scale of the problem in Britain was mapped in a late-nineteenth-century survey carried out of children under the age of 2 years in London's Great Ormond Street Hospital. This found one in three children hospitalised with some features of rickets.[50]

The great John Snow (1813–58) was among the first physicians to investigate the dietary basis of the disease, arguing that alum in bread (used for whitening flour) may have been a critical cause, although Snow also listed poor air quality, poor diet, lack of exercise and 'a scrofulous taint' as contributory factors.[51] Snow tried to discount the less important factors, but rickets has a multi-causal aetiology, so his task was hard. Available remedies included cod liver oil, but these were culturally localised.[52] Many smog-bound cities provided their inhabitants with insufficient sunlight, a source of vitamin D. Rickets was not thought of as an outright killer and so 'attracted little attention from the public health administration'.[53] It was also primarily a disease of the poor. It was not until the 1920s that Adolf Windaus (1876–1959) discovered the role played by vitamin D, for which he won a Nobel Prize. Windaus, it should be noted, also stood out among scientists in Germany by openly opposing the Nazi regime.[54] Even if vitamin D emerged as the specific culprit, causation was still multi-factorial.

The discussion of physiological growth in environments returns us to the earlier discussion of the work of Robert Fogel and other researchers of the biological standard of living. In examining the long trends in physiological growth and resilience, and therefore the general conditions explaining chronic disease, the economist Robert Fogel has presented an evolutionary and environmental perspective. For him, as for many others giving an evolutionary account of physiological development, the genotype determines the potentialities of the organism but environment determines how much of that potential is realised. Early-years development is critical. Nutritional or environmental difficulties occurring during a woman's pregnancy and a child's first year of life lead to later compromises in physiological growth and therefore adult stature. It has been suggested from resemblances in height between relatives that around 80 per cent of height variation is under genetic control, with the rest controlled by environmental factors such as diet and disease exposure.[55] So far about 50 genes and regions of the genome have been associated with height. Although the relationship is not fully understood, evolution and environment are the controlling factors which help explain the biological basis of stature and its triggers. Studies in the 1930s had tried to assess the link between height and heart disease and cancer rates.[56] In Britain height differences have long been used as an important differentiator for social and economic inequalities, with welfare improvements leading to the equalisation of stature between social classes in the second half of the twentieth century. Physical stature has been considered as a proxy measure for health, disease and social welfare generally.[57] A second aspect of Fogel's thinking is metabolic. Human physiology needs energy in two distinct ways, one for physiological growth and one for metabolic expenditure. Put simply, people cannot work, or can work only fewer hours, if they have not consumed sufficient levels of protein.

Fogel's studies of long-term anthropometric trends – changing body size over time – are in part an attempt to explain how the biological standard of living influences physiology and how in turn physiology influences the economy. While the notion of biological standard of living must only be one part of a discussion of living standards, it is nevertheless an important one. Other broader considerations of standard of living include the discussion of functioning and capabilities, introduced by Amartya Sen, and an alternative focused on relativities between groups and social classes proposed by the sociologist Peter Townsend (1928–2009).[58] The advantage of nutrition, Sen has pointed out, is that being well nourished 'may have more or less similar demands on commodities (such as food and health services) irrespective of the average opulence of the community in which the person lives'.[59]

In a sense this is a restatement of part of the McKeown thesis (see Chapter 5), but with attention paid to the feedback of health to the economy. The fact that people have been becoming bigger and stronger, the result of improving nutrition, Fogel says, accounts for up to half of the growth in national income in Britain since 1790. It was not just technology or energy that brought about industrial growth, he asserted, but also improvements in the human capacity to work. Furthermore, nutritional improvement helps account for the long, gradual increase in longevity since 1790 and the reduction in rates of chronic diseases in the twentieth century, including the decline since the mid-twentieth century of musculoskeletal disease, digestive disease, heart disease and cancers. The examples he draws upon for this latter argument, much of it undertaken with Dora Costa, and discussed earlier, are mostly from the USA. There is thus a difference in the time frame that they use and that used in the Popkin version of the Nutrition Transition.

Fogel's pioneering studies have led to research interest in the tracking of stature changes in Europe where historic height data is available, such as army recruitment medical assessments. In Italy, for example, this data shows the height of army conscripts increasing steadily throughout the second half of the nineteenth century, reflecting, it is suggested, increases in food intake due to growth in agricultural production and also better sanitary conditions and primary schooling.[60] One study examining 15 Western European countries from the middle of the nineteenth to the end of the twentieth century, suggests that from the 1870s to the 1970s average height increased by around 11 centimetres, or more than 1 centimetre per decade. As with Fogel's own account – nutrition plummeted in the early decades of the nineteenth century in Britain – there are paradoxes within the data. The authors of this study noted that increases in height were maintained in a period that embraced two world wars and the Great Depression. One possible answer they suggest is that the relative price of food fell and its nutrition content improved, even from 1914 to 1945, a time of major wars in Europe.[61] In some countries food rationing may have improved the nutritional situation of poorer groups, but in others there appear to be quite sensitive associations between fluctuating nutrition and stature. Italians born in 1945, at the end of the war and during a period of severe food shortage, were 3.7 millimetres shorter than those born in 1944 and 7.9 millimetres shorter than those born in 1946 when food shortages were being relieved.[62]

The Dutch case provides the most interesting example so far owing to the very long time perspective employed. Based on skeletal evidence it has been suggested that, in the late Middle Ages and at the onset of the early modern period, the Dutch population was taller than in the first half of the nineteenth century. A spectacular increase in Dutch heights began in the second half of the nineteenth century and accelerated in the second half of the twentieth century. At the end of the twentieth century, the Dutch became the tallest people in the world.[63] Comparing the Netherlands with the USA and England confirms the role of 'bigger-picture' factors, not only the microbiological environments of the nineteenth and early twentieth centuries but the pressures of industrialisation and urbanisation, which developed at varying paces between these three societies. The latter phase of height increases among the Dutch has also occurred in a period of rapid improvement in heart disease rates.[64] In the USA and England, however, increases in height have given way to increases in girth. As noted earlier, Komlos observed that across the twentieth century the US population went from being the tallest in the world to being the most overweight. The explanation was to be found, he said, in differences between the USA and Europe, in particular the 'greater social inequality, an inferior health care system, and fewer social safety nets' in the USA.[65] But the shift from height to girth also moves the discussion away from improving nutrition in 'old' environmental circumstances, such as the improving sanitary environment, to the 'new' environmental circumstances, in which environments are clean of microbes but 'dirty' in cheap processed foods.

One other important factor introduced by Fogel, the use of food for energy, emerged as a feature that was as significant of this new environment as of the old. In the nineteenth century, food – considered as a source of metabolic energy – was expensive. In the twentieth century, food costs slowly declined while the calorie content or 'embedded energy' within food significantly rose. The energy contained in modern confectionery or sugary soft drinks, for example, is much higher than anything obtainable in the distant past. It is this 'energy glut', the overconsumption of high-energy foods, which is one of the significant features of the rise in population weight.[66] From the perspective of the nineteenth century this might be a problem many people might have wished for, but resisting environmental factors now might be as difficult today as resisting environmental factors then. The communities that suffered pellagra in the USA, poor blacks in the main, are the same groups who are most significantly afflicted by the new environmental conditions today.

The highest current rate of obesity is found in Mississippi with African-Americans, in large part owing to their consumption of low-quality food.[67]

The difficulty of policy engagement

We began this account of the Nutrition Transition by implying that it was a recent phenomenon but have found that it has long been observed, dissected and debated. What Popkin and colleagues initially depicted as a modern phenomenon is probably but the latest phase of a longer process. It could even be argued that this is a health phenomenon which began to emerge with settled agriculture, then mercantile trade, early urbanisation, and industrial capitalism itself. At its heart is the long human struggle for dietary sufficiency and against seasonal or climatic-induced shortfalls. As we suggested, Adam Smith and others noted how affluent American colonists could escape what later was termed the Malthusian crisis or trap. The Nutrition Transition, moreover, dovetails with other transitions, but it brings theoretical and public policy complexity in so doing. The Nutrition Transition, we have argued, is not just nutritional but is about the interface of bodies, minds, mouths, markets, culture and 'nature'.

While Popkin has most elegantly set out a central representation of the Nutrition Transition, other interpretations crowd in and alter what the phenomenon is. Fogel and colleagues, notably, pointed to the longer picture of a decline of diet-related ill-health. The evidence from the USA suggests more of an ebb and flow. Popkin's point that a new pattern of disease emerges with dietary change remains essentially valid, but the causation is complex. Mass population weight gain and obesity do appear to be a new worldwide phenomenon; this is neither speculative nor a repeat of the past but wholly modern. And it is partly why the Nutrition Transition has been so effective in capturing and forging public health imagination. For there to be more people on the planet who are overweight and obese than hungry suggests a new configuration of global public health inequality.

Fogel's technophysio model accords closely with our Techno-Economic model (see Chapter 3). In that we argued that economic improvement, commercial marketing and knowledge had produced beneficial effects for human hygiene and the microbiological environment. However, in modern times, according to the subject discussed in this chapter, improvements in food technology, the marketing of high-fat foods and the lessening of the human need to expend energy (because of cars, etc.) are reversing the health benefits. The Techno-Economic model is thus in some disarray.

Be that as it may, a significant challenge is emerging for public policy. For most of the twentieth century, scientific effort centred on the case to grow, produce and distribute more food. The Nutrition Transition questions the continuation of that simple policy formula, calling for a revision of what and how people eat. Yet, while that policy proposal is emerging, the older version stressing the case for more food to be produced is also being revised and reasserted. This is being championed by those worrying about a coming food deficit crisis by the mid-twenty-first century.

They point to data and trends about environmental threats from climate change, soil and biodiversity loss, water scarcity, fossil fuel dependency and population growth.[68] This revised policy appeal to produce more food at all costs is currently the dominant policy position, yet, unless the Nutrition Transition is to be dismissed, the reality is that a new composite policy paradigm is needed. This should address the public health challenge of hunger and underproduction alongside mal- and over-consumption and overproduction. In short, a more differentiated policy package is needed than just producing more food or persuading populations to eat less.

Part of the problem with the Nutrition Transition is that it describes and theorises a phenomenon which is not just about nutrition. It refers to massive changes not just in what people eat but in how food systems operate: turning precious food into cheaper calorie commodities which can be marketed and sold in ways which were unimaginable even decades ago, let alone in the era of Malthus and his pessimistic prognostications. The Nutrition Transition is a cultural and societal transition, not just an eating one. Other forces enable the transition to happen: marketing, logistics, cheap energy and changed lifestyles. One of the strengths of the Nutrition Transition as a concept is that it has captured the imagination of policy-makers. The idea encapsulates what can be seen with the eye, as populations get literally fatter within single lifetimes. It has also reinvigorated a social nutrition tradition within the discipline of nutrition which has for years gradually become more enamoured of biological and genetic explanations and research foci.[69] It has become a standard-bearer for a more critical intellectual stance. Leading nutritionists have increasingly expressed deep concern about the speed with which developing countries' health is being shaped by unaccountable economic forces. And new analyses of different eating styles and food products are beginning to emerge as a result. One is the powerful argument made by the Brazilian nutritionist Carlos Monteiro and others that nutrition can now distinguish between good and bad foods, good and poor diets, useful and harmful forms of food processing.[70]

The Nutrition Transition has thus become a serious intellectual segment in the rebuilding of the public health perspective. Its coherence and weight of evidence have shaken many food companies. Yet, for policy-makers at national, regional and global levels, it has posed different problems. If the Nutrition Transition were purely a health problem, it would be addressed by ministries or bodies concerned about health. But it actually demands responses from across government, across societal institutions and beyond health to economic, environmental and socio-cultural agencies. This rarely happens, because of fragmentation between ministries of agriculture and food, on the one hand, and agencies or ministries championing the environment and health, on the other.

The notion of the Nutrition Transition has helped generate an important new consensus across otherwise fractious governmental and para-governmental bodies. This is a welcome de-compartmentalisation of thinking and effort. In 2003, unusually, the UN's FAO and the WHO joined to produce first a report[71] and then a common strategy centred on the need to address non-communicable disease. The report presented a coherent analysis around the Nutrition Transition, which the WHO translated into its realpolitik as the 2004 World Health Assembly Resolution 57.17, the Global Strategy on Diet, Physical Activity and Health.[72] This was repeated with greater urgency in a UN special meeting in New York in 2011.[73] But such work from the UN is purely advisory. Neither the FAO nor the WHO nor Unicef has leverage over member states. The responsibility lies at national level, where all too often powerful food industry forces resist regulation or intervention. In some areas, such as Europe, there are regional bodies such as the European Union, and trade-related bodies such as ASEAN or NAFTA, which also tend to favour trade rather than health in public policy. The Nutrition Transition is thus addressed by weak policy responses, which tend to be voluntary or dependent on corporate responsibility or appeals to consumers to change. Thousands of projects and voluntary schemes have flowered around the world, as professions and civil society grapple with the immensity of the implications of the Nutrition Transition. As Popkin himself and other analysts have observed, the world continues to get fat, and the mismatch remains between bodies, food supply, culture and environment. How to unspring this lock-in of a mutually destructive sort is a public health priority. The mechanisms for doing so are themes we discuss in the chapters on the Cultural and Democratic Transitions (see Chapters 11 and 12) and in the final chapter (Chapter 13).

10

BIOLOGICAL AND ECOLOGICAL TRANSITION

The 'Biological Transition' is a term used to identify and specify the processes of change that life forms go through in their environments. This transition has been a core concern for biologists and evolutionary scientists since the emergence of Darwinism. While others, notably the eighteenth-century German polymath Johann Wolfgang von Goethe (1749–1832), pointed to the importance of understanding biological change as a central principle of life, only with Darwin, Wallace and others in the mid-nineteenth century did this core principle achieve a due scientific framework and rigour. Whether they are called evolutionary biologists or theoretical or plant ecologists, all these scientists operated within the framework of evolutionary thinking and understanding of the interconnections of life as laid out in the grand systemic analysis of Darwin and his co-analysts.

The US biologist Richard Burian has noted that early in the twentieth century Darwinian ideas fell out of favour (some even spurned them) and biology as a field became fragmented.[1] During the 1920s and into the 1930s, the first step towards a reformulation of Darwinism in the light of developing knowledge was around Gregor Mendel's (1822–84) ideas about genetic inheritance. This spawned the pursuit of what came to be known as population genetics. The biologists Ronald Fisher (1890–1962), J.B.S. Haldane (1892–1964) and Sewall Wright (1889–1988) all used models employing large numbers of mutations with small effects to provide mathematical demonstrations that Mendelian analysis was compatible with Darwinian gradualism. In 1937 the Ukrainian-born but US-domiciled Theodosius Dobzhansky (1900–75) drew these ideas together in one of the major works of what would become known as the modern evolutionary synthesis. This was the synthesis of evolutionary biology with genetics.

In his book *Genetics and the Origin of Species*, Dobzhansky defined evolution as 'a change in the frequency of an allele within a gene pool'.[2] Dobzhansky's integrative work was instrumental in spreading the idea that it is through mutations in genes that natural selection takes place. While the religious opposition to Darwin's ideas was becoming more muted in the land of his birth, in places like the USA it was growing with every passing year. By 1973, such was Dobzhansky's frustration, he penned a short commentary titled 'Nothing in Biology Makes Sense except in the Light of Evolution'.[3] His point was that this was now the unifying theory. Since those days, evolutionary biology has remained fractured, but his statement remains true. The shared framework provided by evolutionary biological thinking may be constantly amended and debated, but its core truths remain around a principle of adaptation shaped by variation, selection and retention of characteristics. That public health has to address and be built on an understanding of this Biological Transition is self-evident. If all life forms can be understood through this transition, then their health must be integrated into its processes. Some writers have stressed the slow evolution of biological change. Others point to its speed. Some focus on the plant and biosphere, the sheer mass and weight of plant life on earth. Others focus on the role of cell division and the evolution of microscopically tiny life forms. Still others focus on the genetic substrate of living processes. Whatever their focus, they all work within broadly the same framework.

The Biological Transition refers to the slow emergence of life from the first free living prokaryotic forms about 3.5 billion years ago to the first individuated colonies (bryozoans) some 480 million years ago.[4] John Maynard Smith and Eörs Szathmáry described the Biological Transition as essentially a long process of staged evolution in biological complexity. These stages bring complexity in numbers, levels of organisation, levels of selection, and interconnection.[5]

For public health, this transition has had particular resonance. It created the human body, on the one hand, and connects that to its environment, on the other hand. This growing complexity, constant multiplication and innovation of life forms outside the body also enters the body, not least through the mouth in the form of food and micro-organisms. In some respects, there is a fusion of the world beyond and inside the human body.[6] Human bodies are permeable and in constant interaction with their circumstances (as was noted in the previous chapter). The human body is both a biological platform and carrier, most overtly as a transmission point of disease, and a collection of historical responses and adaptations. More recently, a mere blink of the eye in evolutionary terms, human-created processes such as industrialisation, urbanisation and other transitions here described have transformed the workings of biology by altering environments. The human presence has developed technologies which have had an immense impact on how bodies fit or do not fit their context. The destruction of biodiversity through industrialisation is one example of how that relationship can be altered. Antibiotics are another, a modern form of intervention which, as is now being recognised, does not halt the biological process of change. Bacteria adapt and circumvent the initial power of the antibiotic, in the process now known as the development of antimicrobial resistance (AMR).[7] Humans bolster their bodily health yet simultaneously threaten it through actions. Humans have become actors and shapers of the Biological Transition not merely its recipients.

Five images of bodies in the biological world

In earlier chapters we examined accounts of how bodies were shaped by environments and noted the importance of genetics. In these accounts, bodies are more or less just physiological carriers of human identity, a legacy of the French philosopher René Descartes's (1596–1650) thesis that mind and body are really distinct, a thesis now called mind–body dualism. Public health has tended to work within this dualistic frame of reference and has persistently drawn upon five sometimes overlapping images when addressing the biological world and how bodies do or do not fit its dynamics. These are:

- bodies in a war zone with the environment;
- bodies exemplifying the balance of nature;
- bodies in symbiosis or intimate linkage with changing nature;
- bodies which are flawed;
- bodies stretched between collective and individual variations shaping health.

In the first, the image is of warfare. It is a powerful and much cited metaphor that extends from the combating of disease vectors external to the body to the body's own internal immunological system.[8] We note the language of the 'arms race' and 'wars against germs', and the case being made for repelling 'bacterial invaders'. This is the dominant image of the biological world in recent history, and is amplified and much loved by the marketing and advertising industries. For them, public health is about fighting the threats, and confronting or battling with the world of what we now know of as germs and bacteria. The goal is to eradicate the source of disease and ill-health. To take an example, one of the triumphs of twentieth-century public health was the eradication of smallpox, slowly but inexorably corralled into non-existence. The only surviving strains are in secure laboratories, it is stated.[9] This image presents a world of 'bugs' judged as dangerous, to be defeated for health. The body is painted as existing in a war zone, what Mackenbach has called 'a fundamentally hostile external environment'.[10] This image is symbolised by the Victorian campaign against dirt, instigated decades before scientific knowledge identified the real 'enemies'.[11] Yet the image is now almost obsolete, not least because, as many scientists have noted, if this is a fight it is one which the microbes and viruses – as well as the insect pests which carry them – will eventually win. Gone are the days when a US Surgeon General could opine that it is 'time to close the book on infectious diseases and declare the war against pestilence won'.[12]

This is not to say that viruses and bacteria have no deleterious effects – far from it, the evidence is clear – but it is to say that there is no final solution, no point at which humans are likely to be able to say that they have won against life changes, no point at which humans triumph over biological processes. Indeed not only are humans part of the biological processes, but their actions alter those processes. Many of the technical remedies used to 'resolve' problems of disease often generate feedback which in a relatively short space of time can neutralise the initially advantageous effects of human actions. This has been the case with TB and antibiotics, for example. Today, medicine and drug companies are more open in recognising how antibiotics are losing their effectiveness as new variants of bacteria or viruses emerge. Despite this recognition, the appeal is still to conquer the biological agents of disease by beating the vectors.

The second image is of the 'balance of nature'. For most of the twentieth century, the prevailing dogma was that disease organisms eventually should evolve toward benign coexistence with their hosts; harmful diseases were interpreted as a transitory state of maladaptation.[13] This image percolates into how public health practitioners see the world of bugs and bacteria. It is something to be accommodated to, rather than confronted. Public health's role, seen through this image, is as steward, the all-seeing eyes which ensure that balances are achieved or restored. Nature is acknowledged as greater even than the formidable firepower of humans, medicine and science. A key notion is homeostasis, the proposition that healthy systems achieve a balance and where all elements of a system have their role, place and multiple connections. The overarching metaphor is of science unpicking the complex interactions which can generate homeostasis in ideal circumstances. Arguably this image was first articulated by the French physiologist Claude Bernard (1813–78) with his notion of humans having an internal, biological environment, a *milieu intérieur*. But the notion was refined and popularised as 'homeostasis', a term coined by the American physician Walter Bradford Cannon (1871–1945). Cannon popularised it in a 1932 book whose title says much: *The Wisdom of the Body*.[14]

This image is now arguably a powerful model for understanding how the body adapts to its immediate environment and conditions. The body is continually challenged by stresses which it can accommodate. Cannon argued that this was 'hardwired', to use a modern term, in humans' core reflexes of 'flight or fight'. The modern account is to see the central homeostatic controls in the nervous and endocrine systems, where bodily regulation is performed. The image implies a benign manager but requires a benign environment which does not overtax the system of internal biological self-regulation.

A third image is synergistic co-evolution, a variant of the balance position. As life has diversified over billions of years, species have developed in mutual, synergistic association. Indeed, no multicellular eukaryotic organism is capable of surviving and reproducing using only its nuclear genes and the gene products it makes. Species require and co-opt the genomes of other species by forming mutualistic and selfish alliances. These mutualistic interactions involve dozens or even hundreds of plant and animal species, all of which are engaging in subtle processes of co-evolution and which would not exist without the existence of such complex interactions.[15] This is the notion of symbiosis, a phenomenon first noted in the late nineteenth century as being when different plants or life forms intertwine to mutual benefit. A ceaseless process of mutualism in feedback loops and change may be described.[16] This image can posit humans as both acting on and shaped by symbiosis in nature, whether wittingly or unwittingly. It does not assume that the body is sufficiently resilient in the environment to over-come external threats. Instead, this image turns outwards towards the condition in which the body finds itself. The image thus refocuses attention on interactions in the external circumstances. Symbiosis is the explanatory mechanism now most often offered by biologists themselves. Health scientists working on tropical diseases, for example, often work to accommodate and reduce the impact of insect-borne diseases not by aiming for eradication but by primary protection, minimising rather than seeking to eradicate the threat.[17]

The fourth image, flawed bodies, follows from one mostly reactionary interpretation of Darwin. Here the picture is of people or classes of people who are born to fail owing to their biological or social inadequacy. In the USA, according to historian Richard Hofstadter, business entrepreneurs accepted 'almost by instinct' the Darwinian idea (in fact originating in Herbert Spencer) of 'survival of the fittest'.[18] In Britain, says medical historian Charles Webster, 'Darwinism came to the aid of a variety of social causes, including the obstruction of state interference in the field of social welfare, opposition to feminism, defence of imperialism and subjugation of inferior races, and support for the traditional industrial order and free trade.'[19] In fact it was not Darwinism per se but social Darwinism, a separate intellectual and political project, which promoted this interpretation and extension of Darwin. Entirely different interpretations of Darwinism to this conservative interpretation were also possible. Some did indeed emerge in the late nineteenth century. One strand imported Darwin into philosophy, evidenced in the work of G.H. Mead and John Dewey in the USA.[20] Another came into biology and other natural sciences in the work of the polymath Alfred Russel Wallace, co-discoverer of natural selection. Yet another emerged in the evolutionary economics of Thorstein Veblen, considered in Chapter 8. For Veblen, evolutionary economics threw biologism into reverse. Because the wealthy leisure class were removed from the pressures of survival they were under no pressure to progress. They became, for Veblen, almost supernumerary to societal advance.[21]

Eugenics, a term invented by Charles Darwin's cousin Francis Galton (1822–1911) in 1883, crossed broader intellectual and geographical frontiers than did social Darwinism. Eugenics was picked up by an extraordinary range of political views, from Fabians like George Bernard Shaw and Sydney and Beatrice Webb to US presidents like Theodore Roosevelt and Calvin Coolidge. Eugenics, concerned with hereditary improvement, differed considerably from social Darwinism, and many of its adherents were 'wholly opposed' to Darwinism.[22] In the USA one strand of sociology, developed by William Graham Sumner (1840–1910), followed the eugenicist route plotted by Hebert Spencer, but in Britain mainstream sociology developed as an ideological reaction to eugenics, as the Oxford sociologist A.H. Halsey outlined.[23] The popularity of this bogus scientific set of beliefs lay in the supposed need to maintain and improve the hereditary human stock. The underlying ethos of eugenics was the protection of the intellectual and social class elite. In fact, the explanation of eugenics was largely sociological, since in Britain, the USA and elsewhere generations of educated middle- and upper-class men and women were attracted to it to satisfy their own self-aggrandisement. According to the historian Richard Soloway, these social milieus 'were culturally inclined to think in socially conscious, value-laden and hereditarian terms'.[24]

H.G. Wells, a prolific writer – of over 100 books – and staunch advocate of ecological thought, was a thinker of genuine depth, and the progressive inspiration for the International Declaration of Human Rights. He was also a eugenicist. A man of lower-middle-class background, he believed that the 'inadequates' of society, as he saw them, should be prevented from having children. Across the world eugenics faded quickly after its legacy and impact were associated with the horrors of the Nazi final solution. It should be noted that many people did question and confront the social implications of eugenicism. One honourable critic was the English chief medical officer Sir Arthur Newsholme, by religion a non-conformist Methodist and thus not wholly part of the British establishment.

The fifth image centres on the sharing of characteristics within biological processes, and stresses the necessity of individualisation of change for long-term evolution. All members of a species, apart from clones, have distinctiveness, yet they are protected by a herd-like sharing of characteristics. On the one hand, this image points to the reality of natural processes giving species shared resilience. On the other hand, it paints a Darwinian picture of populations constantly throwing up variations and idiosyncrasies. The genetic codes contain the 'memory' or legacy of this dynamic. These are fundamental to the possibilities of biological change. Variation enables subtle responses to the environment. What matters for health in this image is how the possibility of individualisation arises amidst herds and helps protect individuality.

A distinction in this fifth image needs to be drawn between genetic or organismic distinctiveness as a biological phenomenon and individualism as a political philosophy and social principle. In the late twentieth century, the language of disease began to be reframed around the political support for individual choice in marketplaces. The argument was that, since all bodies have a unique genetic make-up, their 'owners' have the right to follow their own choices of what to do. One source of this argument was neoliberal versions of economics, while another was the individualisation of risk championed in the growth of risk management techniques (as exemplified in the banks, whose credit crisis shook the world economy from 2008). The latter school of thinking invoked mathematical models to accept that unlikely events can be possible; management is about minimising those risks. If consumers happily spend in lotteries, in the belief that highly unlikely events can happen (winning the jackpot), surely such unlikely events could happen to them with regard to health too. Anyone could be struck down by rare events. The consequences of this argument, nominally derived from a view of biological change, was illustrated in the UK after a paper was published in the *Lancet* in 1998 suggesting that the triple vaccination against measles, mumps and rubella (MMR) was likely to trigger autism in very young children. As a result, many parents refused to let their infants be vaccinated, and population rates of measles, for example, went dramatically up. The editors of the *Lancet* formally retracted the paper in February 2010, after an inquiry which suggested inappropriate collection of evidence.[25]

Two foci: the Microbiological and Ecological Transitions

Having recognised the necessity of seeing the Biological Transition as a whole, within an evolutionary framework, in the rest of this chapter we separate it into two foci. We are not alone in splitting the Biological Transition in this way, but we stress the need to see the Microbial and the Natural Ecological Transitions, the two foci we now explore, as an integrated whole. We have separated them purely for pragmatic reasons, to highlight important distinctions for public health. We focus first on what could be seen as the world of microbiology, the oldest part of evolution, where life literally began to take shape. This is the world of germs, bacteria and viruses, the cellular level of biology. In the following section, we go on to describe the changes in the world of plants and the biosphere itself. That is the world of biodiversity and the enlarging human presence on the planet, the impact that humans have had on the biosphere. In that section of this chapter, we will explore how the changes humans have wreaked on the earth are now in a feedback loop. What weaves these two foci – one microscopic and the other macroscopic – intimately together is the fact that all nature and processes are interrelated. After Darwin and others, we repeat, it was no longer possible to view human health as disconnected from the biology of other forms of life.

The microbiological world

Public health thinking was transformed from the late nineteenth century and throughout the twentieth by the growth of knowledge about biology, virology and bacteriology. The remarkable growth of understanding enabled medicine and pharmacy to tap into different modes of tackling disease, but, as we noted earlier, by the twenty-first century some humility had returned. The capacity of biological processes to move faster than human science reminded public health thinkers that triumph was premature. Cells and the transmutation of cells could be studied, but they should be respected. Darwin had articulated the connection between biology and evolution itself in his work, and in one famous diagram he sketched a 'Tree of Life' suggesting connections (see Figure 10.1). In this metaphor, he was not unusual. Others before and after him also invoked the notion of there being a Tree of Life, a grand connection of biological beings. But was this a tree, in which progress is to be 'higher up' the tree and in a more complex biological form? Or was it a web of life in which connections exist but which should not be assumed to be in a relationship of superiority or inferiority? Darwin himself was unhappy about making that imposition of supremacism. Most biologists since have echoed his sentiments. Darwin's world, of course, was not aware of micro-organisms, the discovery of which came later, so the respect has to be developed in the light of the new sciences of bacteriology and virology.

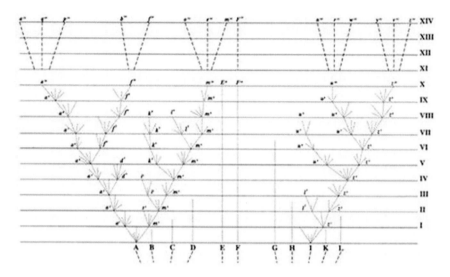

FIGURE 10.1   Charles Darwin's Tree of Life

The search for hidden mechanisms in disease is a long one (see Chapters 1–3). Early sanitarians had no knowledge of what they were. Justly, Louis Pasteur (1822–95) is celebrated as putting microbiology on to its modern footing, although he was not the first to propose germ theory. In the 1860s, Pasteur proved that fermentation of yeasts was the result of the working of what came to be known as micro-organisms. Working with Claude Bernard, he confronted the existing dominant theories of people such as Justus von Liebig. Using microscopes, they could show multiplication in substances such as milk and beer. The implications were critical for health. As C.-E. Winslow, microbiologist and public health thinker, stated, this was because 'milk is second only to water as an agent in the transmission of disease'. Pasteur, Winslow recognised, 'extracted the truth from the mass of good and bad guesses of those who had preceded him'.[26]

Where the Frenchman Pasteur was looking at human foods in Paris, Robert Koch (1843–1910) the German microbiologist was focused on transmissible diseases. He developed techniques to cultivate bacilli, famously identifying that for anthrax in 1877, tuberculosis in 1882 and cholera in 1883. Koch's work led to sterilisation of surgical implements and the notion that ill-health could be contained by stopping transmission by contact. His work was deeply controversial in both Germany and the UK, and met what one modern historian called 'almost fanatical opposition'.[27] The British approach to cholera was effective for entirely different reasons; their pragmatic approach began to improve sanitary conditions such as through drainage and other measures summarised in earlier chapters. Except for local measures they saw no need to follow the implications of Koch's arguments or the continental system based upon quarantine and isolation.[28] The British were politically and economically committed to trade and could not entertain public health impeding it.

In the twentieth century, this pioneering work of Pasteur, Koch and others was built upon, and the modern pharmaceutical industry emerged as the vast and powerful enterprise its corporations now represent. In 1928 the Scottish chemist Alexander Fleming (1881–1955) discovered penicillin after the accident of leaving a culture dish of staphylococci over a holiday. He returned to his laboratory to find the dish covered with a fungus but with the staphylococci in contact destroyed. Prompted by an assistant, he grew the fungus and found that it destroyed certain bacteria. He named it penicillin and published a paper the following year. Little notice was taken, but he continued to try to develop it, finding it hard to cultivate. Indeed, he abandoned working on it during the Second World War, and it was Florey and Chain at Oxford, helped by funds from the US and British governments, who worked out how to produce it on a mass scale. Penicillin was introduced to the market in 1943, in time to treat the wounded at D-Day, initially available without prescription. Fleming, Florey and Chain shared the Nobel Prize for medicine in 1945.

Fleming was only too aware of the ceaseless movement in microbiological life and in 1945 was already anticipating the emergence of drug-resistant bacteria, evidence of which emerged the following year.[29] What he and others had not

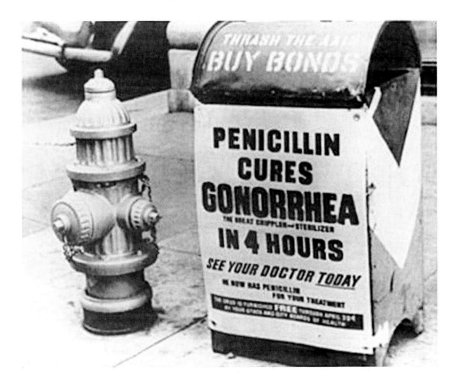

FIGURE 10.2 Advertisement in 1940s South Carolina, USA

anticipated, according to Didier Mazel of the Institut Pasteur in Paris, was multi-drug resistance. It was thought that the appearance of multiple mutations conferring resistance was considered to be beyond the evolutionary potential of a given bacterial population.[30] By the mid-1950s, multidrug resistance had begun to emerge. Within a few decades, despite constant production of new drugs and families of drugs, antimicrobial resistance (AMR) had become a worldwide phenomenon. The terms 'antimicrobial', 'antibiotic' and 'anti-infective' encompass a wide variety of pharmaceutical agents that include antibacterial, antifungal, antiviral and antiparasitic drugs. In the early 1990s, by the age of 15 years US children had received, on average, more than four courses of antibiotics to treat a single disorder, otitis media, a common ear infection.[31] The widespread and often inappropriate use of antimicrobial agents is the single most important cause of the emergence of drug resistance, both in the community and in hospital settings.[32]

The WHO made AMR the focus of its 2011 World Health Day, with the strategy to constrain profligate use in order to maintain drugs' utility and prevent their demise. The WHO pointed out that 440,000 new cases of multidrug-resistant tuberculosis emerged annually, causing at least 150,000 deaths. Resistance to anti-malarial drugs is now widespread. A rising percentage of hospital-acquired infections are caused by highly resistant bacteria. Unnecessary use by farmers to treat animals is another source of concern. Zoonoses remain a persistent threat, for instance through E. coli, campylobacter and yersinia. Antibiotics have been used partly to treat diseases, not least to enable factory farming (battery conditions) to operate, but also as growth promoters.[33] AMR can be passed through meat consumption. The emergence of AMR, the WHO concluded, is 'a complex problem driven by many interconnected factors: single, isolated interventions have little impact'.[34]

This, of all lessons, is why current microbiological thinking is as we recorded above, where it is accepted that the microbiological world can outperform pharmaceuticals and medical science – so far, at least. Brad Spellberg and colleagues from the Infectious Diseases Society of America in 2008 summarised why there needs to be some humility if people continue to posit the situation as a war of microbes versus humans. Simply, it is that the microbes can work faster and smarter (see Table 10.1).[35] Three microbiologists have wittily commented that the 'microbial content of the biosphere approaches 10^{31}, a number beyond comprehension, even when compared to the US National Debt'![36]

TABLE 10.1 Microbes versus humans

Variable	Microbes	Humans	Factor
No. on earth	5×10^{31}	6×10^9	$\sim 10^{22}$
Mass (metric tonnes)	5×10^{16}	3×10^8	$\sim 10^8$
Generation time	30 minutes	30 years	$\sim 5 \times 10^5$
Time on earth (years)	3.5×10^9	4×10^6	$\sim 10^3$

The implications of the current situation are considerable. Pessimists depict a world where 'superbugs' triumph. Optimists at best propose a rebalancing of people in the microbiological world, the need to build and maintain resistance and to reserve the wonderdrugs for major rather than routine use. All agree with the WHO prognosis that infectious diseases are not beaten and are ever present (see Figure 10.3). To some extent, the narrative given is a sobering one, of premature triumphalism mixed with complacency and profligate use of drug technology to pretend to 'beat' disease. And yet the tale of microbiological advance is remarkable, and the understanding of the ecology of the microbial world is awesome compared to the past. One notable illustration is the epidemiology and rapid learning about HIV/AIDS. Even AIDS, devastating though it is, causes far less damage compared with the havoc that was caused in New World populations on contact with Old World pathogens.[37]

The origins of HIV/AIDS are still under discussion, with theories ranging from viral change to transmission from animals sources in Africa. Whatever the route to humans, it began to be scrutinised when cases emerged first in San Francisco among

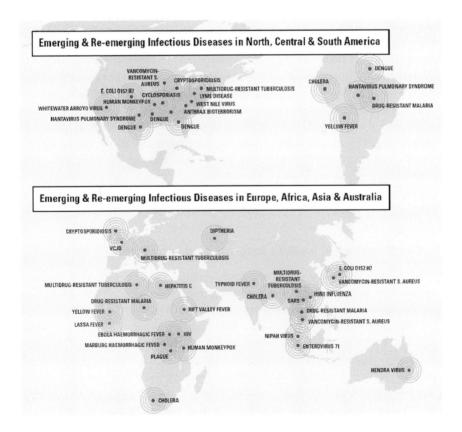

FIGURE 10.3   Worldwide emerging and re-emerging infectious diseases

gay men, leading it to being initially described as gay-related immune deficiency (GRID), then as human T-cell lymphotropic virus type III (HTLV-III) and then as the current term, human immunodeficiency virus/acquired immune deficiency syndrome (HIV/AIDS). The aetiology of the disease is now reasonably well understood, and a huge effort was unleashed led by the developed-country public health, virology and pharmaceutical industries, encouraged by a strong gay population both seeking solutions and championing global action and behaviour change. The story of HIV/AIDS is moving in many respects: the scientific effort, the suffering, the globalisation of its spread, the inadequacy of governmental responses in many parts of the world lacking strong public voice and public health advocates, and the strong self-help pressure of the gay movements worldwide. Although great strides have been made since the first cases were identified in the early 1980s, the level of the public health impact has been immense. The UN AIDS programme estimated that in 2010 there were 34 million people worldwide infected with HIV.[38] Even more worrying was the enormous problem of children being born with HIV or made orphans by HIV. In 2009, according to the UN Joint Programme on Aids, 370,000 children became newly infected with HIV globally and an estimated 42,000–60,000 pregnant women died because of HIV.[39] This population of people infected with HIV is heavily concentrated in developing and poorer countries, suggesting that the developed world with its greater financial resources, overtly active gay communities, and legitimate and reasonably resourced healthcare services has made a difference. This is an example of why we stress in this book the importance of the cultural dimension for health and is why we have an entire chapter on the Cultural Transition and its centrality to Ecological Public Health thinking (see Chapter 11). The public health story of HIV/AIDS illustrates the intersection of biological, cultural and economic factors, in that it was recognised first in economically rich countries but spread fastest and with the most devastating population impact among poor communities and nations. This social framing of public ill-health is also true for how TB is more rife among prison populations and drug-taking groups.

Vaccination: public health's long-running success story?

In her book *Deadly Companions*, the microbiologist Dorothy Crawford examines the place of microbes and viruses in society and modern lives.[40] She shows how the biological miracle interventions of modern medicine carry risks. Microbes are unbeatable because they are us; we are them! Crawford points out that our bodies have 1,014 microbes in our gut, weighing a total of around 1 kilogram. They outnumber our bodies' cells by a factor of ten to one.[41] In fact, most cells in our body are not human but microbial. Our biological history is the interplay between the human body and the microbial environment.

The history of public health often presents the triumph over microbes as advance. Indeed, if one's life is saved, so it can be. Crawford and others suggest some humility, however; our ultimate protection is learning to live with microbes, not to defeat them, or perhaps learning how to defend humans but without the illusion of defeating microbes. This is not a new argument. And in one story within the drama of public health it has been fought out for over two centuries. That tale is of immunisation and vaccination.

The story begins with smallpox. Smallpox has been one of the most devastating diseases afflicting humankind in history. With a fatality rate of up to 30 per cent among those infected, smallpox claimed hundreds of millions of lives until its eradication in 1979. While most diseases were felt more heavily among the poor, by the middle of the seventeenth century smallpox, according to Stanley Williamson, had become 'more unsparing in its assault on the upper classes' while 'tending to decline among the lower classes'.[42] Smallpox vaccination, when it came on to the scene and fulfilled so many hopes for a simple means of prevention, is forever associated with the name of Edward Jenner (1749–1823).

To naturalists, Jenner might be better known for being the first to publish an account of the egg-substitution habits of the cuckoo.[43] He is world famous, however, for being the English country doctor who, in 1796, took the pus from a cowpox lesion on a milkmaid's hand and vaccinated an eight-year-old boy, James Phipps. (He did not have to bother with ethical approval forms.) The term 'vaccination', which comes from the Latin *vacca*, meaning cow, was coined by Louis Pasteur in the 1880s, in honour of Jenner.[44] Six weeks later Jenner variolated, that is to say inoculated, two sites on Phipps's arm with smallpox. The boy remained unaffected. Based on 12 such experiments and 16 additional case histories, Jenner published at his own expense a volume that swiftly became a classic text in the annals of medicine, *Inquiry into the Causes and Effects of the Variolae Vaccinae*, and received a large financial award from the public purse from a grateful government.[45] What did not become so evident in all the enthusiasm was that vaccination might require 'topping up' (Jenner thought it wasn't needed), and if inexpertly done might result in poor efficacy and even harm to the patient. The purpose also needed to be properly explained and undertaken in conditions of at least minimal trust. Given that vaccination required individuals to accept the injection of a medicinal agent into their bodies, lack of attention to all these factors proved disastrous.

Variolation, the forerunner to vaccination, was not new. It had been used in China and India for centuries. It was the concept of personal health converted to public health, to use the language of Lemuel Shattuck (see Chapter 2), the one depending on the success of the other in practical, if not theoretical, recognition of humankind's biological interconnectedness. What Jenner offered was something superior to what there had been in the past. A vaccinated person developed at most a rash and could not spread smallpox to others.[46] Jenner's demonstration of proof, and its positive reception, was decisive; even Thomas Malthus thought that his dire warnings on disease might receive some adjustment in the light of its apparent efficacy. Interest in Jenner's vaccine spread rapidly. Following correspondence with William Jefferson, the US president, vaccination began in that country just two years after its introduction to Britain, using Jenner's own inoculant. Vaccination was made compulsory in the US army.[47] King Charles IV of Spain sent an expedition to the Americas in 1803 to introduce smallpox vaccination to its colonies.[48] Compulsory programmes of vaccination followed in Bavaria (1807), Denmark (1810), Norway (1811), Russia (1812), Sweden (1816) and Hanover (1821). Iceland introduced vaccination in 1816 and made the clergy responsible for it. Each case had different precedents no doubt. In the case of Russia between 1804 and 1810, 8 million Russians were infected by smallpox; more than one in ten had died. Many motivations for this early public health intervention were undoubtedly in play, with fear, one suspects, playing a determinant role.

Smallpox spread in waves in the early 1800s, resulting in the first Vaccination Act in England and Wales in 1840, followed by legislation in Scotland and Ireland. The amending 1853 Act introduced compulsory vaccination for all infants within four months of birth, but contained no powers of enforcement. Responsibility lay with the poor law guardians, the people also charged with operating workhouses. Under the 1867 Act the compulsory elements were enhanced. It became the duty of the guardians to appoint vaccination officers, to enter into a contract with a qualified medical practitioner to vaccinate children and, if required, to do so at the child's home, and to give certificates. The pressure to conform to compulsory vaccination was deeply and bitterly resented by many parents. Almost another half-century elapsed before it was made compulsory in France in 1902.[49] The soundings of alarm in the progress of entire population vaccination programmes had already begun, and they were amplified by complaints of amateurish and ineffective practice, an organisational system in disarray. From 1853, there was open rebellion from noisy sections of the public.[50] Mirroring the public health movement, an anti-vaccination movement based on tracts, books and journals appeared in the 1870s and 1880s, with names like the *Anti-Vaccinator* (founded 1869), the *National Anti-Compulsory Vaccination Reporter* (1874) and the *Vaccination Inquirer* (1879).[51] By the 1880s, the controversy had attracted the attention of Alfred Russel Wallace, Darwin's co-discoverer of natural selection. A man of undoubted scientific credentials, he joined what was already a politicised and polarised debate. He later wrote that that vaccination was:[52]

> the cause of many deaths, and of a large but unknown amount of permanent injury; the only really trustworthy statistics on a large scale prove it to be wholly without effect as a preventive of small-pox; many hundreds of persons are annually punished for refusing to have their children vaccinated; and it will undoubtedly rank as the greatest and most pernicious failure of the century.

In fact, Wallace was not anti-public health; indeed he was a proponent of 'sanitary science'. What he objected to, as a man of socialist leanings, was the flagrant dismissal of working-class sensibilities and concerns and poor medical science and poor evidence. Lacking an unambiguous and trusted account of its effectiveness, anti-vaccinationists mounted a credible critique.[53] Evidence on the effectiveness of vaccination did begin to emerge, but not until the 1900s. Evidence does take time.

More than a century later, according to the US Centers for Disease Control, the use of vaccination had become sufficiently widespread fully to control the disease. Since then, it reported, vaccines have been developed or licensed against 21 other diseases, 10 recommended for use only in selected populations at high risk because of area of residence, age, medical condition or risk behaviours, the other 11 for use in all children.[54] While the science has grown, and there have been numerous social scientific studies on reactions to vaccine-preventable diseases, what has been studied only rarely is how these influence disease dynamics.[55]

If Jenner's discovery had created a new pathway of biological advance, it did not quieten debate. A persistent and vociferous discussion about its theoretical precepts, effectiveness and consequences has continued to this day. One anti-vaccination website canvasses public signatories, trying to achieve of a goal of 1,000,000,000 signatures, a seventh of humankind. (Only 52,186 had been achieved by late 2011!) It has been suggested that the presence of such campaigns on the internet amplifies fears regarding vaccination safety, with many worrying about the vaccines more than the underlying diseases that they protect against. Immunisation depends in part on public confidence in their safety. This is not merely a factor of public reaction to achieve compliance. All vaccinations entail some risk. Alongside this there is a variety of other factors at play, including religious and philosophical belief and freedom and individualism. In the case of immunisation for measles, mumps and rubella (MMR), all these perceptions were inflamed by the association with the risk of autism. The implication is that, as rates of immunisation fall, 'herd immunity' – the microbiological interconnections between human bodies – can be lost.[56]

Vaccination in the early form pioneered by Edward Jenner as a means of prevention and containment of smallpox, widening far beyond smallpox in the twentieth century, has represented a powerful if at times problematic current in biological advance. As with other public health interventions the motivations, like the results themselves, were mixed. Fear drove the spread of vaccination, but fear also provoked opposition to it. The nineteenth-century controversy in Britain, the central point for the diffusion of vaccination practice, was, in the words of one of the chief administrators of twentieth-century global immunisation campaigns, 'disastrous'.[57] This brief account of an at times convoluted story shows the cultural limitations to the Bio-Medical model on a mass scale and how its application often failed to be attuned to public concerns, and for that matter, although the pro-vaccination lobby had difficulty accepting it, evidence-based arguments against.

Vaccination is in a hardly less problematic situation today. In the early 2000s northern Nigeria's Islamic leaders advised followers not to have their children immunised with oral polio vaccine. Fears were spread that vaccination was associated with infertility. The government worked with religious leaders and others to counteract these conceptions.[58] In 2011 the 'hunt for bin Laden', orchestrated by the US Central Intelligence Agency, utilised a bogus vaccination campaign to identify the terrorist. The result, said the *Economist* magazine, was that vaccination campaigns worldwide, criticised by many religious leaders as a 'Western plot', had indeed become such a plot. It remarked:

> If the fake vaccination campaign was a necessary part of the operation to 'take out' Osama bin Laden, it would have been better to leave Mr bin Laden in. One more ailing ex-terrorist holed up in a ratty house in remote Pakistan, watching old videos of himself; this was not worth jeopardising global vaccination campaigns.[59]

The natural Ecological Transition

The term 'Ecological Transition' was introduced by John Bennett (1916–2005) in a book of that name. Bennett was an anthropologist not a biologist. He suggested that the transition had two dimensions: social and technological. In the first he saw humankind's changing sense of nature, and depicted the history of the human species as a process of ideational separation from nature. In effect Bennett saw a progressive denial of the 'natural' in and by humankind. Nature is incorporated into the human frame of reference, in effect subjugating it. Bennett suggested that a specifically human-centred orientation had emerged during the Western Renaissance but was now infused into every civilisation and nation. This process, he suggested, increased with industrialisation. With regard to his second dimension, the technological, Bennett perceived a tendency to seek 'ever larger quantities of energy in order to satisfy the demands of human existence, comfort and wealth'.[60] In this neat depiction of an Ecological Transition, Bennett drew upon earlier work by another anthropologist, Leslie White, whose thinking had been published three decades earlier. His ideas were discussed earlier (see Chapter 7). Whereas White had equated increasing energy use with human progress, Bennett judged humankind's extractive view of nature as an unacceptable human conceit. This difference of evaluation remains important to this day. Nevertheless, there was a common core to their thought. Biology is underpinned by physics and chemistry.

Another conceptualisation of the Ecological Transition comes from an entirely different discipline, social psychology. The psychologist Uri Bronfenbrenner's childhood socialisation theory – his ecological perspective is introduced in Chapter 1 – is to this day an intellectual root of much current social-ecological thinking within public health, as we also saw in the discussion of the Social-Behavioural model. He referred to an Ecological Transition as occurring 'whenever a person's position in the ecological environment is altered as a result of a change in role, setting or both'.[61] Transition for Bronfenbrenner is seen as a process of shifting through and beyond thresholds of experience rather than physics or biology. It is in that respect a 'liminality' approach used by anthropologists and psychologists (from the Latin: *limen*, 'threshold'). For Bronfenbrenner, a child growing up passes across various definable social and physical thresholds, stages of experience and differences in environments. For him, the Ecological Transition was the movement between social worlds rather than biological worlds, yet he meant that this experiential change could be marked by biological processes such as ageing and cognitive development. Already with just these different meanings, the term 'Ecological Transition' has a certain degree of plasticity! Yet it is important for the case we are exploring in this book. It is helpful to return to the founding concepts of the Ecological Transition, captured by the term as first formulated and implied by Darwin and Haeckel. It was the latter who actually coined the word 'ecology'.

Darwin in a sketch in his notebook around 1837 famously articulated the connection between species as spreading like the twigs of a multidirectional branch. In the final version he put into *The Origin of Species*, he turned that first meandering thought into the fan-shaped diagram shown earlier in Figure 10.1. This was more like a bush replete with branches than a tree, although it is known as the 'Tree of Life' graphic. The important issue is that there was no central trunk. Later attempts to depict the evolutionary pattern were bolder, indicating a separation of branches, with a 'top of the tree' position for humans. Ernst Haeckel, the German biologist, drew upon Darwin's sketch and ideas but also upon pre-Darwinian conceptions of human progress in the writings of Goethe and Lamarck.[62] Hence Haeckel's version of the Tree of Life became a substantial tree trunk of evolution and a staged, hierarchical ordering of species (see Figure 10.4). Evolutionary biologists may argue about the scientific appropriateness of the Tree of Life, but it remains a striking metaphor. It allows for the intimate connectivity between all living beings, with implied co-dependency. It also presents a theory of progress, as species differentiate and biological complexity intensifies.

According to Darwin's friend T.H. Huxley, Haeckel aimed at a 'much higher game' than Darwin. His theme was 'anthropogeny . . . the tracing of the actual pedigree of man – from its protoplasmic root, sodden in the mud of the seas which existed before the oldest of the fossiliferous rocks were deposited, in those inconceivably ancient days'.[63] Haeckel was painting a very big version indeed of the Tree of Life metaphor, entering into what Huxley acknowledged as 'more or less justifiable speculation'. Later theorists have tended to drop the tree analogy, instead using metaphors such as a 'web of life' or 'systems'. What matters is that the Ecological Transition represents an attempt to understand the changes in this web of life. Indeed, Darwin first described that web through his notion of the 'entangled bank', his poetic observation of the dynamic interaction of species and habitats which he could observe in an English bank and hedgerow. The point he and others ever since have sought to articulate is of an ecological system in a process which produces inordinate complexity.[64]

The botanist Arthur Tansley (1871–1955) contributed many of the concepts in use in ecology today. Tansley stressed the importance of the changeability of life, in contrast to the view that plants were, as he put it, 'static entities'. Appreciating this dynamic quality of interrelationships, he observed, resulted in a 'far deeper insight'.[65] For Tansley, organisms were complex entities occupying an eco-system. Flora and fauna, abiotic and biotic entities, were all interdependent and inseparable. While he was hardly the first to recognise the enormous impact of the human presence on nature, in his words the natural world was 'touched by man'. He was the first to bring into English a new concept to capture this meaning. Humankind's presence, he said, was 'anthropogenic' (from the Greek *anthropos*, 'human', and *genic*, 'having origin in'). The term has taken centre stage in ecology but was in fact first used by the Russian geologist Pavlov, not Tansley.[66]

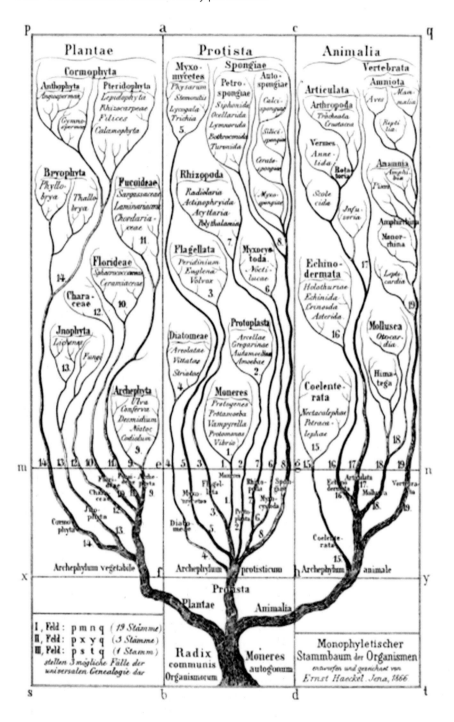

FIGURE 10.4 Ernst Haeckel's Tree of Life: a common origin for plants, animals and micro-organisms

In field surveys, Tansley remarked that the landscape and its flora and fauna were as much the creation of human beings as the product of natural forces. While he took delight in the English countryside, Tansley's interpretation wrenched ecology away from a focus on the natural order of things to the interaction of humans and natural ecology, and how *homo sapiens* alter nature. Ecologists since have interpreted the increasingly anthropogenic texture of nature in far more pessimistic terms than Tansley, suggesting that humans are irrevocably damaging the natural environment. Some accounts of environmentalism paint the origins of such dire thinking as beginning in the twentieth century with the arrival of campaigning groups or legislators. In fact, that deeply pessimistic strand of environmentalism is traceable to the period of industrialisation and before. George Perkins Marsh (1801–82), for example, an American diplomat with wide interests from languages to forests, was one of the first to study how landscape had been altered by the presence of humans.[67] Marsh described how humans irrevocably altered Southern Europe and North Africa, not least through the spread and domestication of animals such as the goat and camel, which destroyed natural flora and aided desertification.[68] This line of study ultimately depicted a co-evolution of humans as change agents in the natural world, a process of change that began in the ancient past and continued to the early settlements, and today takes on a massive scale of change.[69] From this perspective, it is almost assumed that there is little 'virgin' nature left. Indeed it has been assessed that between one-third and one-half of the land surface of the earth has been transformed by human action, and that proportion is growing.[70]

Generally speaking, the anthropogenic process that Tansley's focus encouraged is more or less a reflection of human history, with a direct impact on ecology and sometimes (but not necessarily always) with negative consequences. Hunter-gatherers, the first and longest stage of human development, used and consumed many different foods, browsing across the natural world.[71] With the shift into stable settlements and the cultivation of land, even with the simplest of farming technologies, a process began of the narrowing of dietary habits, for example, and the reduction in the number of plants consumed, as plants were selected for cultivation rather than browsed. That process coincided with the conversion of wild habitat to farmland, heralding a tendency to monoculture and species loss. Settlements created fields, which ended uncultivated land's mix of wild plants and animals, as well as destroying forest habitat through the collection of wood for fuel. Later, population growth added to the process of pollution, overexploitation, habitat loss and fragmentation, and with greater international trade came the introduction of invasive species and new rounds of what is now known as biodiversity loss. As we noted in the Energy Transition, much of the drive to exploit nature was for energy.

Tansley, and subsequently all modern ecologists, have noted how, from the very early years of human presence, their impact on other forms of life was amplified by technology. Animal husbandry improvements increased output of meat and dairy, for example, but disturbed not only plant ecology in grazing ground but relationships between the predator and the predated. Today, the creation of cattle feed lots, intensive pig or chicken farming, vast-scale monoculture and industrial-scale fishing are a further round in this same process. Concentrated food production has centred on a few high-yielding marketable commodities and varieties.[72] Today, one estimate is that humans rely for the bulk of sustenance on around 30 food plants out of the thousands of edible plants which exist, with just nine plants providing over 75 per cent of the total calories consumed by humans.[73] According to the FAO, only 15 of the total crops on the planet provide 90 per cent of total global calorie intake, with three (rice, maize and wheat) as staples for half the world's population. The loss of species is alarming. Since 1900 about three-quarters of the genetic diversity of domestic agricultural crops has been lost.[74] Another study suggests that, whereas humans have eaten 5,000 plant varieties across history, about 1 per cent of total flora, only about 150 of those are now traded.[75] Meanwhile, commercial dynamics have driven a concentration of ownership over traded seed stocks. In 1996, the world's top ten seed companies had 37 per cent of the world market; by 2006, the top ten seed companies had 57 per cent of the world market.[76] Even where calories come in the form of meat and dairy products, the role of plants is hidden, in that the animal has processed the plant for humans. Plant biologists are now concerned about undue reliance on a few varieties of those 30 plants, and their lack of genetic diversity. Until recently, for example, all potatoes grown in Europe came from two samples imported more than 400 years ago from the Americas.[77]

Human ways of eating and producing food have altered ecology not just in the plant world but in all features of the material and biological world. A critical example is water.[78] Seventy per cent of all potable (good drinking quality) water is used in agriculture worldwide, with the majority of that being used for irrigation or animals. The world's eco-systems are being skewed to service humans in a manner which now seriously threatens sustainability. That was the headline from the massive Millennium Ecosystems Assessment global research project in 2005.[79] This skewing is also unequal. Water footprints are a way of measuring water use. On average, every human in the world uses 1,240 cubic metres a year of water, but US consumers use 2,480 cubic metres per capita a year, while in China the average water footprint is 700 cubic metres per capita a year.[80] Water is a critical factor for both agriculture and public health. Human society has historically often treated waterways as a means for disposing of waste, not least human excreta, thus creating health hazards, as we have seen from Chapter 1 onwards. One study estimated that many cities in the developing world discharge 80–90 per cent of their untreated sewage directly into rivers and streams, a hazardous source of micro-organism spread.[81] Increasingly too, humans have channelled water for their own use, both for direct drinking and for industrial and commercial use, directing it away from nature.

Dams are one way in which progress has been pursued, harnessing water power for energy and for human drinking and commercial use. Eco-systems have often taken second place to these motives, but recent ecological thinking stresses the unforeseen consequences of such huge dams. In the 2000s, there was worldwide interest in and concern about the Chinese Three Gorges Dam system, for example. This was a vast project which re-engineered the Yangtze River in a sequence of dams. Construction began in 1992 and was completed in 2006. This necessitated the removal of 1.2 million people (two cities and 116 towns) and ended some rare species of fish, but provided the equivalent of one-ninth of China's then electricity output and in theory brought the historical bouts of Yangtze flooding and deaths to an end.[82] Retrospectively, the Chinese government was reported to admit the seriousness of the ecological impact.[83]

Such grand projects are not new. In the mid-nineteenth century, for example, the 900-mile Ganges Canal in North India was built by the colonial East India Company, partly in reaction to a famine, opening in 1854. It was heralded as a great technical success, bringing water to 2.5 million people by the twentieth century and delivering an enormous return on the capital investment.[84] Since Independence in 1947, India has built more than a thousand further dams, but the disadvantages are now becoming more evident, in the form of displacement of people, silting, deforestation and loss of habitat. Critics of large-scale dam technology suggest that the issue is not the scale of the projects but the loss of community control, which is more possible with small-scale dams and water management systems.[85]

On the one hand, this unequal anthropogenic process is long and old, as the early observers such as G.P. Marsh suggested, but on the other hand the rapidity and scale of change do appear to be of a new order. In the late nineteenth century, British fishermen protested that they were having to journey further to catch fish. T.H. Huxley, an adviser to no less than three British fishing commissions, argued that, in the manner of Malthus, any tendency towards overfishing would come up against a natural check in the diminution of supply before any permanent exhaustion of stocks occurred.[86] Then, this advice was interpreted, to use a colloquial phrase, in terms of there being 'plenty more fish in the sea'. In the twenty-first century, almost all analysts of marine stocks (apart from the Japanese on whales) agree that stocks are in a fragile and generally declining state owing to anthropogenic impact.[87]

Biodiversity is a shortening of 'biological diversity', which has been defined by the UN Convention on Biodiversity (at its creation in 1992) as 'the variability among living organisms from all sources . . . and the ecological complexes of which they are part'.[88] The Convention was an outcome of the UN Conference on Environment and Development, held in Rio de Janeiro, Brazil, but that was the result of campaigns and research from the 1970s.[89] The full extent of biodiversity is unknown. New species of plants and animals (particularly small species and soil life) are constantly being discovered. But, fast as they are discovered, the rate of overall biodiversity loss continues. In some respects, the consequences of this loss might be immense, but the precise impact has to be speculative. The overall picture, however, is that there is a decline in biodiversity in all three of its main components – genes, species and eco-systems. There are suggestions that species are currently being lost at rates that exceed the natural extinction rates of the past by a factor of somewhere between 100 and 1,000.[90]

Climate change is almost certainly a new phase of ecological change, perhaps a deciding transition for millions of species and for the human experiment of recent centuries. Its projected impact is constantly being calculated, with sobering results

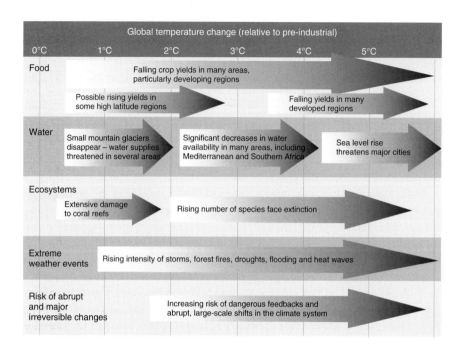

FIGURE 10.5 Expected impact of global temperature change on food, water, eco-systems and climatic events

in the main. Figure 10.5 gives a summary provided by the Stern Report of some major effects for food, water, eco-systems, weather and extreme events as temperature rises.

Responses to evidence of the Ecological Transition

The immensity of the Ecological Transition, whatever its foci (microbiological or natural ecological), is now being clarified. What to do about it is less clear. Strategies are emerging, but so far with inadequate scale of effect. We detect at least six approaches:

- *Denial and inaction.* The first is that there is not a problem or, if there is a problem, it does not matter. There are many climate change deniers, for example. Often the debate is constructed on narrow lines, becoming more about ideological and economic division than about science. There are people who deny that biodiversity loss is significant, or that economic progress has inevitable consequences.[91] Others see the Ecological Transition as the natural order of things, or that events beyond current human control might be the deciding variables. Thus sunspots are deemed to cause climate variations.[92] Some argue that the cost of tackling the effects of the manifestations of the Ecological

Transition far exceed the benefits of doing so, even if one could do anything or could afford to pay for it all.[93]

- *Legal or institutional change.* The second position is gradualist and statist in focus. The UN Convention on Biodiversity, for example, was agreed at Rio in 1992. It is an equivalent strategy to the WHO's 2003 Tobacco Framework,[94] for example, or the FAO's Voluntary Guidelines on the Right to Food.[95] The thinking here is that slowly, surely, evidence needs to be built up on the Ecological Transition or sub-sets such as climate change, water stress, soil loss or marine pollution. Building the evidence base enables a consensus to be forged at the global level. This is the role of the Intergovernmental Panel on Climate Change, for example. The creation of a global framework takes time, hard work and much diplomacy, but it can then act as a shared set of values and guidelines for how to monitor a problem and ensure that governmental action is in accordance with the spirit of the international agreement. National governments can then enact legislation as appropriate, and the consensus is translated in the real action at the local or national level. Whilst the advantage of this approach is the building of 'common sense' as a template for the legitimacy of action, its disadvantage is slowness and that it can be obstructed by minority interests or furious and well-funded lobbying by vested interests. This has happened, for example, over climate, where parts of the energy industry have actively worked to sabotage global action to restrict carbon emissions.[96]
- *Build eco-systems into everyday life.* The third strategy is more radical; it accepts that there is an ecological impact from human activity but proposes that it could be reshaped to incorporate ecological protection or enhancement.[97] Thus supporters of biodiversity can argue that a way to protect, for example, forest biodiversity is to treat it as a source of food and to eat (and thus value) that biodiversity. The FAO has a division which supports agrobiodiversity, and there are good case studies of indigenous peoples being encouraged to protect local species which they had eaten and used in the past but were moving away from continuing to do, in the pattern of change described by the Nutrition Transition (see Chapter 9). To have such traditional foods reassessed as important can lead to renewed respect for local biodiversity.[98] Taken further, this approach suggests that modernity itself will need to be redirected. Mass urban life will have to be remodelled on ecological principles.[99] Cities of the future will have to be 'greened' and become more ecologically resilient and adaptable than they currently are.[100]
- *Conservation.* This fourth approach is perhaps the oldest. It is to create parks and sanctuaries for nature: to put metaphorical, legal or real walls round nature to protect it, and to enable its ecological interconnectivity to continue. In the early twenty-first century, for example, an estimated 12 per cent of all land is in some kind of protective system of governance.[101] Most national governments have some system of nature conservation, and it is a strategy already well adapted to the emergence of multilevel systems of governance from the global (e.g. UN) to the local (e.g. local nature reserve, or your garden).

- *Cost eco-systems services into market forces.* This approach is to pay for nature, usually by internalising externalised or unaccounted costs. It is the application of ecological economics to the market system. In 2007, the G8+5 leading world governments' environment ministers met in Potsdam, Germany, and agreed to 'initiate the process of analysing the global economic benefit of biological diversity, the costs of the loss of biodiversity and the failure to take protective measures versus the costs of effective conservation'.[102] This initiated an intergovernmental process to cost eco-systems and biodiversity, with a policy report published in 2010 about how to factor such costs into mainstream economics. In this approach, eco-systems are judged to be 'natural capital'. Ecological phenomena and impacts become spoken of as 'public goods'. The strategy is to encourage ways to integrate biodiversity conservation into policies and decision frameworks for resource production and consumption. Thus this strategy takes its policy and intellectual place alongside the strategy for the enhancement of human capital considered in the Economic Transition (see Chapter 8) and the social and cultural capital that is considered in the Cultural Transition (see Chapter 11).

- *Economic and technological optimism.* This sixth strategy differs from the deniers. It accepts that ecological change is occurring and perhaps accelerating, but concludes *not* that there is nothing to be done (or that action should be resisted), but that 'Something Will Turn Up'. This is the modern version of Charles Dickens's Mr Micawber's motto in *David Copperfield* (first published in 1849). A technical fix will be found by some unspecified persons or bodies at some unspecified time in the future. The best route to this happy outcome is almost always deemed to be market forces plus a judicious mix of investment and incentives (which need neoliberal guidance as to governance, of course).[103] This too is an old strategy. It recalls Voltaire's story of Dr Pangloss in *Candide* (published in 1759), his parody of the Enlightenment philosopher, who experienced dreadful trials in his life but still to the end knew that 'All is for the best in the best of all possible worlds.'[104]

The implications of the Ecological Transition

A formidable picture emerges for public health from the scale and breadth of this transition. A burst of scientific understanding enables humanity to appreciate both the vastness and the complexity of the connections in the natural world of which humans are a part. Ecological thinking rightly can claim to offer a better, more integrated and more comprehensive way of looking at humankind and health in context. Figure 10.6 is one simple overview which attempts to capture this set of interrelations, taken from the UN's Millennium Ecosystem Assessment.

The Ecological Transition requires public health thinking and action to see the connections between the biosphere and the ecosphere, between the microbial world and the world of flora and fauna. Across all this vast web of life, or Darwin's

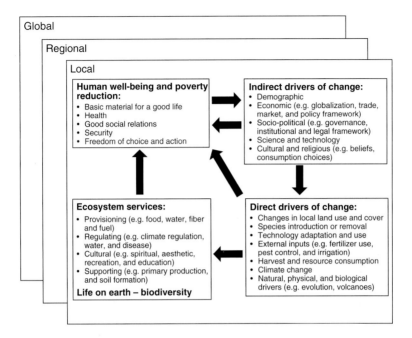

FIGURE 10.6   Millennium Ecosystem Assessment drivers of change

entangled bank writ large, human activity has become a powerful and shaping force. Currently, it looks as though the role of human activity has been damaging, both in its extermination of other species and in the rebounding impact on itself, in the form of zoonoses and microbial resistance, for example. The unprecedented loss of biological diversity from anthropogenic causes has profound implications for human health. One way that biodiversity loss threatens health is by exacerbating risk and incidence of infectious diseases. The primary reservoirs for many pathogens are species that dominate in biodiversity-poor settings. In contrast, it has been argued that where biodiversity is strong the species which spread disease feed from a wider variety of hosts, most of which are poor reservoirs for the pathogens, resulting in lower infection prevalence.[105] A point stressed in this chapter, from all the reports and studies, is that human health and experience are now being threatened by an unprecedented scale of biodiversity loss. All life is literally entering a new phase in evolutionary history, with some arguing that 'tipping points' might be emerging.[106]

There are grounds for optimism too. It is possible to conceive of risk reduction for humans and how we upset the mix of plants, planet and animals. People are already aware of the cultural element to the Ecological Transition: the loss of green space, the reliance on natural systems, the limits to material resources, covered in previous chapters. One of the most useful insights from the biologists and ecologists, however, dispenses with the myth of the balance of nature; this is a romantic notion, well intentioned, but not adequate as a metaphor for describing the complexity and dynamics of change. Perhaps an important lesson from considering the Ecological Transition is to respect the limits of knowledge and the limits of nature. It is not endlessly resilient; it can be destroyed. It warrants protection, just like the public health. This is a destruction not of the 'out there' but of the conditions on which humanity depends. In the end, there is little distinction between the environment, nature and humankind. They are in one web of life. but one element – humankind – is wreaking remarkable damage, perhaps ultimately on itself.

This chapter has re-entered a core set of arguments about Ecological Public Health. We have suggested that health has a rich tradition of ecological thought on which to draw. The Ecological Transition invokes diverse models of health. At least two of our five models (see Chapter 3) have particular relevance. The Techno-Economic model now looks naive, from an ecological perspective. The Bio-Medical model, which draws upon the medical gifts of nature, has recognised that it is spoiling those gifts. Antibiotics were discovered by humans in nature rather than invented, and are now in danger of being squandered, as the experts in the field opine. What emerges from this chapter is a theme central to this book, to which we return at its end. How can public health engage more sustainably, i.e. durably and well, with the complexity of nature's dynamics?

11

CULTURAL TRANSITION

Is there a Cultural Transition?

The term 'Cultural Transition' is hardly a conventional term in the social sciences, let alone public health. Yet here we argue that changes in culture are intrinsic to the public health, which is why its professions and agents need to make the cultural dimension of life central to their activities and thinking. Culture is not a 'bolt-on' to public health but intrinsic, particularly expressed in the Social-Behavioural model (see Chapter 3). We have, throughout Part II, examined how what appear to be simple explanations subtly invoke cultural assumptions or messages. In this chapter we explore what we mean by the Cultural Transition.

To understand the Cultural Transition requires engaging with literature and thinking which are not normally included in public health training (by which we mean education in any field of work which has a public health remit or professional accreditation). Yet, in the late twentieth century, public health bodies gradually had to engage with aspects of culture – or more particularly the cultural industries, such as the advertising or marketing sectors. These use social science knowledge and deep financial pockets to manipulate or encourage behaviour for commercial rather than health reasons. The role of advertising, for example, is now proven to have an impact on children's food choices.[1] As a result public health bodies are in the position of reacting to the legacy of other forces, always put into a 'catch-up' position, picking up the pieces from, and trying to compensate for, the actions of others. This can make a mockery of health promotion or ill-health prevention.

Social scientists, particularly sociologists or social anthropologists, are distinctly chary about treating culture, whose meaning we explore below, as something that we can define at one point in time and then proceed to measure differences at another point in time. The Belgian-born French social anthropologist Claude Lévi-Strauss (1908–2009) believed that the underlying cultural structures to any human society – whether in kinship systems, myths and rituals or through artefacts such as masks – are evidence that the human mind always and everywhere works in the same way. The underlying structure of society he proposed as therefore persistent.[2] By implication, history and culture are either ephemeral, the blink of an eye in human developmental terms, or else of very long duration.

Some psychologists, conversely, are less bothered by the notion of cultural change, even over very short periods of time or at the individual rather than societal level. One common use of cultural change in this sense is the notion that people go through 'stages of change' in their ideas and beliefs. In effect, people are said to have a personal culture or lifestyle which can be mapped and modified. The health task is thus one of shifting existing personal culture to a healthier one. In one version of this approach proposed by psychologists, people are said to start out as 'pre-contemplators' with no intention to change, then to become 'contemplators' who intend to change, then to become actors who adopt new behaviour patterns if irregularly, and finally and hopefully to become 'maintainers' who behave consistently and regularly.[3] This approach has been implicit in much public health practice, for example in work on people with alcohol, tobacco or drug dependencies, and in the use of social marketing today. Some writers have suggested that this approach complements the social-ecological model of Bronfenbrenner (see Image 5 in Chapter 1).[4]

Other psychologists vehemently disagree with this approach and its assumptions, scorning it as theoretically lightweight. The influential Canadian-born psychologist Alan Bandura wrote that this approach offers no more than a 'series of arbitrary pseudo stages'.[5] He contrasted it with what he judged a genuine stage progression theory of cognitive change offered by Swiss developmental psychologist Jean Piaget (1896–1980). For Bandura change, if it occurs, happens in environments; habits are deeply resistant to change. These are thus genuine, often heated areas of debate. The degree of disagreement tends to undermine the view by the US National Cancer Institute promoted in its widely read *Theory at a Glance* booklet.[6] This was aimed at medical or public health practitioners, suggesting that one can 'pick and mix' the right social psychological theory for the task in hand.

In contrast, the advertising and marketing industries overtly apply theory sparingly. That said, they are, in their own way, toughly evidence-based. They have to account to clients. Their essential task, for a fee, is that of changing the cultural order or cultural environments in order to cue changes in behaviour. Their work ranges from trying to get children to consume more soft drinks or switch to a different line of products, to promoting cigarettes. Although the promotion of smoking is banned in many societies, in less protected societies (i.e. much of the world) it flouts the WHO's global framework convention that promotes bans.[7] Despite the public health evidence of tobacco's harm, the giant companies continue to sell and push their products. The advertising bans restrict what they can do in some markets, but, as British American Tobacco, one of the giants, openly states, this merely restricts which of the five golden Ps of marketing – product, price, packaging, promotion and place – it devises its marketing mix around. In mid-2011, it had this statement on its website: 'We see this as marketing for a new era, where product brand communication is primarily based on one-to-one permission marketing to adult smokers, in much more focused, narrower channels, with tight standards for age verification.'[8]

Given the track record of the advertising and marketing industries undermining health, public health advocates have been typically sceptical about these 'cultural industries'. Kelly Brownell and Kenneth Warner have argued that from the mid-1950s tobacco manufacturers and their marketers established a consistent template of response, or script, in response to criticism. The list included casting aspersions on public health research (in modern language, calling it 'junk science'), making insincere public declarations of concern for consumer health, employing massive, sometimes covert, resources to lobby politicians and governments, offering self-regulatory pledges, and finally lodging responsibility for unhealthy consumption in personal choice rather than company policy. The same script, they say, is being used by food companies to counter responsibilities for the obesity epidemic, albeit food is not tobacco.[9] Certainly, with obesity, as with many other public health problems where wealthy industries confront public health forces, there are abundant examples of policy groups and NGOs being created or emerging with the aims and/or sponsorship of an industry under threat. By their critics they are termed business interest non-governmental organisations (BINGOs). Their implicit task is to promote the suggestion that public health concerns are overplayed, that this creates unnecessary worries and self-defeating, moral panics, and that public health groups themselves are self-interested.

Public health advocates are generally sceptical of advertising and marketing. But commercial marketing industries are a fount of ideas, policies, programmes, methods and measures on health with growing political influence. What is termed social marketing is an attempt to emulate the methods of commercial marketing and apply them to socially benign goals. The subtitle of one book in this genre asks rhetorically 'Why Should the Devil Have All the Best Tunes?'[10] The debate about whether the cultural industries can be suborned to work for public health is not new. In 1930 John Dewey referred to the 'publicity agent', the marketing expert, being 'the most significant symbol of our present social life'. The reason why, he continued, was that, while there were individuals able to resist, 'sentiment can be manufactured for almost any person or cause'.[11] The counter-argument was offered by journalist and commentator Walter Lippmann (1889–1974). He said that the world had become too big, too complex and too fast-moving for people to interpret it with much accuracy. Democracy was being subverted, and the solution was for the government to act to bring about the 'manufacture of consent'.[12] Manipulation of the public could be presented as being in the public's own interest. The argument about mind control is essentially a recognition that culture can be moulded and changed, and that it is possible for powerful forces to do this. From George Orwell to social marketing, a debate exists about the morality and direction of attempts to mould culture.

We use the term 'Cultural Transition' to mean and refer to something bigger than attempts to change culture by vested interests. Our concern is to highlight long-term shifts in people's thinking, as societies move from feudal and highly ordered entities to more fluid and industrial or post-industrial forms. This transition was commented upon by many, prominently by Karl Marx and Max Weber, as we see in a moment, but also by J.S. Mill. For Mill it formed part of the Enlightenment. In 'periods of transition', Mill said, people give up their old beliefs 'and not feeling quite sure that those they still retain can stand unmodified, listen eagerly to new opinions'.[13] We are interested in how that cognitive change occurs and the direction given to human experience. For us, this cultural dimension to the human condition is one of our four dimensions of existence (see Chapter 1). What people think and how they order their lives have been subject to long-term historical change. Many writers have pointed to the transition from simple to complex societies, from feudal to post-modern, from rural to urban, from a collectively formed to a more individualistic ethos. People often refer to cultures as 'ancient', 'primitive', 'pre-modern', 'modern' and more recently 'post-modern' (an 'exasperating term', says Bertens[14]). The terms are attempts to grasp differences at the human experiential level. Like Lévi-Strauss, we do not subscribe to the notion that primitive societies are not sophisticated; he was correct and clear on this. Anthropological evidence suggests so-called primitive cultures contain rich meanings and knowledge.

By the Cultural Transition, we refer to a process of change from a world where people live such lives full of rich symbols and understanding (within relationships and meanings largely shaped by their dependency on nature and by their immediate surroundings and hierarchical forms) to a world where the complexity of lives is decoupled from nature and its constraints. A new mode of living has infinite and more loosely linked permutations of meanings, relationships and modes of communication. The Cultural Transition is a move from a world characterised by the local, the staple, the inherited, the communal, the tactile and the parochial to a world with more fluid sets of cultural possibilities. In the rest of this chapter we explore that.

Part of the problem in speaking about the Cultural Transition in these or any other terms is the enormous difficulty in saying what culture is. The word is packed with connotations. No fewer than 164 different definitions of the word were identified by the US anthropologists Alfred Kroeber and Clyde Kluckhohn even by the mid-twentieth century.[15] The British cultural analyst Raymond Williams in his magisterial *Keywords*, a lexicon of cultural terms, noted that 'culture' is one of the two or three most complicated words in the English language.[16] The word 'culture' comes to us today with ancient agricultural connotations, from the Latin *cultus* referring to tillage of the soil and thence to both French and medieval English. With such fluidity and definitional span, are we even right to posit a Cultural Transition, let alone propose that it is important for public health?

We are here proposing culture to mean how people live their lives, their patterns of self-understanding and identity, and their habituated behaviour and the 'rules' by which they shape and interpret their lives. Culture is the shorthand for shared bodies of experience and meaning in daily lives, their interpretative values, the signposts by which people give meaning to what they perceive and experience.

Culture is thus the interpretative dynamic filter through which men and women address family structures, birth control, divisions of labour, inequalities in existence, and more, in short much upon which public health centres. A culture provides the rationale and format for their understanding and behaviour in a world where health outcomes and healthiness define what people experience.

As many writers have noted, it is useful to distinguish between collective or public culture and culture expressed at the level of the individual. We entered this distinction at the beginning of this chapter. The collective consciousness is the interpersonal world. The private culture is part of one's biography. Both inform each other. This is the entangled bank of culture, to apply Darwin's metaphor. Already in this short introduction to the notion of the Cultural Transition, we note divergent views of what culture is, how and whether it should be shaped, and the difficulty of unravelling its complexity. The rest of this chapter gives an overview of major schools of thought and arguments which we judge to be relevant to public health.

Mapping the Cultural Transition

The Cultural Transition is both ideas and material factors working in combination. A writer who has attempted to explore cultural change over time and across countries in this vein is Ronald F. Inglehart, a political scientist at the University of Michigan. Over decades, Inglehart with a consortium of colleagues worldwide has sought to map the shift in culture, particularly the changes in values, what people think important and what they hold in common. He both advised and helped establish the European Union's regular Eurobarometer, by which the European Commission monitors citizens' views on diverse policy issues. At the global level, in six World Values Surveys, in 1981, 1990, 1995, 2000, 2005 and 2010–12, Inglehart and colleagues have documented a pattern of changing values coinciding with the Economic Transition. The surveys have covered a variety of countries and levels of national income.

From these studies, Inglehart has proposed that societies go through a movement from traditional to modern values and thence to post-modern values. The studies have shown, he argues, that values can be plotted on two axes. One is the shift from values moving from 'survival' to 'self-expression'. The other ranges from 'traditional' to 'secular-rational' values. Figure 11.1 gives a picture of countries plotted on these axes and falling into different cultural groups, drawn from two World Values Surveys.

Inglehart and colleagues have linked these shifts to the process of democratisation.[17] In this respect, the studies are consistent with key thinking on the Economic Transition. Superficially, indeed, Inglehart's work is reminiscent of Rostow's stages-of-growth thinking, celebrating the West as the apogee of development, but the similarity is superficial. Actually, as Figure 11.1 shows, Inglehart identifies clusters of countries across the dimensions explored, rather than unilinear stages of growth. The data exhibits non-linear relationships between wealth and well-being. By 2000, he was concluding:[18]

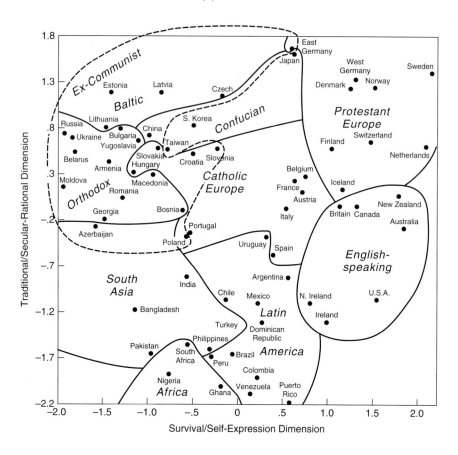

FIGURE 11.1 Locations of 65 societies on two dimensions of cross-cultural variation: World Values Surveys, 1990–91 and 1995–98

As one would expect, rising income levels go with rising levels of happiness and life satisfaction. The peoples of rich societies are happier than those of poor societies. The overall correlation is very strong (0.68). But beyond a certain point, the curve levels off. As we move from low-income societies to high-income societies, there is a steep increase in subjective well being. But the impact of rising income stops when we reach the threshold of $10,000. Beyond that point, there is practically no relationship between income and subjective well-being.

This is a devastating conclusion, suggesting that the Economic Transition shows diminishing returns, and that the onward march of progress might be illusory. It has reinforced contemporary discussion about happiness and well-being,[19] and questions whether Western styles of living are cultural progress. Comparative national studies of opinion and belief began in the 1960s.[20] Opinion research has grown over the last half-century but remains fraught with difficulties. Abstract concepts like 'democracy', 'corruption', 'religiosity' or 'nationalism' can be asked about but may well generate entirely different responses to the same words from different people in different places. For Inglehart *et al.*, this raises a deeply theoretical issue: that the analysis of cultural change is really a continuing social scientific debate about differences between the analyses offered by Karl Marx and by Max Weber (1864–1920). This is a debate not just about the dynamics of cultural change and whether culture advances in a linear sequence or by ebbs and flows, but about whether social science can offer society optimistic, pessimistic or pragmatic conclusions about the direction in which culture is going. It heightens questions about whether industrialised societies are turning into new cultural forms, as is argued by the post-modernist theorists, or whether they are locked into existing forms of material inequality, with diminishing returns.

In Marx's view, industrialisation provided the central dynamic to modernisation. Capitalism is corrosive of all existing cultural systems but creates new cultural relations, which has positive possibilities (as long as the oppressed working class gets a voice and a fair share of wealth). As Engels and he dramatically remarked in the *Communist Manifesto* in 1848:

> All fixed, fast-frozen relations, with their train of ancient and venerable prejudices and opinions, are swept away, all new-formed ones become antiquated before they can ossify. All that is solid melts into air, all that is holy is profaned, and man is at last compelled to face with sober senses his real conditions of life, and his relations with his kind.[21]

This oft-quoted passage would doubtless require different language today, less Shakespeare, now judged as elite culture, and more Seinfeld, modern televisual culture.

With Weber, culture is influenced by modernisation but is a factor determining industrialisation. In his study of *The Protestant Ethic and the Spirit of Capitalism*,[22] first published in 1905, Protestantism is depicted as the force which helped unleash capitalism while at the same time the bureaucratic forces of capitalism retain the residues of a secularisation of traditional values. Inglehart backs the argument that culture is linked to economic change, arguing that:[23] 'Economic development is associated with pervasive, and to some extent predictable, cultural changes. Industrialisation promotes a shift from traditional to secular-rational values, while the rise of post-industrial society brings a shift to more trust, tolerance, well-being, and post-material values. Economic collapse tends to propel societies in the opposite direction.' But he adds certain riders. Modernisation does not follow a linear path. Secularisation is counterbalanced by moral and spiritual values retained from the past. Cultural change is path-dependent, that is to say shaped by existing cultural forms such as Catholicism, Confucianism and Protestantism, as was illustrated in Figure 11.1.

For some writers today, the Cultural Transition is a proxy for Westernisation. The assumption is made that only in the West is there tolerance to a diversity of views and that a capacity for people to question ways of existence only thrives there. In a celebrated essay and subsequent book, the US political scientist Samuel P. Huntington (1927–2008) identified culture as central to the notion of a clash of civilisations at the turn of the twentieth to the twenty-first century. The term stemmed from a perceived threat to the West, a notion that progress is a fixed march towards US or Western styles of thinking and rationality. These Huntington associated with Islamic culture. He summarised the importance of culture in this 'clash' in an early paper thus: 'It is my hypothesis that the fundamental source of conflict in this new world will not be primarily ideological or primarily economic. The great divisions among humankind and the dominating source of conflict will be cultural.'[24] This thesis has often been read as the cause of the division and conflict between the West and the Islamic world, particularly in the era unleashed by the US presidency of George W. Bush. Dieter Senghaas, a German political scientist, countered that there are two main errors in the Huntington thesis. The first is that the main clashes are within civilisations rather than between them. The second is that Huntington views the clash as occurring entirely within culture, thus failing to acknowledge that the causes of such clashes have economic roots. The main source of such clashes, Senghaas said, is modernisation, which inevitably produces conflict.[25] The so-called Arab Spring of 2011 perhaps indicates a rather different interpretation, a desire for democratic participation, equality under the law, and distributive justice from within Islamic cultures. This is a reality which fits more easily within Senghaas than Huntington.

Neither industrialisation nor modernisation should be confused with Americanisation, not least since the USA overtly champions traditional values within the identity of what it is to be an American. For Inglehart, if anything, the twentieth-century Nordic societies represent the 'cutting edge of cultural change'.[26] For Inglehart, both Marx and Weber are right to some degree. Material factors such as wealth can determine the pace of value change, but also existing sets of belief are not easily swept away, and indeed form the context for diverse models of modernisation. Modernity is not unilinear. Marx and Weber assessed the cultural framework of capitalism as a social system, and although both of them considered particular forms of consciousness arising from capitalism they did not accept these forms at face value.

In the case of Weber he was describing 'occidental reason', in effect the culture and reasoning processes of the West. This was the favourable setting for the development of capitalism. The sociologist Richard E. Nisbett, writing recently, agrees: 'Most Westerners, at any rate most Americans, are confident that the following generalisations apply to pretty much everyone.' He lists what these are: 'people want to be distinctive', 'people are in control of their own behaviour', 'people are oriented towards personal goals of success and achievement' and 'people strive to feel good about themselves'.[27] In the East, by contrast, people are wary of being wholly distinctive and 'out of sync' with their parent culture. People find value and meaning through group not just individual goals. Nisbett says there are stark cultural differences between West and East, the former with an individualistic orientation, the latter socially collectivist.

Such culturalist arguments are painted here with enormously large and somewhat anecdotal brushstrokes. They appear to support Max Weber's *Protestant Ethic* thesis that economic development occurs on the basis of cultural factors. Individualistic striving thus begets capitalism. Ha-Joon Chang, the Korean-born Cambridge (UK) economist, notes how one philosophy of the East, Confucianism, discouraged people from taking up professions like business and engineering that were necessary for economic development. He also points out that, in the mid-nineteenth century, the Germans were described by the British as being indolent and slow, too individualistic and unable to co-operate with each other. The Japanese, early in the twentieth century, were described by Western visitors as lazy. His conclusion is that culture affects economic development, but likewise economic development affects culture. Cultures change and can do so rapidly. No one any longer suggests that the Germans and Japanese are lazy, because the stereotype – or is it the reality? – has changed. In the case of the very different cultures of Japan, Germany and his own country, Korea, many of the behavioural traits that were supposed to 'explain' economic development (e.g. hard work, timekeeping, frugality), he argues, were actually its consequences rather than its causes.[28]

The implication drawn here supports the propositions made in this chapter. Culture may be enormously complex but it is also malleable. Capitalism refashions cultures, much as Marx predicted but in ways which he could only begin to surmise. If cultures can modernise, in the manner described by Marx or Weber, they can also, as we see, unravel.

Social capital: a bridging concept too far?

A theme in this debate is whether the individualistic and fragmenting tendencies of Western culture can be countered by socially binding institutional dynamics and whether these can be engineered to generate more social cohesion. Public health thinkers have joined this debate, assuming that higher social solidarity creates better health; we noted this argument in the Epidemiological Transition (see Chapter 5). The social capital literature is growing rapidly, with already more than a thousand citations on the US National Library of Medicine and National Institutes of Health database PubMed. A review of this literature is beyond the scope of this chapter, and therefore we will concentrate on the essentials only.

The concept of social capital has a mixed history, as we shall see, but the general focus of most discussions of social capital in health is US-originated. In addressing the question of social capital, US social scientists have routinely turned to their own society's past, in particular the research and analysis of Alexis de Tocqueville (1805–59), the French aristocrat who articulated an early sociological analysis of the USA in the 1830s.[29] Here, said Tocqueville, was a new society with strong civic associations, a culture of 'everyday democracy', yet horribly marked by slavery (an observation frequently sidelined in US celebrations of Tocqueville's study). In Tocqueville's account, civic associations are strong in the northern US states, inhabited by Protestants, and weakest in the South because of slavery.

Taking up Tocqueville's account, political scientist Robert Putnam has today looked for the reasons why social bonds are said to be in decline. Putnam suggests a number of reasons, including the movement of women into the workforce, rising residential mobility, a host of demographic changes, including fewer marriages and more divorces, and the 'technical transformation of leisure' which individualises leisure-time.[30] The unifying concept in his analysis he acknowledges to be one already extensively in use by social scientists 'in several disciplines'.[31] This is the now popular notion of social capital. Beginning with the publication of a 1995 essay, 'Bowling Alone', this term has spread rapidly through the social sciences, leading to a veritable industry of social capital research, some of which, as we have suggested, seeks to make links between social capital and patterns of health and in some cases the environment also.[32]

Tocqueville never used the term 'social capital'; it is more recent. One of the first to do so, John Dewey, the US philosopher and educational theorist, observed that improving a child's command of language provided 'the keys which will unlock to the child the wealth of social capital which lies beyond the possible range of his limited individual experience'.[33] For Dewey, social capital was a metaphor for knowledge and education, a topic we return to later in this chapter. And by 'capital' he meant stock. In the 1970s, French sociologist Pierre Bourdieu (1930–2002) resurrected the term, but from a different source, although he too was particularly concerned with the educational implications. He identified social capital as one of three dimensions of capital (economic, cultural and social), each having its own function within a capitalist society. Loosely informed by Marx's understanding of economic capital, but applied to the French educational context, cultural capital and social capital form part of the overall framework of what Bourdieu called 'symbolic capital'. This provides legitimacy for the unequal division of economic, cultural and social resources in society.[34]

For Bourdieu these were not freely floating attributes but stored in bodies, minds, property and ownership relations. Cultural capital is a competence or skill that cannot be separated from its bearer. Objects or technologies may function as a form of cultural capital, in so far as their use or consumption presupposes a certain amount of embodied cultural capital (for example, the skills to read an operating handbook). In societies with a system of formal education, cultural capital exists in an institutionalised form. When people receive qualifications, their embodied cultural capital takes on an objective value. Similarly, social capital is established in groups and is exclusive to them; assessing or measuring social capital requires inquiring into power and its unequal distribution, said Bourdieu.[35] Families or groups have a volume of capital under their control. In Britain, for example, to have attended one of the major private schools and/or Oxford or Cambridge University, the educational background of a large number of the British establishment, is to be provided with a fast track to success. A review at the start of the 2000s found that 77 per cent of high court judges, 81 per cent of permanent secretaries (the head civil servants of government ministries) and 83 per cent of ambassadors had been to either Oxford or Cambridge, despite this being the lot of only 2 per cent of British students.[36] In some cases these forms of non-economic capital are overt; they may also be hidden, perhaps visible only to those who share the attributes, which used to be called sharing 'the old school tie'.

Putnam's use of the term is fundamentally different from that of either Dewey or Bourdieu. Putnam drew from three sources: firstly, the Scottish philosopher David Hume's analysis of materially based economic reciprocity (which informs much of social cognitive science today); secondly, Tocqueville's own observations on civic associations in the early USA, noted above; and, thirdly, the neoliberal Chicago economist Gary Becker's notion of 'human capital', defined as technical knowledge held by persons.[37] By implication this is a far more utilitarian and stark notion of education than that offered by Dewey. Putnam defines social capital: 'By analogy with notions of physical capital and human capital – tools and training that enhance individual productivity – "social capital" refers to features of social organization, such as networks, norms, and trust, that facilitate coordination and cooperation for mutual benefit.'[38] Whereas for Bourdieu social capital is a cultural characteristic shaped by socio-economic inequality, expressed through power and inequality, for Putnam it is politically neutral and held in common. In fact he even describes it as a public good 'like clean air'. The implication is that society cannot have enough of it. 'Stocks of social capital, such as trust, norms, and networks, tend to be self reinforcing and cumulative.'[39]

'Social capital' is being offered as a term to describe a form of cultural 'stock', and on that basis it is possible to measure and compare it through time and space. Ronald Inglehart, whose polling work we summarised above, describes social capital as the 'Tocqueville–Putnam thesis', adopting its use for his own research. For him, 'membership in voluntary associations is strongly linked with stable democracy'. He thus implies a mutual dependency between strong social capital and democratic institutions and vice versa.[40] Others have measured social capital across Europe, finding that, in general, trust is not declining, with the UK as an exception which has become more like the USA.[41]

Today the term 'social capital' is ubiquitous, a conceptual shorthand. It is used extensively in social science, in public health research and in political discourse. But questions remain owing to the different interpretations of the term, even by Putnam himself, who admits that while the term 'capital' has 'a felicitous ring' the debate around it has alerted him to its 'negative externalities'. He acknowledges that some forms of social capital are destructive, to say the least. The Ku Klux Klan, he cites, has been a persistent form of social capital. (We note it is one of course exclusively 'owned' by white people.) Having circulated the notion as real, Putnam then made recommendations for future investigation: social capital needs to be assessed with regard to different tendencies. These include: its formal and informal aspects; 'thick' versus 'thin' strands of social capital (by which he means the difference between 'nodding acquaintances' and stronger relationships); inward-looking and outward-looking social capital (such as the distinction between exclusive and non-exclusive groups); and bridging versus bonding social capital (the first of which extends between groups and the second within groups). Social capital, Putnam warns, is 'multidimensional', and therefore 'we must take care not to frame questions about change solely in terms of more social capital or less social capital'.[42] This warning is ubiquitously disregarded, we note. Unlike Bourdieu, and despite the belated subtleties, Putnam's use of the concept still looks bolted on to an unexplicated theory of society and cultural dynamics.

Although social capital theory speaks in the language of neoliberal economics, US economist Samuel Bowles had remarked that in this field the concept has only limited impact. Economists, he says, use even simpler socio-cultural constructs such as 'the self-regarding individual'. Furthermore they are completely uninterested in 'the process of cultural transmission – who acquires what trait from whom, under what conditions, and why'.[43] This is damning criticism of the cultural sophistication of economists by a leading economist, which we share. Nevertheless, while economics might ignore culture, economic processes certainly influence culture. The examples Bowles gives include the framing of social psychological processes, the altering of extrinsic and intrinsic motivations, and the evolution of social norms and cultural learning processes. These are subtle processes for which social capital is too superficial a notion. Elsewhere, he and his colleague Herbert Gintis have argued for the rejection of the concept, if not the focus, of social capital research. They wrote:[44]

> Capital refers to a thing that can be owned – even a social isolate like Robinson Crusoe had an axe and a fishing net. By contrast, the attributes said to make up social capital describe relationships among people. As with other trendy expressions, 'social capital' has attracted so many disparate uses that we think it better to drop the term in favor of something more precise. 'Community' better captures the aspects of good governance that explain social capital's popularity, as it focuses attention on what groups do rather than what people own.

Capital, says Bourdieu, is always rooted in some form of ownership, and some are always excluded. But is Bowles and Gintis's suggested alternative term – 'community' – any better? In conventional meaning, community too implies a socially unifying identity. Certainly communities may appear to be consensual, but they are also conflict-ridden, encompassing multiple, sometimes overlapping or sometimes divergent, identities. And these identities and allegiances shift over time. The early twentieth-century German sociologist George Simmel (1858–1918) argued in his *Web of Group-Affiliations* that society and groups are expressed and constituted through dualisms, conflicts and contradictions.[45] A person's individuality is located at the centre of many different influences; people are defined by each new group they join or are affiliated to. A homogenised view of social bonds therefore will always imperfectly render the differentiated relationships found in 'communities', to use Bowles and Gintis's expression. The attempt to measure and compare these bonds may even have a capacity to mislead, and undoubtedly such exercises will almost certainly understate the drivers of their complexity. In the twenty-first century, the period of late modernity, virtual social networking means people become members of groups whom they might never meet in person, and they take actions based upon assumed unity of purpose where none might otherwise exist. The Arab Spring and the English riots in 2011 were all in part prompted by membership of electronic social networks.

Do these concepts help public health analysts better understand the complex linkages between culture and health? Co-operative social network dynamics in human culture appear to be a distinctive trait of humankind, since the norm of co-operation is not found, or is found only in a limited form or else it is hard-wired rather than socially formed, in other animals. While this capacity is said to define human uniqueness, the social norms of mutual support and family structures are in constant flux. Social capital research, particularly the new field which links social networks to health outcomes, provides some means to map how culture and health interact. The focus on culture is valuable, if the focus on 'culturalist' explanations, without properly tying them to broader determinants of social relationships, including what we term the four dimensions of existence, is not. If history shows anything, it is that social norms of co-operation are fragile and can be broken by events. As the Swiss economists Ernst Fehr and Urs Fischbacher have observed, there is a decisive lack of knowledge regarding the social and the economic determinants of social norms, yet it remains obvious that social norms reflect the socio-economic environment. Even so, they note, 'empirically as well as theoretically we still know little about this'.[46] Social researchers, they say, are still inquiring into this problem.

Is the problem that social capital was devised to address a cultural problem, or is the source of the problem elsewhere? Perhaps the fraying of working-class culture in Anglo-Saxon societies like the USA and the UK has more to do with their socio-economic policies, expressed in reducing levels of trust, than in intrinsic cultural aspects but which culture also expresses. If descriptive social analysis has some utility, but has drawbacks, perhaps there is another mode of analysis which is even more effective in constructing a social narrative about what the problems are and how they might be addressed. Fictional representation can be as powerful as, perhaps even more powerful than, sociology. It investigates at the 'level of meaning', as Max Weber recommended. It tells a better story, obviously. Just as the nineteenth-century novels of Charles Dickens provided a window on the urban underclass of Britain, so too the US television series *The Wire*, set in economically depressed Baltimore, USA in the early twenty-first century, exposed the causes of endemic drug use in black communities, the collapse of working-class employment, and the stresses on the local state and the education system. It achieved in drama a degree of acuity which largely unread academic accounts do not. Dickens, we noted, was an active member of the public health movement. David Simon, the writer of *The Wire*, makes the case for a similarly impassioned but thoroughly analytic analysis of context, culture and economy for the USA today. *The Wire*, he said, formed:[47]

a meditation on the death of work and the betrayal of the American working class . . . it is a deliberate argument that unencumbered capitalism is not a substitute for social policy; that on its own, without a social compact, raw capitalism is destined to serve the few at the expense of the many.

The Wire, in other words, and like the works of Dickens, was a depiction of the social capital of people *without* capital. That said, not every community is devoid of strong community bonds, and many communities, if they have other resources, might not even need them. In some societies, strong social bonds or high levels of social solidarity may be a sufficient substitution for low levels of income, provided it is evenly spread. Culture is always changing, in transition to new cultural forms, altering the context for public health. We now look at a more daunting, and certainly more difficult, analysis of the scope and tenor of cultural change.

Cultural Transition: the view from Frankfurt via America

A towering theoretical perspective on culture and on the Cultural Transition has been provided by a school of German social thinkers called the Frankfurt School. Their collective work – sometimes excruciatingly difficult – spans more than eight decades. Established in Frankfurt in 1923, a group of interdisciplinary social theorists collectively known as the Frankfurt School, more formally the Institut für Sozialforschung (Institute for Social Research), introduced Sigmund Freud's theory of the unconscious into a new, eclectic philosophical mix with Marx and Weber. It has redefined cultural study. Under the banner of 'critical theory' (a term which drew from Marx's notion of dialectical critique), the Institute was led for much of its history by Max Horkheimer (1895–1973), together with a clutch of brilliant, if to the Anglo-Saxon world sometimes abstruse, social theorists. The best of these were probably Walter Benjamin (1892–1940), who committed suicide having escaped the Nazis when he was about to be returned by Franco's Spanish authorities to Vichy France, Theodor Adorno (1903–69), who returned to Germany after the Second World War spent in the USA, and Herbert Marcuse (1898–1979), who had escaped but remained in California till his death.

The experience of exile and fleeing to the USA reinvigorated the Frankfurt School's thinking, which had been halted by the Second World War. Forced to adjust their continental perspectives to what they saw in the dynamic US economy and culture, they took on a more empirical outlook. This spawned a blisteringly critical, distinctively un-American view of that country's emerging cultural system. In their joint and seminal 1947 book *Dialectic of Enlightenment*,[48] as much a report on the fate of philosophy as on the cultural conditions of the USA, Horkheimer and Adorno examined the failure of the Enlightenment's expectations of social progress. They argued that the Enlightenment's drive to reason had turned it into the opposite, transforming instruments of knowledge into tools of domination. For Horkheimer and Adorno, science and technology had created new means for mass destruction and cultural death. The potential for live, creative culture was being subverted by the mass, standardising influence of the new corporate 'cultural industries'. The long struggle for democracy and social enlightenment was thus being usurped by new demagogic forms and actual despots.

In the sunny, apparently idyllic setting of California, it was the subsequent writings of Herbert Marcuse which captured most attention, particularly among students. In his book *Eros and Civilization*, written in 1955, Marcuse posited a distinction between the repression of the instincts necessary for any civilisation, and what he termed 'surplus repression' enforced by a society of exploitation and class domination.[49] In *One-Dimensional Man*, published a decade later, he argued that modern capitalism transforms dissent into the technical problems of the social system, smoothing economic and social inequality through cultural incorporation and employing consumerism to bolster wasteful production and promote acquisitive personal competition and environmental destruction.[50] For Marcuse, the cultural dimension of existence had become a hugely significant force in modern society. It was no longer a small matter but fundamental to modern life.

As this analysis was being formulated in exile, some of the original Frankfurt School, ill at ease with the US's brand of cultural commercialisation, chose to return to Germany. Back in Europe, from the late 1960s, they passed their Enlightenment baton to a new generation. Most significant among these is Jürgen Habermas, who shifted the scope of the Frankfurt School analysis to the long-term Cultural Transitions of modern capitalism. Habermas (born in 1929) completed his first major work in 1961, an analysis of what he referred to as the 'public sphere', the discursive and representational space formed during emergent capitalism, particularly in Britain. In the transition to capitalism, said Habermas, following the analysis of Walter Benjamin, one aspect of culture – art – became a commodity, no longer remaining part of the Church's or court's 'publicity of representation'.[51] Art thus entered the public sphere despite being a commodity. Its cultural significance lay in wealth. For Habermas, a key feature of modernisation was the formation of civil society, separate from the State and commerce, principally composed of the new middle class. The emergence of civil society, he says, accompanies the formation of a depersonalised State authority. For Habermas, the public sphere declines almost as soon as it emerges, shaped by corporately formed mass culture and the onset of public administration which controls society's institutions that help steer culture. Thus the promise of democratising the public sphere is repressed and channelled. What started as an open discursive space is closed down or commodified or subverted. Habermas thus reconnected his social critique to that of Adorno and Horkheimer.

Habermas saw the Cultural Transition as occurring on two levels. In the first, one sees changes in the structure of rationality through the process Max Weber had called the 'disenchantment of the world'. 'Precisely the ultimate and most sublime values have retreated from public life either into the transcendental realm of mystic life or into the brotherliness of direct and personal human relations.'[52] Here, the locked-in primarily religious belief systems of society are disestablished. Religious belief becomes private, whereas earlier it was everyday, communal and directive (keeping people within its boundaries). The monasteries of the mind are dissolved by an intellectualisation driven by external pressures and seismic events. In the second transition, Habermas suggests there is progressive rationalisation of what he called the 'lifeworld'. By this he did not mean the 'lifeworld' as sketched by the German philosopher Edmund Husserl (1859–1938), better known as the father of phenomenology, who had also used it. Husserl's notion of lifeworld was an individual one, a world of private consciousness and perception. For Habermas, by contrast, lifeworld means the inter-subjective, cultural sphere of shared meanings and interpretations. This becomes rationalised in the sense of it becoming subject to reason. It becomes self-reflective and a conscious process. It happens through language and is openly expressed. People can articulate their lifeworld. It can be made conscious and be chosen not imposed. Here, Habermas described a process of human communication becoming free of narrowly restricted contexts by the enlargement of the public sphere of actions. As the rationalisation of the lifeworld has occurred, said Habermas, people have become able to reflect upon tradition and to distance themselves from the world of tradition, which thereby has lost its quasi-natural status.

In these two processes of modernisation, Habermas argues, Western culture has been able to become more secular, and modern societies have become more rational, driven by the influence of the empirical sciences, autonomous arts, and new principles-based theories of morality and law.[53] This new version of Frankfurt thinking drew upon a strand of progressive American philosophical thought which was not explored by his Frankfurtian predecessors, specifically the school of American pragmatism associated with the names of Charles Sanders Peirce (1839–1914), William James (1842–1910), John Dewey (1859–1952) and George Herbert Mead (1863–1931). Their ideas are illuminating on culture.

American pragmatism was initiated by the startlingly fresh amalgam of science, semiotics and philosophy provided by Charles Sanders Peirce. William James, one of the founders of modern psychology, was probably more feted and more influential in Europe than the USA, although this influence was later to wane.[54] John Dewey was America's most distinctive public intellectual in the early twentieth century, comparable in influence to J.S. Mill in Britain, and providing an analysis of, and influential counterweight to, America's growing corporate and conservative tendencies. While the focus of each varies (even down to disputes over the meaning of 'pragmatism' as a term), they all began from a common basis in European philosophy and in particular a vital understanding of the implications of Darwin's discoveries for the analysis of the human psyche. Note, it is Darwin rather than Freud. In Chicago, Mead (who despite his brilliance never wrote a book, and is now known only for his lecture notes published posthumously!) integrated Hegel and Kant's idealist perspective on human progress with the social and psychological implications he drew from Darwin. In fact, said Mead, the doctrine of Hegel and Darwin was 'the same'. What Darwin achieved was to show how human development had arisen on a naturalistic, materialistic basis. Until then it was thought that humankind's structures of mind and identity were constructions of thought alone.

As he observed: 'It must be confessed that Hegel's philosophy was an affair of thought for its own sake and failed to come out of the philosophical chamber into the living world where it should give man the method of living.'[55] In other words the 'living world' of Darwin's naturalism required a full extension into philosophy, sociology and psychology which Darwin had not been able or motivated to do; his interest was more biological. Axel Honneth, a younger Frankfurt scholar, has observed that Mead converted the Darwinian model of the organism responding to its environment to a social plane. While social Darwinism adopted a conservative biological reading of Darwin, the US pragmatists turned Darwinian insights in a societally progressive philosophical direction.

Pragmatism as a theory is quite unlike what one would expect from the conventional use of the word. It draws from an understanding of human practical-cum-conceptual development. Pragmatism developed into, on the one hand, the exploration of ordinary human problem-solving processes and, on the other hand, into a system for generating a more complete scientific understanding. The first is based on common sense (in effect a form of low-level practical reason). To quote Axel Honneth again, 'it is precisely in situations in which actions are problematicized during their performance that humans make cognitive gains'.[56] The other direction taken by the pragmatists was the philosophy of science, providing a methodology for understanding nature. A distinction is being made between everyday understandings as culture and the more formal structure approach to generating knowledge from scientific investigations. The value of the pragmatic perspective for public health evidence is considered in the final chapter.

For Mead, the key distinction in life was between 'I' and 'me', by which he meant one's internal life and the public persona. The 'I' is not immediately aware of itself; the 'me' is the version of oneself from the perspective of an outsider. This Mead called 'the generalised other'. Sense of self is always engaged with sense of the other, outside oneself. Identities are always in a process of development or emergence. We are always interacting with others. The cultural dimension of life is thus constantly in flux, being read into one's internal life, and subject to change and growth in a way that is directly analogous to processes in the natural world, of which humans are a part. There are linkages between identity formation, the processes of inter-subjectivity, and social existence. These are real processes which frame human lives. This exchange is formed in language, shapes moral development, and interacts with the external environment. Patterns of societal change are embedded in social psychological processes and in the natural environment. Patently, we are not isolated atoms in the world but members of changing social processes and reflecting and recreated identities. Culture is embedded in this process. The American pragmatists thus raised the question: what is the relationship of the personal to the environment?

Habermas picks up these themes from the pragmatists. The lifeworld is an inter-subjective, culturally transmitted and linguistically assembled reservoir of meanings and patterns of thinking and being. The rationalisation of the lifeworld implies the drawing together of a society where people make decisions through discussion or 'deliberation'. Thus Habermas breaks with the older European intellectual traditions with their older models of human agency, be they Marx's proletariat, Hegel's world spirit or Kant's subject-centred rationality. Unfortunately, says Habermas, the ideal conditions for the lifeworld exist only as a potential. The reason is that, in late capitalism, the Cultural Transition is a contest between the lifeworld and the *system* – the organised structure of societal functions: administrative, economic and social. The relationship between the lifeworld and the system, he says, is incipiently one of colonisation, with the system taking over the lifeworld; in effect the interpersonal and personal space is captured by stronger forces. For Habermas, the lifeworld is always in transition, always adapting, always renewing itself. Culture is contested space.

The constant churn and creativity of the public sphere and of the lifeworld occurs in new ways today, compared to the past, but the relationship of the lifeworld to the system is one of ever-present tension. In this regard, for Habermas, like Weber before him, societies are managed through political domination. Order is imposed.

> Political domination has socially integrating power only insofar as disposition over means of sanction does not rest on naked repression, but on the authority of an office anchored in turn in a legal order. For this reason laws need to be intersubjectively recognized by citizens; they have to be legitimated as right and proper. This leaves culture with the task of supplying reasons why an existing political order deserves to be recognized.[57]

To sum up, in the eyes of the Frankfurt School past and present, culture is not simply a creative add-on to society, a discussion about art (although it explained the development and fate of art) or just the product of the so-called creative industries, whose role, said the earlier generation of Frankfurt theorists, was simply to corrode individual creativity. Today, culture is both an essential and a growing arena of contest. It is both industry and politics, and it is particularly a matter of language. Positively, according to Habermas: '[n]o one possesses exclusive rights over the common medium of the communicative practices we must intersubjectively share'.[58] Language and human communication is therefore not a kind of private property. It is the area where contest normally occurs in societies where there is a modicum of freedom.

Where does this description of some of the insights from Frankfurt, via the USA, offer value for public health? In our discussion of the Economic Transition (see Chapter 8), we were reminded of how capital, Nature and labour are core elements for understanding economics. That is the old conception of economics, which the neoliberal market economists have downplayed, reducing economic processes to capital and the market, as we saw. In a not dissimilar fashion, the Frankfurt School view of the Cultural Transition returns social theories to older traditions of philosophy, based on notions of liberty, moral choice and self-development, all shaped and constrained by wider social and moral forces. For Habermas, politics will only be reinvigorated by the promotion of deliberative democracy and strengthened legal and juridical systems. Therein lies an opposition to the various versions of neoconservative thinking which have reshaped the West through the Washington Consensus and the triumph of Chicago School market economics.

One of the most powerful thinkers among modern conservatives, countering this Frankfurtian critique, is the US sociologist Daniel Bell (1919–2011). He coined the term 'post-industrial society'. In his 1976 book *The Cultural Contradictions of Capitalism*, Bell gave a direct riposte to Habermas's view of the tensions within the social structures of late capitalism. Bell said that it was all too simplistic, that 'it is all too easy to say, as many radicals do, that all of this is a consequence of "capitalism"'.[59] While Bell saw Habermas's analysis of the legitimation problems of capitalism as essentially 'correct', he did not agree that the administrative or cultural system has the corrosive qualities ascribed by Habermas. On the contrary, said Bell, the problem of capitalism, its 'cultural contradictions' of the book title, relates to the fact that the original cultural drivers of its success, as identified by Weber, in the form of the Protestant ethic, and Tocqueville, have lost their appeal. People have become consumerist and lost the initial (worthy) drives to work and be diligent. For Bell, as for some US conservatives, modernity is the problem; it threatens to undermine the origins of its success. The answer to the corrosive effect of modernism (not capitalism), according to Bell, lay in the revival of religion. In lamenting the loss of a society where people diligently go to work and to church, and act within culturally conformist rules of the day, this critique stands Max Weber on his head. Instead of religion and moral standards fuelling capitalism and industry, today religion is called upon to act as a brake on the cultural forces that capitalism has now released. This is the analysis that writers such as Putnam, outlined above, implicitly share.

A more radical rejoinder to Habermas's arguments (although Habermas described them as essentially conservative) is that the Cultural Transition remains a legacy of the Enlightenment. This has been proposed by a diverse group of scholars, many of whom trace their intellectual lineage to another German philosopher, Friedrich Nietzsche (1844–1900). Nietzsche saw history as shaped by the search for power; everything is about power and its resistance.[60] Only a type of super-philosopher, an *Übermensch*, can stand outside that process to give perspective and observe the titanic forces at work. Among the many analysts who follow Nietzsche's accounts of power, perhaps the French historian of ideas Michel Foucault is the most prominent.[61] For Foucault, social life is determined by power. There is no autonomous space of civil society or lifeworld, as Habermas argued. Everything is shaped by power. According to one critical account, Foucault's version of the rise and development of civil society 'is negative from the start'.[62] There is no public space, no creative opportunities for release from the tensions articulated by the Frankfurt thinkers. Everything appears a modern and systemic rolling out of a new form of absolutism. Whereas the Frankfurt School described culture as a dialectical process of opposing forces, mediated by inner and outer realities, for Foucault everything is a construction of the powerful. So strong is this conception of power, one which appears in the very pores of society, that historian Lauren Goodlad has observed that the notion of culture itself 'has neither an integral place nor an adequate correlative in Foucault's method of analysis'.[63] Culture is a myth.

It is no surprise that the exchange between these two thinkers, Foucault and Habermas, which stretched across the wide landscapes of European cultural philosophy, received no easy resolution or even meeting of minds. Cultural thinking to some extent remains split into camps of rival followers, with different schools of analysis and research broadly identifying with one or the other camp. Foucault died an untimely death from AIDS, an ironic fact for the theorist of 'biopower' who had argued that the body is the site of the ultimate contestation between self and external power. Nevertheless, the impact of Foucault in reminding public health analysts that bodies and physiology have a cultural significance is important and remains. The work of sociologists such as the Australian Deborah Lupton has explored this cultural dimension to the meaning of human physiological frailty and how culture frames the body.[64] This is a line of thinking which resonates with the feminist critique of body-centrism and the heightened awareness of the impact of male-dominated notions of beauty and body size, and how women can internalise these cultural norms as oppression.[65]

Culture and behaviour change

The importance of the above debates for public health is simply that for the last century or so, in the name of public health, people and organisations have tried to change human behaviour, to help the public with the consequences of either its own actions (unhealthy behaviour) or its acceptance of unhealthy circumstances (unhealthy environments). As we summarised in Part I, there are multiple images and models of what is meant by public health. Two models in particular have resonance for the discussion of the Cultural Transition: the Techno-Economic and the Social-Behavioural models. Both raise and attempt to answer a core challenge for public health, the problem of control. Who is in control of culture? Who and what can reshape behaviour and its determinants for health? Is this even possible? Or are people dupes of their circumstances?

In the Techno-Economic model, cultural change is driven by a tacit alliance of economic development and growth of knowledge. Culture is viewed as malleable, something to be altered in the name of progress. The prime example given by the economic historian Joel Mokyr, for example, is the linkage between the marketing of hygiene products a century or so ago, the emerging scientific knowledge of germs, and the establishment of new social norms to shape behaviour and drive consumption of those products.[66] Thus women were exhorted to have cleaner homes, to buy new domestic and personal hygiene products which would aid the smell and look of their homes, to change how they and their families viewed their bodies and bodily functions, to alter and 'modernise' their sense of self as homemakers, and to reshape what was considered a beautiful functioning home and domestic sphere. Thus, the Cultural Transition seen through the

Techno-Economic lens is of a kind of sanitary enlightenment, the process of giving new rules for everyday living, and of science and marketing framing new norms for what is deemed acceptable and 'righteous' behaviour.

The Social-Behavioural model begins with an assumption of a knowledge deficit. From the early nineteenth century, this model has been invoked to help people improve their health literacy. They are assumed to be broadly ignorant and suffering from a lack of solid knowledge. The rules of everyday living that have to be instilled, it follows, are the transmission of simplified expert knowledge which will improve the public health outcomes by changing cultural norms. Trying to persuade people to wash their hands before and after going to the toilet or when preparing food is culture change. Discouraging spitting in public to combat TB is also culture change. Another example is the late-twentieth-century global effort to improve diet through the slogan to eat 'five [portions of fruit and vegetables] a day'. The origins of this health education programme, now worldwide, are found in the epidemiological evidence from the British epidemiologists Richard Doll (1912– 2005) and Richard Peto that raised consumption of fruit and vegetables had a direct impact on rates of cancer.[67] This knowledge was then translated into 'marketing' terms via the five-a-day slogan, set at that level partly to accommodate the realities of low consumption by Californians.[68] It was also created by a partnership between the US fruit and vegetable industry and the public health authorities. Whatever the commercial impetus, public health professionals tend to take comfort from the evidence thus far that such attempts to change culture can work, if suitably funded and resourced.[69] However, to evaluate such programmes as successful is to ignore wider forces going in precisely contrary directions. The five-a-day message has had to compete with huge marketing budgets for processed foods, just as the message to take more exercise is countered by the message to view cars as cultural icons.

A difference between the two models is the role of the State and commercial actors who benefit or stand to benefit. In the Techno-Economic model, the public impact may be incidental rather than deliberate, whereas for the Social-Behavioural model the intent is overt and planned. The Social-Behavioural model is essentially health education without the technical or economic imperatives.

Advertising and marketing shaping the rules for everyday life

The WHO has taken an increasingly concerned position on the role of the marketing of 'unhealthy' products, particularly food. Its scepticism was shaped by the half-century-long struggle to control the marketing of tobacco products, a line of goods about which there is little health doubt; they are very bad for health. Food is more difficult, where the debate about whether there are good or bad foods is more complex; is the public health concern over particular products or total diets? There is little doubt that commercial marketing contributes to the obesity epidemic. As one international group of researchers has observed, food marketing to children is massive. Expanding through communication channels, composed almost entirely of messages for nutrient-poor, calorie-dense foods, it is increasingly global and therefore difficult to regulate by individual countries.[70] Large food processors, for obvious reasons, resist the notion that any of their products might actually be harmful for health and have pushed the 'total diet' approach. In 2006, the WHO grasped the nettle and laid out an approach and range of measures that could be considered by national governments to constrain the marketing of non-alcoholic drinks and foods to children.[71] These ranged from regulation to controls by other forms. The focus on children is and was significant. Both sides of the arguments agree that children are vulnerable to influence, yet marketers frequently deny that they ever target them. Increasing alarm about food companies shaping young consumers' views of food – as fun, cool or desirable – has led to a new generation of public health campaigns to set standards by which marketing can be either regulated or at least monitored or self-regulated. Supporting the creation of such standards, the WHO's assistant director stated in 2006 the importance of ensuring that 'children everywhere are protected against the impact of such marketing and given the opportunity to grow and develop in an enabling food environment'.[72]

In 2011, the sum spent globally on advertising of all goods and services, not just food or drinks, was an estimated $466 billion, with unregulated internet advertising rising rapidly inside that total, to £72 billion in that year.[73] Measured advertising expenditure grew by 50 per cent in 1995–2009 worldwide, according to one academic drawing upon industry sources.[74] In 2011, an estimated $148 billion was to be spent in the USA alone.[75] Figures on advertising, let alone wider marketing expenditure, are notoriously hard to obtain. The figures just cited were from WPP, one of the industry global giants, presumably reliable, and gold dust for the industry as it jostles for business and trends. The figures are also hard to collate in a coherent manner and should be taken as approximate. What matters is that new regions are coming into the global advertising and marketing arena, with the Far East growing in particular as it develops economically. Advertising spending is fragile, however. The Arab Spring of 2011 reduced advertising spending in that region by an estimated $1.4 billion, for example.

The picture on marketing expenditure is made more complex by the emergence of new forms which have relatively low budgets such as viral marketing, the deliberate creation of 'news stories' which attract consumers to view or hear them, spreading by consumer-to-consumer interaction and transmission. Another form is product placement on TV programmes and in films, where manufacturers (usually it is they) pay for their product to be displayed, with the logo or name prominent. The product is enhanced by the script. Yet another aspect of marketing is the rise and rise of public relations (PR). This is the cultural industry which manages the public face of sponsors. In a world hooked on to the internet and where image is all, PR has become intrinsic to the business model. PR may be itself a misleading term. According to a study of the industry by David Miller and William Dinan, British academic researchers who run the Spinwatch website, the word 'propaganda' is more appropriate, because 'it implies the unity of communication and action. It is communication for a purpose.'[76] In their view, 'spin' includes the work of not just PR agencies but policy think tanks and research

teams who suggest they are neutral, disinterested parties but are de facto communications arms for concealed commercial interests. As a result, the distinction
between journalism and PR has been blurred. One study suggested that in the
USA in 1980 there were 45 PR workers for every 36 journalists, but by 2008 this
had risen to 90 PR people for every 25 journalists.[77] This study pointed to the
emergence of monopoly press ownership and a collapse of independent journalism, alongside the rise of corporate media communications. The newspaper is
a medium in rapid decline, its place taken by electronic media with their more
robust, less capitalised business model.

The critique of the socially negative role of marketing is not new. Herbert Marcuse, as we outlined above, was arguing in the 1960s that Western societies were
becoming 'one-dimensional', with protest and oppositions to consumerist capitalism being diffused and even incorporated.[78] Half a century on, is that criticism true?
In the USA, while independent cultural media channels for debate such as local
papers have declined, new channels have emerged, notably through the internet
and telecom-based mobility. These are now powerful media for cultural debate,
but power over them has continued to centralise. Advertising funds much of the
internet by placing advertisements with websites. Facebook and Twitter are private
corporations, funded by advertising. Facebook, for example, struck a deal in 2011
with Diageo, the global alcohol giant, based upon the success in boosting some of
its brands by up to 20 per cent in the USA.[79] Diageo is reported to aim to spend
almost 20 per cent of its media spend on digital marketing, out of global marketing
total spend of over $1 billion per year.

The critical issue is the direction of change: is it good or harmful for health? For
Inglehart and colleagues in their global exercise of tracking values, the big cultural
shift is towards secularisation, rationality and democratic values. But these values are
accepted as being in tension with the cultural legacies in societies from their former
existences. Thus the Arab Spring of 2011 – when a wave of democratic impulses
went through the Middle East, destabilising authoritarian regimes and exposing
tensions with religion-based opposition – was a struggle to shake off existing cultural controls and authorities and to battle over which cultural set of rules should
replace them. Political cultures can be confronted, but religions and moral belief
systems are more resistant than others, according to the Inglehart analysis. Edward
Said (1935–2003), the Palestinian-American cultural analyst, disagreed with this
interpretation. Modern life is characterised by a clash, he countered, between versions of ignorance.[80] Said argued that there is no unilinear march towards social
progress in cultural matters, yet one can be clear about the criteria against which
one can judge the changes and differences between and within Cultural Transitions. In this, he was with Inglehart.

Technological impact on culture

The twenty-first century is already hugely affected by the internet, and the emergence of instantaneous communications. But is this new? In the mid-twentieth

century Marshall McLuhan (1911–80) was already pronouncing that the 'medium is the message', which is to say that the technological form of the means of communication was a shaping factor in the substance of that communication.[81] McLuhan offered a neat technological account of the Cultural Transition, suggesting that human exchange has moved from movable type (printing) to electronic media. This has enabled modernity to spread. This argument is an amplification of Walter Benjamin's thesis from within the Frankfurt School that art had lost its gloss and uniqueness through multiple reproduction. The ubiquity of copies of Leonardo da Vinci's painting *Mona Lisa* – in posters on walls worldwide – means that it is impossible to be dominated in the same way by elite notions of beauty and sensibility.

The new technologies of computers, the internet and mobile phones are now cheap and increasingly accessible. Mobile phones have spread through the Far East and Africa despite low incomes. Even small farmers can use mobile phones to better decide when to sell their products and fit propitious times and prices on commodity markets. The impact is remarkable. Relatives around the globe can keep in contact. News can spread through micro-communities. New correspondences emerge through media channels which did not exist a few years ago. Facebook reached half a billion members within less than a decade of its founding. Vertical communication from authorities to the mass populace thus is giving way to more horizontal, person-to-person communication. That is the common interpretation and glossy perspective.

In reality, these democratising tendencies of the new technologies occur within limits and can be under pressure to adapt. The technologies are owned and gate-kept by governments and corporations. They are subject to licences. There are furious political battles about the legitimacy of patents and information sharing. Lawyers increasingly are active in tying down what companies see as 'intellectual piracy' of content, whether of films, music, visuals or writing. Behind the apparent liberation of communication within culture is an unprecedented global reach of intellectual property rights (IPR). Whenever a mobile phone is turned on, the company knows where the person is, and all calls and emails are tracked. No one is anonymous or in a crowd in this new world. And yet the communication possibilities are experienced widely as liberating. Health promoters are now turning to telecoms to aid health. A new sub-discipline has emerged in the form of health informatics, where emails or texts are sent to patients to remind them to take their medicine or to act appropriately or to motivate people to exercise. Smokers are supported in cessation by motivational information delivered in one's hand or on to the computer via emails.

The impact of new technologies, we suggest, can be overemphasised, but equally it should not be dismissed. Previous technical revolutions such as printing, motorised or rail transport and mobility, telegrams and telephone, the fax machine, the postal service and the television (discovered in the late nineteenth century but rolled out as a mass communication in the mid-twentieth century) all form the changing technological infrastructure of the long-term Cultural Transition that this chapter suggests is so central to the public health project. Each round of new technology may shape consumer behaviour. New technologies may indeed become remarkably cheaper, such that even people on low incomes can use them. The ability to transmit information to peers may be democratised but, following the Frankfurt analysis, one should not slide into thinking that this ability to share information non-hierarchically is inevitably democratising. What is new is the ubiquity, pace, scale, transportability, immediacy and accessibility of the new digital technologies. The technical object can easily become both a medium for communication and a signifier of and vehicle for cultural identity and transition.

Health education as cultural intervention

What can public health do to engage with this complex issue of culture and the Cultural Transitions? Indeed, is there anything that can be done other than the small-scale, given the powerful interests which own and shape the technology? Public policy and public health have often both been challenged that they have no place in this cultural terrain. There are no grounds for them to intervene or act. The relationship between health and culture is and should remain private, say neo-liberals. It is up to the individual or family or community to tackle any problem, or indeed to accept if there is a problem. Leave it all to consumer choice in the marketplace. This strand of thinking has been displayed to counter public interventions for centuries. In the 1810s, a debate raged about education in England and whether schooling should be extended beyond the elite and the Church. James Mill (1773–1836), the father of the better-known J.S. Mill, lambasted the established Church for its line that education was for churchmen not the working classes. He took the more liberal, utilitarian line that good government requires an informed and educated citizenry.[82] His son J.S. Mill later encapsulated the issue as: 'It is better to be a human being dissatisfied than a pig satisfied; better to be Socrates dissatisfied than a fool satisfied.'[83] While utilitarians countered religious conservatives, economic liberals countered activist liberals. As so often in England, the outcome was a melange of different principles and strands of thought. In England, pragmatism and idiosyncrasy tended to rule.[84] On the Continent, things were different.

The argument about whether there should be an institutionalised secular form of schooling went on across Europe in the nineteenth century. In Germany, under the patrician leadership of Otto von Bismarck (1815–98), the decision was taken formally to invest in wider schooling for its future State elite through the *Gymnasium* system. England instituted formal schooling on a mass but limited scale only in 1870, triggered partly by concern that it was lacking a sufficiently technically educated workforce for its industry to compete with that of Germany and the USA.[85] This illustrates the difference between English liberalism and continental conformism noted by Max Weber.

In health, the same mixture of advocacy and activism applied. The city of Manchester, which had appalled both the Frenchman Tocqueville and the German Engels, had established a board of health in 1796, following disease outbreaks. It had no real powers, no money and though some political influence almost no political or legislative weight. The Manchester and Salford Sanitary Association, with the Ladies' Sanitary Society later alongside it, was founded in 1852 'to promote attention to Temperance, Personal and Domestic Cleanliness and to the Laws of Health generally' and 'to induce general co-operation with the Boards of Health and other constituted authorities in giving effect to official Regulations for Sanitary Improvement'.[86] The target audience was the working classes, and the message was the benefits of sanitation and temperance. As well as this voluntary educative work, some members believed that the Association should put direct pressure on the local authorities of Manchester and Salford to formalise the cultural mission. They gathered facts on overcrowding, poor water supply, ventilation and sewage. Sanitary reform thus had two central dimensions: health education and sanitary-environmental change.

This argument about the role of learning goes beyond formal schooling or leaflets on washing, nutrition and drinking – all things debated upon in those years. It highlights how culture is learnt, transmitted and shared, and how the norms of daily life are imbibed and collectivised, but also confronted and changed. For public health, these question are still alive today, as the debates on obesity show. How is it that populations have become fatter? Is the core to the fattening of the world's population just the economic dynamic of food costs, overproduction, cheap prices and the ubiquity of food? Or is there not also a cultural as well as an economic dynamic? Is it not also the responsibility of people to keep themselves slim and fit? The low costs and ubiquity of food have altered cultural 'rules' about when and how to eat. People can indulge themselves daily, not just on feast or celebration days. The role of marketing and advertising is to shape culture by reframing the rules of daily life. Individual consumers are faced with an unequal cultural power between themselves and commercial interests. This was why the Mills, father and son, shifted their positions from being in favour of market institutions alone.

J.S. Mill's views are often misread. *On Liberty*, his most famous work and the one he thought was his enduring legacy, has been cast as 'libertarian' and thus supportive of the ideas of a 'free market' as defined by latter-day libertarian think tanks in the late twentieth century among others. According to this view, promoted by the Californian Reason Foundation and many others, J.S. Mill was 'a moral Libertarian'.[87] Advocacy of libertarianism takes many forms. Some are erudite and speculative studies such as Robert Nozick's,[88] and others just catchily titled but crude such as *Nanny State: How Food Fascists, Teetotaling Do-Gooders, Priggish Moralists, and other Boneheaded Bureaucrats Are Turning America into a Nation of Children* by David Harsanyi.[89] Mill would have disowned both. The author of *Political Economy* and *Utilitarianism* had his feet firmly planted in early Victorian social thought but had ingested almost the entire panorama of Western philosophy. In the course of his very active intellectual life, he advocated a mix of utilitarianism (his own term), political economy, feminism, personal freedom, social justice and social and economic democracy. *On Liberty* is a testament to Mill's promotion of diversity in opinion, independence of outlook, the value of education for collective improvement and, most of all, the belief in social progress. The book has to be read in the light of Mill's other writings, not independently of them and in contradiction of them. His views on censorship, of pornography for example, have to be read on the basis of his views on the oppression of women.[90] Indeed, he argued that the experience of social oppression might result in habituation to oppression and thus a form of hidden 'moral coercion'. Late in his life, according to one account, he held hopes for 'a post-bourgeois social order [which] involved a gradual transition to collectively owned, democratically managed worker co-operatives, enabling the elimination of an "idle" capitalist class'.[91] In its fuller picture, therefore, *On Liberty* is neither a manifesto for unbridled selfishness nor obeisance to corporate culture, about which economic libertarians are themselves customarily silent. Indeed, it is the opposite.

The cultural battle over health behaviour is long recognised and widespread. The campaigns to stop spitting in public (to address TB), the appeals to alter sexual behaviour (HIV/AIDS), the rules to wash hands before and after going to the toilet (food-based infections and diarrhoea), and the bans on smoking in public buildings (lung disease), as we have seen, are all examples of public health agencies – sometimes in alliance with other forces, sometimes not – uniting to reshape culture. There are many techniques and schools of thinking upon which public health bodies draw to create new cultural norms, ranging from 'hard' interventions such as laws, regulations and fiscal measures to 'soft' ones such as advice, leaflets and education. There are different and well-established strands of thinking about cultural change and public health. Most centre on notions of learning and education. They also go to the heart of what is discussed in the next chapter on democracy: how can the State help citizens without excessive constraint? How can liberty be enhanced while not allowing some people or groups to be disenfranchised? And is this a function for the State in the first place? And, if not, whose responsibility is it?

Health education as cultural schooling

The Social-Behavioural model of public health relies extensively on cultural change in its toolbox of methods and interventions. It straddles the world of facts and habits, proposing that the delivery of facts will lead to or at least help the aligning of behaviour with rationality. The innocent version of health education is simply this: give people information and the tools for their education, and health will be better protected and enhanced. This strand of thinking stems from the Enlightenment but spreads across the political and policy spectrum, from liberalism to State-centric socialism and from top-down authoritarianism to patrician action, from Immanuel Kant to Ivan Illich, from James and J.S. Mill to John Rawls. In this spread of positions, there is a common reiteration of the value of health education. Everyone needs to be educated, and citizenship requires some regularity of input to ensure that the mass of a population can engage in the mass economy and civil society from a perspective of some literacy. Thus there is a notion that health education is about the building of health literacy.

In this respect, who could possibly oppose health education? Yet they do, or rather they argue about who should do the educating, and for what ends, measured by which values, and by whom it should be delivered. Is it through a benign

State, or enlightened commercial companies delivering information according to corporate responsibility values? Or should the process be left to families? If so, is it the role of mothers or the wider family and community to lead this cultural cascade of information transfer? Or should the process of acculturation to healthy social norms be left to more neutral teachers? If so, who monitors and sets their frame of reference? And is the 'target' population only children and the new generations, or a process of constant updating of adults too?

These questions get translated into moral and practical concerns about schooling and are constantly fought over in politics. In sexual health education, for example, there is often a clash in almost all societies, in all religious traditions and in all modes of schooling. An overview of 68 reports on global trends in sexual health education concluded that this line of education 'had a long and chequered history, its fortunes waxing and waning with the changing of governments and the tide of public opinion'.[92] Sexual health education means many things, ranging from 'Just Say No' campaigns encouraging sexual abstinence, to explicit information on sexual behaviour and historically taboo discussions about sexual practices and their various sexual risks. Not only is the degree of success thus variable but the very notion of health education is itself malleable. It can be direct and interventionist or distant and 'take it or leave it'. It can even be a plea for ignorance, if it takes the form of discussing matters by euphemism rather than directly. The critics of health education argue that getting more information is a proxy for allowing the people in authority to shape young minds; usually their concern is about the State. Thus the idea of health education, which at first sight seems to be beyond contention, is actually contentious. Its appeal as being on the 'soft' side of culture change is somewhat thin. Health education, far from being beyond ideology, is as ideologically framed as other more apparently hard interventions such as regulation, taxation and bans.

Health education as social psychology

If health education generally draws upon the theories of pedagogy and schooling experience to target mass behaviour, in the 1950s a new variant emerged shaped by a concern to alter deviant behaviour and to use the relatively more scientific, newer versions of psychology to do so. Although Freud and psychoanalysis had a huge impact on advertising and marketing, shifting Freud from the clinical couch to Madison Avenue, it was not until health education started to draw on the more laboratory-derived lessons of psychological sciences that behaviour change took on a focused and direct cultural dimension.

The case for targeting behaviour change had been raised in the 1950s by people such as Sir Richard Doll in his work on tobacco and Jerry Morris (1910–2009) on the value of physical activity for health. The case for health education had now been given modern legitimacy; the challenge was how to change population behaviour. The school of psychology then in the intellectually dominant position was behaviourism, in part reacting to the perceived excessive theorising of Freudian psychoanalysis. The philosophical approach to psychology championed by William James in the USA and the instinct-oriented experimentalist psychology of William McDougall (1871–1938) in the UK were difficult to translate into operational form. They were too loose or perhaps too sophisticated in their thinking, when what was needed was means–end science. These early schools of psychology were anyway rejected by the behaviourists. Their rise stemmed from their assault on the unscientific credentials of psychoanalysis, best summarised by the German-English psychologist Hans Eysenck (1916–97) in his 1953 *Uses and Abuses of Psychology*. The new scientific behaviourists argued that the mind was complex and that behaviour could more easily be altered by changing circumstances using reinforcement of 'good' behaviour and the punishment of 'bad' behaviour. There was no need to impute deep motives or theorise the legacy of evolution in instincts when behaviour and how humans relate can be shaped by conditioning. One does not need notions of consciousness or instincts to reframe motives and behaviour.

B.F. Skinner (1904–90), professor of psychology at Harvard University, advocated operant conditioning, the application of rewards to sanction the undesirable. Skinner argued that psychology showed how behaviour, reasoning and even language were all subject to positive and negative conditioning, and that these conditioning mechanisms could be identified and shaped to promote societal improvement on liberal lines.[93] He summarised this combination of behaviour control and happiness politics in his novel *Walden Two* written in 1948, an extension of Henry David Thoreau's 1854 Massachusetts lakeside musing about the meaning of life and how a good society could be made.[94] Culture need not be mysterious, the behaviourists (in all variants) argued. It was malleable, given the right levers and collective purpose.

That clarity of behaviourist message for culture change was altered by the more complex thinking of cognitive and developmental psychologists. They stressed the complexities of lifelong learning and how competing forces send different signals to shape behaviour and how these interact with inherited mechanisms and genetic potential. A leading example was the Swiss child psychologist Jean Piaget (1896–1980). Piaget argued that cognitive development goes through stages and that learning cannot occur until the person is ready. Infants go through discernible structures of change as they grow into children. By implication, there is no point in educating children beyond the stage of their development. Piaget's work was immensely influential in the classroom, particularly early-years schooling, but other cognitive psychologists had a more direct impact on health education. One was Albert Bandura, professor of psychology at Stanford University in California, the father of social learning theory.[95] Bandura (born 1923) started as a behaviourist but became a social learning theorist who accepted the subtleties of mental processing. The cognitive psychologists began to link context and environment with cognitive processes, enabling a more nuanced approach to health education. As Bandura wrote: '[a] comprehensive approach to health promotion requires changing the practices of social systems that have widespread detrimental effects on health rather than solely changing the habits of individuals'.[96] Gone is the crudity of Skinner or the idea that individuals are in control of their destiny. Thus, at the end of the twentieth century, psychology edged back into the more philosophical terrain of earlier psychologists such as William James. The major change was the re-emergence of biologically oriented psychology, invoking genetics and the predispositions to learning endowed by evolution.

Health education as social marketing

Social marketing is now the common parlance and substitute for what used to be called health education. It is the application of marketing techniques and insights to public purposes, often paid for or certainly approved by public authorities. Modern writers about social marketing draw their legitimacy from the apparent effectiveness of commercial marketing and the deep unfashionableness of 'traditional' health education measures such as leaflets, advice and information. It invokes the weight of psychological theories as applied in the commercial world to offer the promise that, if the public purse shaped marketing messages and means to the pursuit of public goods, health improvement would follow.

A key exponent is the US social marketer Alan Andreasen. His argument is that marketing itself is today a normal and uncontroversial part of the economy. Social marketing thus merely works with the grain of economic normality. Given that the commercial world is now the 'normal world', there is no contest between public and private spheres. Health problems in society are by implication either due to or in part due to a deficit of positive messages for health. Social marketing fills that gap. Andreasen and colleagues say that if there is no public sponsor there may be a mutual benefit between public health advocates and commercial organisations. An example he gives is of boys and girls clubs in the USA working with the soft drinks industry.[97] There is a meeting of interests, with civil society bodies tapping into deeper sources of funds and, for industry, an opportunity to meet corporate responsibility goals while selling more soft drinks. The focus is on individual change because, as Andreasen has written, 'it is *individuals* who make change happen'.[98]

This approach to social marketing is easy to dismiss as cynical or thin commercialism and politically naive. Social marketing, however, has more sophisticated positions and advocates. One argument is that it can be used to reinforce health messages from authoritative voices by translating what otherwise can be seen as 'top-down' and worthy messages into forms appropriate to the target audience. Too much health education is patronising and insensitive to the interests of people on low incomes, for example, and the skill of the marketer is to understand people's real lives and interests, so as to tailor behaviour change messages to their world not the health educators' world. From this perspective, social marketing is a refined tool for public health, based on nuanced understanding of social segmentation. It is about meeting consumer needs and wants and framing health to existing rather than idealised situations.[99] In this sense, social marketing is not new, merely continuing the best work of more traditional forms of health education, but under a banner which has been rebranded and into which new funds, new techniques and new communication channels have been drilled. There is, however, a gulf between these two terms: social marketing and health education. The one is based on the view that the market can do almost no wrong, while the other reserves the right to state that the market may be or is part of the problem. This is a terrain of cultural dispute.[100]

An example of this gulf comes from one of the biggest social marketing campaigns ever conducted in the West, the 'VERB™ – It's What You Do' campaign in the USA. This was a trademarked campaign to encourage US young people aged 9 to 13 years to be more physically active. It was run in 2002–06 by the authoritative US Centers for Disease Control and Prevention (CDC), based in Atlanta, Georgia.[101] For the CDC, 'Social marketing campaigns apply commercial marketing strategies to influence the voluntary behavior of target audiences to improve personal and social welfare.'[102] The evaluation of this huge campaign showed a heightened awareness among 81 per cent of 9- to 13-year-old Americans, who were reported to have engaged in about one more session of physical activity in a typical week than those who were not aware. Awareness varied, with 63 per cent of black American children having awareness of the social marketing. The campaign was funded on a vast scale by conventional health education standards. It received $125 million to start up in 2001, $68 million in 2002, $51 million in 2003, $36 million in 2004 and $59 million in 2005, totalling $339 million. The CDC verdict was that, with adequate investment, health marketing 'shows promise'.[103] Unfortunately this national campaign did not make the link to nutrition nor engage with the dominance of car culture on which the CDC has been a fount of data. In a perhaps veiled acknowledgment of this glaring omission, the campaign co-ordinator at CDC said 'it was a pleasant surprise that we had any behavior change', noting that the third of a billion spent on physical activity marketing paled into insignificance compared to the billions spent on food marketing in the USA.[104]

Another example of social marketing was the English experiment Change4Life. This was a social marketing campaign set up by the Department of Health as part of its strategy to tackle rising levels of obesity, focusing on children and families, particularly those at risk and in low-income brackets. It was awarded £75 million across three years.[105] A fun brand image was created; commercial partners in the media and industry were won, and a witty package of lightly toned materials and messages was created to encourage behaviour change – eating less but better, and taking more exercise. Eight different types of behaviour were targeted including reduced intake of saturated fat, sugar and snacks and a reduction of sedentary activity. After one year, participating retail shops and stores marketing fruit and vegetables with the Change4Life branding reported an average of 10.6 per cent increased sales volume.[106] Change4Life built upon the slow legacy of long-term health campaigns such as five-a-day, another US import. Nonetheless, public funds promoting fruit and vegetables in a country where roughly £0.5 billion a year is spent on food advertising, almost all for processed food, was welcomed. The work of social marketing in the UK was championed by the National Social Marketing Centre, hosted initially by the National Consumer Council.

In France, the big experiment in social marketing is the EPODE project set up to tackle childhood obesity in the 2000s. EPODE (Ensemble Prévenons l'Obésité De nos Enfants), or in English 'Let's prevent childhood obesity together', was set up to tackle childhood obesity. It began in northern France but spread through France, and was picked up in Belgium, Spain, Greece, Mexico and South Australia, with an international alliance being created. In each case it is adapted to local conditions. The key feature of EPODE is the behaviour of the children in the context of the whole family, the environment and social norms at the community level (town or village). It incorporates positive appreciation of balanced diets, while stigmatisation either of obese and overweight children or of 'unhealthy' products is avoided. At the national level, EPODE operates as a public–private partnership between a non-governmental organisation (NGO), a commercial communication agency, corporate partners (which fund the initiative with local authorities) and a scientific committee.[107]

For many years the programme's efficacy and scientific legitimacy mostly rested on one early study. In the second phase, 2004–08, in the EPODE pilot cities, the prevalence of obesity and overweight among 5- to 12-year-old children showed signs of decline.[108] Another review concluded that, at the national level, childhood obesity was no longer increasing, except in particular settings, but that the investment in the EPODE cities reinforced this trend. It was noted that additional efforts were needed to reach people in a situation of social vulnerability.[109] Overall it is difficult to answer the question as to whether the undoubted improvement shown by the data was due to the EPODE methodology or some other factors. A problem was that little is known about qualitative changes in behaviour or how far EPODE towns differ from non-EPODE towns, and about the impact of other national and local initiatives. Other problems have been raised in an independent programme evaluation.[110] Funding is mostly private and non-transparent. Leadership of EPODE is not held by the public sector. Local authority actions are symbolic resources for the promoters and owners of the EPODE brand and the corporate sponsors. This allows large commercial sponsors to speak of their corporate social responsibility when otherwise their products and practice appear contradictory to health. In 2010 Nestlé spent 'well over half a million Euros each year' on its sponsorship of EPODE and related initiatives, and it referred to EPODE as 'one of Nestlé's flagship collaborations'.[111] In the same year Nestlé's profit, according to the company website, was US$35.7 billion.

Like the US VERB initiative, EPODE says little about a world in which food marketing is so powerful. On the contrary, the explicit principle within EPODE is that no food or food category should be stigmatised. EPODE and its various international variants constitute a respected private–public partnership, attracting support from the European Commission, and emulation in countries as far apart as Mexico and Australia.[112] But the question might be asked how much more effective it would be if the restrictions placed upon it were lifted and a more environmental focus was present.

Social marketing is also being applied to one of the thorniest public health difficulties, smoking. Health education has grappled with behaviour change for decades, but today anti-smoking campaigns have turned to social marketing for hope.

In the UK, the longest existing campaign has been No Smoking Day, an attempt to have one instance of high-profile, non-judgemental encouragement to smokers to seek help to stop. The first No Smoking Day was held in 1984, and the evidence base dates from then. Smoking prevalence in the UK was then 36 per cent of adults, tobacco advertisements were shown on television and were permitted in magazines, and smoking was allowed in cinemas, on buses and on the London Underground (railway). In the same year, there was a major fire in the busiest Underground station, King's Cross, which precipitated a culture change in Underground behaviour. Smoking was banned on the Underground, and a huge effort was made to keep the trains and stations clean and dust and detritus free. This triggered a culture change. Although the dangers of cigarette smoking were widely known, until then smoking prevalence varied little by socio-economic group; it was accepted as a cultural choice across all social classes. Yet, within 30 years, that culture changed, smoking rates declined, and this has been widely greeted as a public health success story.[113] By 2010, there were clear differences in behaviour across the social classes. No Smoking Day capitalised on the change in culture and, with other anti-smoking organisations, led it. There has been a decline in smoking, but far less among working-class communities, a class dimension evident across cultures.[114]

In the UK, smoking also became more common among young people, especially young women, and varies considerably by ethnicity. This is the background to UK No Smoking Day now describing itself as a social marketing exercise. Is that just a rebranding of the actions it was doing anyway? Social marketing can easily be the new name for existing practices, sharpened up perhaps but nothing particularly new. The cultural dimension to this public health problem was clearly factored into the WHO's 2003 Framework Convention on Tobacco Control. This recommended that governments deliver social protection from commercially driven change agents. It favoured the 'hard' end of available measures, in contrast to the general espousal of 'soft' measures in social marketing. The Framework Convention recommendations included:[115]

- increasing taxes on tobacco;
- action on smuggling;
- bans on advertising, promotion and sponsorship;
- bans on the use of misleading terms;
- changes to packaging;
- protection of citizens from smoking at work and in public places.

In well-regulated contexts the health impact of tobacco is likely to decline. Growth in tobacco sales, and consequently associated levels of tobacco-related mortality, is appearing in India, China and other parts of Asia, where it has been suggested that attributable deaths will increase from 1.1 million in 1990 to 4.2 million by 2020.[116]

Social marketing has been taken up enthusiastically by public authorities, even up to the level of the World Bank.[117] Much of it has a plainly utilitarian bent. Health promotion is used to stem rising health costs, on the basis of the simple argument that, if commercial marketing can shift culture, so can social marketing.[118] Whether social marketing can resolve the complexities of the Nutrition, Epidemiological or Energy Transitions seems doubtful. The wiser advocates of social marketing know this, but politicians have fallen for the snappy and 'cool' marketing messages, perhaps because they now inhabit that world themselves when campaigning for election. Without deeper explanation and considerable reservations, social marketing is often merely hyperbole, another formula for communicating health education messages, some of which hit their mark and others of which do not. For Andreasen, a big problem is how to market social marketing; it is an industry.[119] For us, the problem with social marketing, as with the analysis of social capital earlier, is that it operates with little serious social theory of how belief is formed. Nor do many of its theorists face up to the scale and negative impact of commercial marketing or what might be called, to coin a phrase, anti-social marketing.

Personal responsibility for health is always part of the picture, even if it emerges more as a matter of assertion than of analysis.[120] Lacking a social theory of how individual behaviour is formed, social marketers have been accused of relying too heavily on strategies aimed at changing individual behaviour and paying too little attention to environmental factors.[121] This point has strongly been made in the developing world in relation to the crisis of HIV/AIDS. Tackling sexually transmitted diseases requires acute understanding of cultural norms. If social marketing is part of Western 'normality', its applicability depends on the spread of that marketing-led approach to daily life.[122] One cannot discount the possibility of positive gains from the use of marketing and advertising. Providing enough money is spent, campaigns can grab public attention. [123] They can create more positive beliefs and attitudes. What is easily forgotten once the marketers have packed their bags and gone on to other campaigns, following the funds, is that there is no effective reinforcement – to use the psychological term – to maintain those beliefs and behaviour after the campaign has concluded. As one observer has suggested, the evaluation literature has been 'more concerned with immediate behavior change than sustainability of effects'.[124] That insight is not lost on the real commercial world, which is why brands receive endless reinforcement, known in the trade as 'buffing'.

Mild cultural change via nudge

Anxious to avoid the accusation of being too interventionist, some governments and companies have been enamoured of an approach known colloquially as 'nudge'. This thinking was promoted in a book of the same name.[125] The authors, Richard Thaler and Cass Sunstein, define their approach as at the soft end of interventions. Hard measures such as taxes, bans or regulations are to be avoided. Nudge thinking accepts people as volitional, conscious beings making choices. People do not need or want constraint. Nudge encourages rather than forbids, entices rather than controls. The way to change behaviour, argue the authors, is to nudge people in the right direction. Nudging uses:[126]

any aspect of the choice architecture that alters people's behaviour in a predictable way without forbidding any options or significantly changing their economic incentives. To count as a mere nudge, the intervention must be easy and cheap to avoid. Nudges are not mandates. Putting the fruit at eye level counts as a nudge. Banning junk food does not.

What can it do for health? Reviewing the approach, the UK House of Lords Science and Technology Committee recognised that nudges are designed to 'prompt choices without getting people to consider their options consciously, and therefore do not include openly persuasive interventions such as media campaigns and the straightforward provision of information'.[127] Nudge is thus even softer than social marketing or traditional health education. As we wrote elsewhere, nudge is being presented as new when it is not, effective for public health when its evidence base is so far thin, and a means for avoiding the self-defeating, heavy-handedness of the State.[128] The intellectual origins of nudge thinking are interesting, with a strong position on the role of culture. Nudge draws upon the notion of social norms and the 1930s social science argument that social norms set the framework within which behaviour occurs.[129] This insight was incorporated into US advertising dicta, fused with what they had already adapted from Freud and the depth psychologists.[130]

What *is* new, in the form in which it is championed by Thaler and Sunstein, is the injection of the psychological view of behaviour into neoclassical economics, a world in which it was previously thought that rational consumers make informed choices and that these drive markets. As we noted in the discussion of the Economic Transition (see Chapter 8), the notion of human behaviour being emotional and irrational at times in economic choices was made by Adam Smith and J.S. Mill among others. It is not a new notion, although behavioural economists publicly go along with the image. These free market origins, in its modern version, are used to explain why consumers make the 'wrong' choices: hence the attraction of nudge for governments of different political persuasions in the UK in the 2000s and 2010s.[131] Nudge simplifies delicate political issues. Instead of blaming the 'wrong' consumers for the 'wrong' choices, or alienating powerful manufacturers and retailers, governments could downplay the complexity of real-life contexts and focus upon the immediate cues for consumer choice.

The UK government backs nudge thinking, and social marketing such as that via Change4Life, outlined above, despite having been presented with a more complex analysis by its own Government Office for Science. In a widely lauded report by the chief scientist's Foresight Programme, a more complex account of obesity was given. This offered a systems analysis rather than just a behavioural analysis.[132] It said that biology, the environment, economics, supply chains, family and communities, psychology and society are all woven together as factors jointly framing choice. No one channel of influence on its own is likely to succeed to change obesity rates. Nudge thinking instead strips away this sophistication and reduces obligations on policy-makers from having to change many factors to focusing only on a few, and these only in a light-touch way. No boats are rocked. No interests need to be threatened. No commercial interests need to be given different economic rules. No prices need to be altered. Above all, the politicians will not be accused of acting on behalf of a 'nanny state', a dread of neoliberal bound politicians. Thaler, a Chicago economist, is associated with the billion-dollar Fuller & Thaler Asset Management (with the by-line of 'The Behavioral Edge' and the rubric 'Investors make mental mistakes that can cause stocks to be mispriced; Fuller & Thaler's objective is to use our understanding of human decision making to find these mispriced stocks and earn superior returns'). Thaler argues that more regulation will not solve the problems created by Wall Street; only better information will do. 'Don't ban and mandate; just nudge.'[133]

Social norms are important, of course, and are important in the account of the Cultural Transition offered here. Social norms are the threads which bind social groups together, but which also divide groups from each other. One would expect surely that, if these were to be nudged, there would be reactions, complications and implications. Yet the nudge theorists imply that there is no reaction. All is presented as simple and emotional; complexity is banished as markets are pursued. In our view, this is oversimplified, not elegant, thinking. We agree that the relationship between norms and behaviour is intrinsic to the public health, but it raises issues of habit formation, power, genetic vulnerability, and individual and group behaviours, let alone the legacy of decades of marketing power and pricing messages. Nudge is no threat to those who pour out cultural messages to consume more fatty, salty, sugary foods, for example.

Society-wide cultural change: breastfeeding

We saw earlier (see Image 8 in Chapter 1) that action to encourage the breastfeeding of infants became a cause célèbre once it emerged that food company interests were working actively to undermine mothers. The tendency to bottle-feed infants gained momentum across Western countries in the twentieth century and with it the politicisation, or denaturalisation, of something that is potentially physiologically and emotionally beneficial for mother and child. In contradiction to the viewpoint expressed by international public health bodies, it has been argued that breastfeeding is not natural but socially constructed.[134] A more realistic viewpoint might be that it is both natural *and* socially constructed. From an evolutionary perspective, breastmilk contains all that a child needs for normal physical and mental development, while it is also an essential supportive medium whereby the child's immune system samples the normal family diet and gradually navigates environmental challenges. An Ecological Public Health perspective, in contrast to an 'oversocialised' approach, would look to find a convivial interrelation between culture and biology, not so much to create emotional pressure on mothers to breastfeed, as might occur in a social marketing campaign, but rather to remove all possible obstacles to them doing so.

Norway has tackled this dilemma by developing an integrated campaign which not only encouraged mothers to breastfeed but worked hard to remove the forces which discouraged it. In the 1970s, Norwegian breastfeeding rates were similar to those of England and Wales (in 1992, 62 per cent[135]). It was necessary that the campaign should create environments which assumed and accepted a culture of breastfeeding, rather than hectoring women to do it, give advice and support, and remove the power of commercial interests by blocking marketing directed at mothers. Norway banned the advertisement and marketing of breastmilk substitutes. In 1994 the breastfeeding rate in Norway was 98 per cent. In the same year it was 57 per cent in the USA.[136]

This might appear to be the action solely of the State, perhaps even a 'nannying' State. But behind such actions is the power of social movements trying to reverse a new cultural order whereby breastfeeding is undermined by commercial and cultural constructs which weaken it. Often these operate at an international scale, and health workers in developing countries find themselves hindered by the public relations campaigns of infant food companies. The creation of the WHO/Unicef International Code of Marketing of Breastmilk Substitutes, introduced in 1981, is a powerful means for managing these new commercial intrusions into health culture. Codes are important, but they require constant monitoring to have a full effect. Although 77 per cent of countries in the world, say the International Baby Food Action Network, which has a presence in 67 countries, have taken some action to implement the Code, monitoring and enforcement are still inadequate, particularly in countries where both laws and legal systems are weak.[137]

The Norwegian campaign was enormously successful. Of course, Norway has consensual cultural properties not found so readily elsewhere. Nevertheless the contrast from the US-sourced ideas of social marketing and nudge is clear. Mothers were not seen as the problem, to be 'segmented', and their behaviour principally was not regarded as needing to be changed. On the contrary, the 'problem' was found in the cultural and economic parameters of Norwegian society as a whole. This was the stigma shown towards breastfeeding women, the promotion of breastmilk substitutes, and the lack of care and advice that women need at a delicate, but joyous, time of their lives. Rather than putting pressure on the women to perform according to State advice, the pressure was released, dissipated and spread.

This promotion of breastfeeding in Norway fits the Ecological Public Health model in all aspects of interrelatedness. It engages with the biological world (obviously), seeks long-term changes in the social world, that of institutions, and attempts to restructure cultural expectations, not just of those directly affected, the mother and child, but of all society. There is also an impact on the material world, that of nature and the economy. The promotion of breastfeeding marks out the limits of commercial intrusion into everyday life.

The Cultural Transition and health

Our analysis of culture and the description of the Cultural Transition suggest that culture has to be a significant public health arena of action and inquiry. The theorists we have reviewed suggest that culture is not just a matter of ideas, artefacts, events and thinking which happen in universities, theatres or museums alone.

Culture is living. It includes people's habits, social processes, everyday rules for life (norms), and what the psychologists call 'cues', the prompts that are so regular they are the real social enforcers. Culture is the collective set of meanings through which people have identity and self-image. This approach to culture is alive to differences and divisions. Not everyone shares cultures. Your culture may not be ours. As was shown in the analysis of social capital earlier, patterns of exclusion can be perpetuated. Culture can limit people's worlds. The eighteenth-century Enlightenment approach to education was to break these received wisdoms and to allow a broadening of interpretation. This was the model of thinking upon which public health activists drew. If the health of the people was to be improved, culture needed to alter too.

Today, in the world of social marketing and 'nudge' thinking, culture has taken an Orwellian tone, in which commercial and public worlds are subtly merged and where the critique of private or commercial interests determining or subverting public policy in favour of public health is easily diffused. Commercial interests and the public interest are merged; tensions are erased. In this process, the notion of individual freedom is constantly invoked to put limits on public health interventions. Public cultural space is redefined as individual space. Health education, which was already looking rather ragged as a public health strategy, is now hopelessly constrained by the primacy of commercial power. Backed politically at the highest level, it has increasingly been rendered subservient.

Is it then meaningful to talk of the Cultural Transition in relation to public health? We believe it is. Our view is that Cultural Transition from peasant and rural societies to urban modernity is highly significant. Our analysis of cultural change is that it is not fixed or unidirectional or uniform. The picture of the Cultural Transition which we find essential for Ecological Public Health understanding is of culture as a bundle of tensions and possibilities. Inglehart and colleagues give one account of how values have changed, as we saw earlier. We expect further developments in coming years to provide cultural surprises. Yet how people think and interpret their worlds is clearly a factor in health behaviour. All the variants of health education summarised above tacitly acknowledge that culture is critical for public health. Our disagreement is that culture is more than cognition and how people think and translate their thoughts for health. Culture, as we have described it, provides reference points through which people act and think. If culture changes, then thought and behaviour change. In the past, when culture was obeisant to dominant authority (often religion or local powers), it was more rigidly coded. But, in the era of the internet, multiple modes of behaviour are more possible and thus have to be factored into health thinking. The cultural has always been an arena of overt action for public health change agencies. As we show in this and other chapters – through examples such as stopping spitting, encouraging washing, advice on diet, all strong messages with considerable public health evidence and implications – public health is about culture change.

This chapter has raised difficult issues about choice, control and the direction of health and behaviour. This has been a tale of serious debates about the accountability and governance of the forces which shape culture. In considering the avenues available to public health, it has highlighted an important tension between soft and hard approaches to cultural change, different interpretations of the role of consciousness and the material world in culture. We see the Cultural Transition as interdependent with other transitions rather than independent. The cultural aspects of human experience should not be separated from how society deliberates on its choices about progress and futures. Culture and democracy are entwined, which is why we now turn from the debate about manipulation and choice to one about participation and social engagement for health.

12

DEMOCRATIC TRANSITION

The Democratic Transition refers to the process of moving from a society and economy dominated by pre-ordained authority in the form of Church, State, tribe, family, monarchy or any other form of often unaccountable power, to one where the population plays a more active role in that society and governance. For some writers, the Democratic Transition can be located at 'a precise moment in time in which a regime makes a qualitative leap in levels of democracy, either from an authoritarian regime to an electoral democracy or from a semi-autocratic regime to a more democratic system'.[1]

This image of the Democratic Transition as 'a qualitative leap' is one version of progressive political change; it lends itself to that version of democratisation as sudden change of social structures, often associated with bloodshed, revolts and revolutions. On the other hand, it is also reasonable to see democratisation not just as a series of abrupt stages (or one stage) but as a progressive sequence, an evolving process. Indeed, many political analysts have described societal democratisation as longer and more fluid processes, involving different strands of struggle to change the boundaries of existence. These include: the rules of government; the nature and range of institutions; forms of administration, bureaucracy and co-ordination; and the relationship between State, citizen, commerce and expert knowledge. Emphases in this version of the Democratic Transition are by no means homogeneous. They vary from a focus on liberty (e.g. in liberalism), tensions between the classes (e.g. in Marxism), income spread (e.g. in social democracy), rights of different groups (e.g. in female emancipation), the position of minority or ethnic groups (e.g. in racism), labour representation (e.g. through trade unions) and a welter of 'special' rights and obligations (e.g. towards children or vulnerable groups).

Becoming healthier is linked to the lessening effects of autocracy (imposed power) and a push for democracy (pressure from below). It is questionable if it is possible to call a society democratic if major impediments infringe the potential of particular social groups to live good and healthy lives. Patterns of health may be one of the critical tests for how democratic societies are. The democracy of ancient Greece and the early post-colonial democracy of the USA coexisted with slavery, it should be remembered, and modern Indian democracy still struggles with the legacy of caste systems. The fates of democracy and public health are intimately entwined. Both are processes and about lives; both can be evaluated and judged; both are shaped by value systems. A central issue for both, too, is often the role of the State, which is frequently the means by which accountability and representation of the people are voiced, and through which health improvement first spread across whole societies and bind previously segmented social groups into the same framework. As has been discussed in previous chapters, for the nineteenth-century utilitarians the State was seen as a body which served the public interest, although it might be commercial organisations which serviced markets and provided the goods and services that delivered progress. Whatever the operational arrangements, the test for success for utilitarians was the achievement of Jeremy Bentham's 'fundamental axiom, it is the greatest happiness of the greatest number that is the measure of right and wrong'.[2]

Utilitarians wanted society to be changed and improve the lot of the people. They argued that institutions were a critical mediator in balancing economic development and health development. It has been argued more recently that such institutional differences between countries, specifically the economic, political and social organisations that societies have chosen or ended up with, are a main factor behind income differences and the standard of living between countries.[3] Utilitarianism began as a modernising project, with only theoretical equality between people through the happiness maxim, but became, with John Stuart Mill, a democratising project: hence the importance of the Greek word – *demos*, 'the people', and *kratos*, 'the rule'. And, like all aware people, the utilitarians knew that societies could be changed by people power. They wanted an orderly State against the background of European history littered with revolutions, uprisings, civil wars and the toppling of former authorities, with demands from 'below' recasting or constraining the actions of 'above'. And the multiplicity of forms that democracy has taken has kept political theorists busy analysing and categorising.

The political theorist David Held's review, for example, identifies ten major models, included the Classical era's Athenian democracy (limited to freemen, and excluding women and slaves, who were the majority!), republicanism (centred on the pursuit of liberty for citizens), and twentieth-century forms such as pluralism (with multiple actors competing for power within corporate capitalism) and deliberative democracy (which stresses the active participation of citizens).[4] Key themes and tensions cut across these different models: how to articulate the public good and will; how best to reflect and represent public wishes; how to govern with and for the people; how to balance the collective and private interests; how to ensure freedom with respect and restraint. These themes have long roots, back to political dialogues first recorded by Athenians such as Aristotle and Socrates but played out too in the English Civil War or French, American and Russian revolutions, or the Latin American struggles to shed the European and North American colonials, right to the tumultuous events of the collapse of the Soviet Union in the late 1980s and the Arab Spring of 2011. The list of democratic upheavals is immense, recognising too that any historical process can go backward as well as forward. What first had the appearance of fundamentally democratic shifts, in France and the USA in the eighteenth century and in Russia and China in the twentieth century, became the settings for very different forms of centralising power.

Here, however, our concern is less with the momentous points of transition and moments of democratic struggle or tension – important though those are – than with the long historical shift in all societies from simple to complex, from being bound by tight received social rules to looser ones, and the impact for health. We use the term 'Democratic Transition' both to capture that long process of emancipation – which enables all lives to be seen as notionally of equal worth (the reality is more complex and less egalitarian) – and to tease out how health plays an important and noble part in that pursuit of democratic freedoms, however defined.

In the political literature, the notion of the Democratic Transition has a particular meaning. It refers most often to the shift taken by authoritarian regimes to voting systems of governance and openness. The principles of democracy are said to be shaping society around the interests of all the people, not just elites, holding leaders to account, introducing more open systems of governance, attempting to distribute power in a new way, and conferring new entitlements. A lot of this recent literature was shaped by the ideological issues of the post-Second World War period, the politics of East versus West, the developed versus the developing world, the communist versus the capitalist. In fact, the Democratic Transition has deeper historical roots and includes tensions between the employer and the working person, the landholder and the landless, the property owner and the property-less. For the great political philosopher John Locke (1632–1704), human progress was defined by the pursuit of what he called natural rights, which were to life, liberty and estate (property).[5] Locke and the other theorists of natural rights such as Thomas Hobbes (1588–1679) were debating the limits and rights of law-making and power distribution. They set the terms of political debate to this day, centred on the application of reason, but with rights being primarily expressed through forms of property: one's own labour, one's own disposable goods.[6] Locke argued that 'the state of nature has a law of nature to govern it', which is that 'all being equal and independent, no-one ought to harm another in his life, health, liberty or possessions'.[7] Locke, for instance, argued that if a king infringes natural rights it is legitimate for the people to overthrow him. Such arguments had become real in mid-seventeenth-century England in the great Civil War, culminating in the execution of King Charles I. This period of internal strife is often depicted as the moment when England made the transition to parliamentary democracy. In fact, the execution of the king led to a period when Parliament itself became the battleground, with the emergence of the leader of the supposedly more democratic forces, Oliver Cromwell, taking on neo-monarchical powers, which in turn led to the re-entry of the royal family on his death. The development of modern democratic institutions follows from the securing of the right not to have one's property arbitrarily taken away.[8] But it is also a process of ceaseless change, debate and reshaping of intellectual and power boundaries between different social forces within societies.

The Democratic Transition thus raises questions about the institutions whereby democracy can be maintained and developed. A core thread across all the tensions described earlier – work, land, property, habitation, income, obligation, human rights, etc. – is the issue of accountability. The Democratic Transition is partly about making government and the bodies which shape the conditions of life more accountable, through voting, institutions, the law or all of these. The demand for the franchise, to vote for one's leaders, is only part of the struggle to get the State to support the weak and to restrict the overweening power of landowners or (today) giant corporations. Democratisation means the creation of a way of living in which people do not live in fear of disease and contagion, or at least where accountable societal mechanisms are formed to protect them, where lives can be more valued and fulfilled, and where employees can seek redress outside the relations of power and employment and improve the conditions of work. The 'Democratic Transition' as a term is shorthand for that democratisation project. This is about the quality and fullness of life. John Stuart Mill, writing in 1861, posed a question: 'If we ask ourselves on what causes and conditions good government in all its senses, from the humblest to the most exalted, depends, we find that the principal of them, the one which transcends all others, is the qualities of the human beings composing the society over which the government is exercised.'[9]

The struggle to get formal processes of legitimation, participation and representation is thus woven around an issue which we have shown in this book to be critical for public health and all health improvement. But there is no one blueprint for democratisation. Societies have varied in how they do this, where they end up at any given point of time, and how deeply the democratic forms are shared or last. There are 'thick' and 'thin' models of democracy just as there are thick and thin approaches to public health. To take examples from the previous chapter, 'thick' might be an integrated set of interventions, from bans on smoking to help those with a dependency on tobacco, while 'thin' might be 'nudge' approaches to behaviour change, which change only the arrangement of choices confronting the consumer.

Political theorists have often focused on the nature of the State in the democratisation process. This reflects a Western perspective. Those societies in Asia or Latin America for whom democratisation has meant struggles to throw off the colonial powers take a different perspective. The Democratic Transition should not be taken as a shorthand for the changing relationship between State and citizen. Important though that is, we think it is more useful to use a more pluralist model of democratisation, in which the forces competing for policy and societal influence include the State not just as a homogeneous entity but as a fragmented State – local, national, international – and diverse civil society manifestations not just individualised or even massed citizenry. Alongside them is an equally diverse but powerful set of commercial and corporate interests ranging from small businesses to giant multinational corporations. Indeed, the latter are arguably now far more important in reshaping daily lives than many states. In this looser conception of democratic tensions, we do not accept that the State is either benign or intrinsically authoritarian. The State is a set of governing institutions over a defined physical and policy territory. Almost by definition, to be a State requires the people to identify and accept (even if under duress) that the State exists. Equally, corporations derive legitimacy only from being 'incorporated' and given legal entity status by one State or another. The State is important (but not god-like) in that it generally is expressed through systems of law. The State also has economic dimensions. A State, says the economist Mancur Olson, is 'first of all an organization which provides public goods for its members, the citizens'.[10] To attach the word 'citizens' to a State implies that democratic values predominate; hence it is a State defined in a relatively recent form. However, Olson goes on to say public goods might come in the form of military expenditure and that this form of public good might not be welcomed by all. Laying aside the use of the term 'citizens', he may just be right. Classically defined, the State is the organisation which aims to monopolise violence, even if the object of that violence is the 'citizenry'. Our notion of the Democratic Transition for discussion of public health, therefore, assumes some fluidity about the social forces which compete for influence over the State and influence over health. Through the process of argument, battles for influence, and accountability, public health features centrally, but the relationship between health and democracy is not necessarily simple.

Is the Democratic Transition relevant for public health?

Even using a minimal definition of the term, few if any democracies existed before 200 years ago, and those that did claim to be, such as the USA, as already noted, were slave states, with the historical analogue being ancient Greece rather than anything that might appear on modern political rankings. To speak of the Democratic Transition and the link with public health requires clarification of two basic questions. The first, most obviously, is what is meant by democracy; the second is what are the primary drivers of the Democratic Transition. The second question is actually the easier to answer, since this can be culled from history; the question of defining democracy is probably hard to resolve, not least since it is a process rather than an end state of affairs. As Bernard Crick, a political scientist, noted, analysis of democracy takes many directions. One is to explore it as a principle of government; another is as a set of institutional arrangements; and another is more cultural, a type of behaviour. These different strands of analysis 'do not always go together'.[11]

It has been suggested that public health improves with democracy. A 2004 study by Spanish epidemiologists, led by Álvaro Franco, used the annual rankings by Freedom House, a US non-profit body set up with the encouragement of among others Eleanor Roosevelt in 1941, which produces a set of indicators for each country, to measure against health. The epidemiologists compared those rankings with health data sets from the UN Development Programme's Human Development Report and IMF data. The study concluded that there was a direct and statistically strong link between level of democracy and public health gain as measured by life expectancy, infant mortality and maternal mortality. Even allowing for incomplete data for some of the 170 countries reviewed, the authors concluded that 'the highest levels of health were in free countries followed by the partially free countries, and the worst levels of health were in countries that were not free'.[12] They continued: 'Democracy shows an independent positive association with health, which remains after adjustment for a country's wealth, its level of inequality, and the size of its public sector.' This study received support from a study looking at Eastern Europe, where it was argued that the countries that were most successful in making the transition to democracy saw some of the greatest gains in life expectancy, albeit with periods of setbacks and with staggered benefits.[13] A further study, advised by Amartya Sen, gave particular attention to China. It pointed to the complexity of the health–politics nexus and the difficulty of identifying independent and interactive influences in both directions. Nevertheless, it was argued, if the case for a democracy dividend in health was difficult to prove the lack of democracy certainly seemed to be a negative factor. Poor openness and accountability in the Chinese handling of the 1958–61 famine and the 2003 SARS outbreak were cases in point.[14] Other reactions to the Spanish study were quick and intense.[15] It was pointed out that some authoritarian states had excellent health indices, including Cuba and even China. Another critique was that what they were really measuring was level of wealth and standard of living. The validity of the Freedom House index was also questioned.

Freedom House was first set up in the light of fascism, later switching its focus to communism. Freedom House today defines a free country as 'one where there is open political competition, a climate of respect for civil liberties, significant independent civic life, and independent media'.[16] Since 1973, Freedom House has published the *Comparative Survey of Freedom*, which rates the level of democracy or 'freedom' in independent states and some disputed and dependent territories. The 2010 edition covers 194 countries and 14 related and disputed territories. Over the years Freedom House ratings have relied on a published checklist of political liberties and civil rights, but it has never been explained how this checklist was actually used. There are alternative indices produced by other bodies.

One among many is that produced by the Economist Intelligence Unit (EIU), the research division of *The Economist* magazine, established in 1843. Its Democracy Index claims to offer a more complete picture.[17] The Democracy Index's researchers argue that surveys like Freedom House do not encompass sufficient or sensitive enough measures for determining how substantive democracy is or its quality. Their own index is based on five categories: electoral process and pluralism; civil liberties; the functioning of government; political participation; and political culture. These together form a conceptual whole. They further note that democracy is more than the sum of its institutional parts. A democratic political culture needs to be legitimate to be sustainable. It thus needs an active and participative citizenry, since neither passivity nor apathy, obedience nor docility, is consistent with a democracy. Furthermore the matter of democracy goes beyond the characteristics of the State and the form of government. Full democracy requires an active civil society in which opinions are freely expressed. Nevertheless, the EIU researchers acknowledge that even these notions might be considered to offer an incomplete picture. Measures of economic and social well-being are excluded. It might be added that such indices fail to measure what for us should be critical issues: the state of public health, measures of health disparity or inequalities, or ecological measures.

No existing democracy index currently encompasses aspects critical for public health; even so their contents are revealing. The Freedom House index, the oldest, shows that the overall trend is positive. The 2010 EIU index, however, indicated a recent retreat, which it says was largely due to economic factors. It showed that almost one-half of the world's states were democracies, although the number of 'full democracies' was only 26, while a much larger number, 53 states, rated as 'flawed democracies'.[18] Unsurprisingly European – or European-derived – societies were ranked the most democratic. Of the 26 full democracies listed, 16 were European, with the top four slots being occupied by small Nordic countries. The majority of states, encompassing the majority of humanity, lived in 'hybrid' or 'authoritarian' regimes. The implications for public health are immense, as is already obvious for the medical or public health workers who work in such states (Cuba excluded).

The notion of democratic rights, if instituted only through a narrow or formalistic style of democracy, might not result in large improvements in health and well-being if such arrangements glaringly lack the presence of the type of social institutions required for the full performance of democratic principles, such as independent trade unions, protection of the rights of minorities, or equality before the law. Indeed, some authoritarian regimes – to return to an earlier argument by critics of Álvaro Franco and colleagues' study, above, ranging from some communist states such as Cuba to populist authoritarian capitalist states such as Peron's Argentina – may have been better at protecting the interests of groups like the uneducated poor or industrial workers than formally democratic (but in practice elite-governed) regimes which represent only the wealthy. The use of indexes and the like may act to downplay genuine historical and political differences and patterns of change.

This problem is by no means limited to states with new or weak democratic arrangements. Even states which laud the quality of their democratic arrangements may, for a host of reasons ranging from the funding systems for political parties to elite control of communications media, skew both taxation and benefits towards either the economic elites or interest groups or the constituencies which put them into power, while also ignoring major parts of the population, many of whom may have a vote but no voice. Such warnings about the potential for 'flawed democracies' might seem new but are not. They precede mass suffrage by more than half a century. In *On Liberty*, J.S. Mill warned that universal enfranchisement might result in the majority usurping the rights of the minority.

Much of the discussion of the Democratic Transition is US in origin, although the language of rights and its twentieth-century endorsement originated from non-US sources. The British political activist Thomas Paine's two-part booklet *The Rights of Man* (1791) endorsed France's Declaration of Rights and was influential in the construction of the US Constitution, although his opposition to slavery muted the extent of his influence. Today Thomas Paine Park stands opposite the New York City Department of Health building on Worth Street, Manhattan, a fitting reminder of the link between democratic activism and the creation of public health institutions. At the beginning of the Second World War, the celebrated author H.G. Wells wrote a letter to *The Times* attached to a draft 'Declaration of Rights', setting out a set of written principles to clarify what people were fighting for: not only legal entitlements, but a set of values. The Declaration was translated into 30 languages and sold thousands of copies. His book *The Rights of Man: or, What We Are Fighting For?* was published with a revised version of his 'Declaration of Rights'.[19] Wells sent a copy to his friend President Franklin Roosevelt, and on 1 January 1942 the allied powers belatedly included the protection of human rights among their official war aims. After some further lobbying, this goal was reflected in the founding charter of the UN, the Universal Declaration of Human Rights, in 1948.[20]

Thereafter, the USA allotted itself the historic role of promoting democracy worldwide, although in fact some of this project operated as a barely concealed weapon, often using CIA funding, in the political contest with communism.[21] Walter Rostow, whom we discussed in the Economic Transition, for example, thought it important that developing countries should be encouraged into higher levels of consumption as part of the journey down the democratic capitalist road, although he did also have some reservations. The policy package included not just US-style democracy but US democratic myths. As one American political study group concluded about the promotion of democracy, 'it cannot simply be a coincidence that the rise of American power over the past two hundred years has corresponded with the expansion of democracy worldwide'.[22]

This conflation of the USA, democracy, consumer-oriented markets and progress has also been questioned. Having an honourable tradition of pursuing democracy is not a permanent state of affairs. Political freedoms can be won but also lost. In that respect, there have been perpetual questions of over the applicability of the USA as an (or the) exemplar for others. Nevertheless, a popular viewpoint in US school textbooks, the view that the USA leapt from colonial bondage to full democracy and freedom, can be countered too. In health terms, the USA scores not so well, so considerable are the health inequalities between rich and poor, and black and white.[23] Looking at freedoms more generally, for a quarter of its over two centuries of existence the USA was constitutionally a slave state. For three-quarters of its history, it was a country racially segregated and then subject to voting property qualifications in some states. To its credit, Freedom House, a body which audits democracy worldwide, recognises that what it applies to others it needs to apply to the USA. Freedom House has stated of the USA that its most recent period is one in which 'a black man today has a one in three chance of being behind bars at some point during his lifetime'.[24] This account punctures US pretensions, perhaps warranted given growing inequality and the decline of trade unions over recent decades, used as indicators.[25] In truth, few self-describing democratic states have unblemished records; our point is not to single out the USA – a similar exercise can be done for the UK, our own country – but to point to the need not to put democracy into an absolutist frame of reference; more simply, some humility is warranted.

It can be a long struggle to get a right into law within a country, let alone expressed within international bodies and signed by enough countries to give the right some political weight. Another struggle often then ensues to get that right implemented and built into daily life. Therein lies the distinction between thin and thick democracy, between rhetoric and reality. Democracy takes time, and is a ceaseless process. A tightrope has to be walked between using the pursuit of liberty as an ideological banner to the extent that it becomes trite or rhetorical, on the one hand, and making it so tightly binding that the long process of democratisation gets lost in short-term ideological judgements or indicators, on the other.

The long process of democratisation

What then is democracy? In the example of Britain and many other countries which take their political roots from Britain, such as the Commonwealth and the USA, political mythology often locates the struggle for democracy with Magna Carta, a statement of the balance of forces between king and barons in the thirteenth century. Today, both those parties would be seen as disproportionately autocratic powers within their national or local boundaries. Magna Carta was the agreement hammered out, written and signed in 1215 at a celebrated meeting of king and barons at Runnymede meadows near Windsor Castle. The document established the right of Englishmen – albeit only some Englishmen – to limit the arbitrariness of the royal State, particularly in the matter of habeas corpus (Latin, meaning 'you may have the body'), whereby persons unlawfully detained cannot be ordered to be prosecuted before a court of law. In this regard, myth trumps reality, as no such result occurred.[26] Magna Carta did, however, begin a process of eroding the power of the monarch and began the curtailment of the monarch's right to be arbitrary. For that reason alone, it is taken as a seminal document codifying the beginnings of democratisation. Even those who later threw off the English yoke see it thus. A copy resides on display beside the American Constitution in Washington, DC.

In reality, Magna Carta barely touched the lives of the mass of the population. It was a reordering of power between the powerful. Mass democratisation in England strengthened with religious freedoms, notably with the break from the power of the Pope and the Roman Catholic Church. Historians such as Max Weber and Richard Tawney championed the analysis that this shift was central for the emergence of industrial capitalism across Northern Europe.[27] The Roman Catholic Church at the point of the Protestant break in the sixteenth century was both immensely wealthy and intellectually and legally powerful. Whittling away religious power over daily life was a long process in England.[28] Religious persecution and sectarianism were rife across Europe at that time. In England, most historians agree, for ordinary people, not just landowners, it took centuries more to reach new levels of tolerance.[29] In 1689 a new Bill of Rights – after civil wars, executions, persecutions and repressions within England – again defined the limits of royal power, and the Toleration Act in the same year gave rights to religious dissenters. The first of these secured property rights and eliminated confiscatory government.[30] The outcome was hardly an extension of the franchise but rather a restructuring of political institutions that severely limited the monarchy's powers and correspondingly increased those of Parliament.

A further milestone, over a hundred years later in 1789 (the year of the French Revolution), was the establishment of British legislation covering the existence of friendly societies, giving civil society an independent legal form and the right to act commercially. A further step was the repeal of the combination laws, which had banned workers meeting together, and this repeal gave some legal rights to early trade unions.[31] In 1832 the Reform Act increased the total English electorate from 492,700 to 806,000. This apparently large increase in fact took voting rights only to about 14.5 per cent of the adult male population, with women completely left out.[32] The fact that it dealt with the requirements of sectional interests – the rising industrial middle class – is indicated by the implementation of the New Poor Law in the following year, which instituted market principles into the structure of the labour market and the relief of poverty. As the Hungarian émigré to Britain Karl Polanyi (1891–1976) once observed, this made human society subservient to the economic mechanism.[33] It was not until 1918 that women over 30 years of age obtained the right to vote in Britain. They received it in 1920 in the USA, and, for a State which has prides itself on its democratic accountability, in Switzerland only in 1971.

The point is that not all of these and many other subsequent legislative Acts (Garrard provides a short but comprehensive list[34]) – which were by no means the sole democratising force – were always democratising in effect or in intention. The democratic process was and is also uneven. What the Acts did was widen the legal basis for independent belief or action, define and confine both the limits and the arbitrariness of State power and, later, resolve some of the pressures of Britain's rapid economic development. This process was, in effect, institutional modernisation, not Democratic Transition. The case for social democracy began from the 'inside' of utilitarian thought through the writings and campaigning of J.S. Mill, and by the influence of these ideas in explaining events before people's eyes, as the stresses and strains of class relationships and the material, social and health inequalities of industrialisation became obvious.

The Democratic Transition occurred by drawing political benefits from economic and political elites and at the same time in part reshaping the membership of such elites. The threat of revolution – occurring elsewhere in Europe – was certainly a motor of change,[35] but other factors helped. According to economic historians Alessandro Lizzeri and Nicola Persico, Britain's economic growth made new institutions affordable, while the ideas of Jeremy Bentham and James Mill – considered at various points in this book – helped coax 'the machinery of government to serve the public purpose'.[36] Another driver was the urgent demands for what economists now call 'public goods', in effect the sanitarian movement determined to protect public health. Public health was thus not merely the outcome of democratic change but a pressure for it. The new arrangements of local government set up in the nineteenth century for public health were in part a means of addressing long-standing local corruption but also a means of institutional modernisation to address rampant public health crises such as adulterated food, drains and water supplies. Although central State spending did not grow overall in the nineteenth century, it certainly grew in local government. It was there, until the 1970s, that public health responsibilities lay and were accountable. Local government spending rose from 17 per cent of total government spending in 1790 to 41 per cent in 1890, reflecting spending on public health infrastructure like sewerage systems, filtered water, and paved and drained roads.[37]

In this respect democratisation and health development – what we referred to as the Sanitary-Environmental model of public health (see Chapter 3) – was a two-way transfer. Pressure to take action changed the nature of local government, diminishing the role of patronage, while the extension of the voting franchise provided a social basis for more effective measures and debate about what was needed. Lizzeri and Persico observed that 'the plight of British cities with its attendant increase in the value of public goods caused an overflow in the dissatisfaction with the old political order, thus tipping the political balance in favour of reform'.[38]

This close attention to the multiple forces of change – demographic, social, economic and health, for the most part acting to move in a similar direction – provides a counterpart to the more romantic view that democratic change occurs on the basis of ideas or the effectiveness of heroic democratic forces. Enlightenment figures from Immanuel Kant to J.S. Mill were so enamoured of the power of reason that they could at times see ideas (notions of liberty and rights) as prime drivers of democratisation. Others have given more rooted analyses, painting democratisation as the incremental outcome of numerous social groups and interests, and as an ebb and flow of social pressures.[39] Even these broader analyses of the Democratic Transition place great emphasis on values and beliefs, but they are not taken as in themselves determinant. Leaders of movements might pronounce high ideals, but members may have more prosaic meanings. Although Europeans like to think that their democratic concepts and institutions stem from European civilised values, the economist and philosopher Amartya Sen has observed that the value of freedom is not confined to any culture. All cultures have strands of aspiration to liberty in some form. For Sen the significance of democracy is that it contains what he refers to as 'three distinct virtues'.[40] These are its intrinsic importance, its instrumental contributions, and its constructive role in the creation of values and norms. Democracy is one of the important factors that makes the difference in the structure of the social and economic life. He makes the additional point that democracy is able to offer citizens social justice only if it functions well. Notional democracy can be corrosive. Institutional forms alone cannot guarantee effective practice. It is in this wider analysis that health plays such an important part and in which values are played out.

If Sen's views take into account many societies, and begin from within political economy, another prominent view on the interplay between social justice and democracy derives from the more US-focused account of John Rawls (1921–2002). Rawls rejects utilitarianism as a regulative principle for society and instead focuses on resolving the long-standing conflict in democratic thought between liberty and equality. For Rawls the key feature of a democratic society is that citizens are free and equal in a context of fairness. There are two basic principles. In the first each person is seen to have the same claim to a fully adequate scheme of equal basic liberties. In the second he stipulated that these must be '(a) to the greatest benefit of the least advantaged, and (b) attached to offices and positions open to all under conditions of fair quality of opportunity'.[41] Although Rawls starts off within a classical liberal theory of justice, like J.S. Mill he moves away from it. He is thus critical of welfare-state capitalism (Rawls was from the US city of Baltimore, which saw a rapid decay in its economy and loss of population), which tends to produce a demoralised welfare class. He thus favours either a property-owning democracy based on broader principles of ownership or, like Mill, democratic socialism based on co-operatively managed firms. Of course, it is something of a utopian picture, a social democratic derivative of liberalism, just as the ideas of Robert Nozick, considered briefly in Chapter 1, travelled in entirely the opposite direction.[42]

The short account we have given here is of the Democratic Transition as an evolving, continual process, not a static or fixed state of affairs. Why public health matters in this rolling process is that people's aspirations for their children's and their own lives to be unencumbered by ailments and the random blight of disease help define what democracy is. The state of public health, the concrete expression of health within families, communities and indeed whole societies, informs the collective sense of human dignity and achieved quality of life. In part, the discussion of democracy is also a statement about what it is to be human, what obligations people have to others, how collective decisions are made and what role individuals, from those on high to the humble, have in setting the direction for society. The health of the people and the subtle as well as voting democratisation of society and economy are entwined.

Health institutions, rights and laws

Immanuel Kant may have set this discussion running and J.S. Mill may have fleshed it out for the modern age of market capitalism, but the more significant drivers of global Democratic Transitions perhaps lie in the outcome of the Second World War. The global ambition for more democracy was codified in Article 21 of the Universal Declaration of Human Rights, issued by the United Nations on 10 December 1948. Its words were simple and elegant. 'Everyone has the right to take part in the government of his country or through freely chosen representatives.'[43] (Since the Declaration also refers to 'the equal rights of men and women', the 'him' in this case implies both sexes.) The Declaration of Human Rights also makes it clear that, through such control, the population of a State should have the opportunity to shape the forces that determine its lives. Such an ideal implies something far more than democracy as simply a plebiscite – voting for one political elite as opposed to another – and implies that the institutions of society themselves need to take into account the needs of the mass of the population. Thus it is possible to speak of 'thin' or minimalist versions of democracy contrasted with 'thick' or maximalist versions.[44] John Garrard has suggested that the form of democracy, real or pretended, is now a function of 'normative' advocacy.[45]

Since the passing of the Universal Declaration of Human Rights, health rights have been symbolically important in democratic discussion. Many strands of international action trace their origins to the Declaration, and there are now numerous important international commitments which follow (see Table 12.1). Many such

TABLE 12.1 Some UN international commitments with public health relevance

Occasion	Date	Relevance
Universal Declaration of Human Rights	1948	Right to health.
UN Covenant on Economic, Social and Cultural Rights	1966	Social rights.
Creation of World Intellectual Property Organization (WIPO)	1967	Patents.
Stockholm Conference on the Human Environment	1972	Environmental protection.
World Food Conference (Universal Declaration on the Eradication of Hunger and Malnutrition)	1974	Eradication of malnutrition.
Ottawa Charter on Health Promotion: 'Health for All'	1986	Health promotion.
Convention against Illicit Traffic in Narcotic Drugs and Psychotropic Substances	1988	Drug trade.
Convention on the Rights of the Child	1989	Children.
Innocenti Declaration on Breastfeeding	1990	Breastfeeding.
UN Framework Convention on Biological Diversity	1992	Biodiversity.
UN Fourth World Conference on Women and Beijing Declaration and Platform for Action	1995	Women.
UN Habitat II and Istanbul Declaration	1996	Built environment and housing.
Kyoto Protocol	1997	Climate change.
Millennium Development Goals	2000	Global poverty and inequality reduction targets by 2015.
World Summit on Sustainable Development (Johannesburg)	2002	Sustainable development.
WHO Framework Convention on Tobacco Control	2003	Smoking.
Global Strategy on Diet, Physical Activity and Health (WHO and FAO)	2004	Recognition of coexistence of lifestyle diseases.
UN Resolution on Right to Safe and Clean Water and Sanitation	2010	Sanitation.

declarations focus on the individual, protecting the person from some hazard or making an aspiration for their lives, and as such intellectually derive from Mill, Kant and Rousseau's notion of the social contract.[46] Some of these declarations, however, are more collective in orientation in that they aspire to reframe conditions within which health can prosper. Examples are the 2000 Millennium Development Goals and the 1974 World Food Conference Declaration. Other declarations address not human but environmental obligations; an example is the 1992 Convention on Biodiversity.

The growth of global resolutions, treaties and conventions such as are given in Table 12.1 is not just a feature of modernity. Nor was a statement of human rights necessary to justify the case for co-ordination of international public health action. In fact, the creation of co-operation to tackle cross-border health threats has a long history, encouraged not least by centuries of fear about contagion and plague (see Chapters 1–3). Navies and armies in particular became repositories for developing knowledge about health threats, despite low levels and paucity of scientific knowledge in today's terms.[47] The spread of modern public health thinking as requiring international co-ordination, however, accelerated rapidly with industrialisation and the growth of mass international trade.[48]

Following early British legislation, public health laws and regulations were among the important shaping factors in developing international diplomacy and technical contacts to halt the spread of infectious disease. Although nation states had responded to disease incursions through national quarantine policies, the development of railways and faster ships were among the technological advances which meant that national quarantine systems were becoming less effective. National arrangements were not only failing to halt the spread of disease but creating discontent among manufacturers and merchants, who suffered economically from quarantine actions and thus pressed for co-ordination. The French government initiated and hosted the first of 14 international sanitary conferences in 1851 to standardise international quarantine regulations against the spread of cholera, plague and yellow fever. However, the development of regulations in different countries was influenced by prevailing social values, particularly considerations on the relation of the State to the citizen. Nations also championed different conceptions of causation and intervention, as we have shown in previous chapters.[49]

Lengthy debates at the 1851 sanitary conferences focused mainly on cholera. Among the topics discussed were microbial versus miasmatic causes of cholera and the relative merits of hygiene, sanitation and quarantine to control or prevent its spread. Agreement was only infrequently reached. Elizabeth Blackwell (1821–1910), the pioneering British-American feminist doctor (whose sister Emily had been the first female member of the American Public Health Association), attended the subsequent 1891 London conference and saw such divisions at first hand. She noted how French delegates warned of the centralising zeal of 'English hygienists'. How is it, they asked, that England, 'first in the field of sanitary science', along with its wide gamut of laws, regulations, agents and so on, still saw no diminution in its annual rate of mortality? They explicitly questioned the British approach.

Blackwell's own answer was that such measures were not enough. The success of public hygiene depended on the public, she said, and on 'general education as well as the education of specialists'.[50] She remarked that no laws or regulations will suffice 'when the habits of the people generally do not promote their application'. In other words, 'mind as well as matter must be considered in the subject of sanitation'.

If agreement was not guaranteed, the international sanitary conferences at least provided a forum for medical administrators, researchers, epidemiologists, surveillance specialists and others. The International Statistical Institute, founded in London in 1885, began publishing an international list of causes of death in 1893.[51] Such efforts were followed by numerous attempts to forge international agreement on other public health themes. For illicit drugs, the effort to establish an international framework began in 1909, leading to the 1912 Hague Opium Convention. At this, the USA and China were fiercely prohibitionist, while European countries, which had been using cocaine for medical purposes in the First World War, took the opposite view, wanting to regulate not ban the trade.[52] In fact, cocaine had only just become perceived as a public health problem in the USA, it being virtually unavailable until the early 1880s. Coca had become a staple ingredient, albeit in small amounts, in cola drinks, the best known of which was Coca-Cola. This distinctively American and now most global of products was formulated by John Pemberton, an Atlanta pharmacist, because alcohol prohibition in that city had removed his previous product, Peruvian wine cola, from the market. Coca-Cola was sold as a non-alcoholic 'pick-me-up'. Stronger concentrations of cocaine, of course, achieved physiologically more than this. The public reaction to the drug, when it came in the form of a Federal ban, drove low-potency products off the market and resulted, in the case of the Coca-Cola Company, in their product's reformulation. Coca production itself, however, was left virtually untouched. An illegal cocaine market thus erupted based on the continuing, but illegal, availability of pure cocaine.[53] In Britain in the early twentieth century cocaine had been available over pharmacy counters in London. It was even on sale at Harrods, the famous department store, later fined as the authorities tried to stamp out the trade under wartime emergency powers, and then through legislation.[54] Drug policy has remained controversial and ineffective, if not self-defeating, ever since. It is estimated by the OECD that the international drug trade is worth approximately US$400 billion annually, of which US$300 billion is laundered. The money filters through the world's approximately 72 tax havens and Western financial institutions, feeding corruption and mayhem.[55] Drugs policy is hardly the best example of either national or international policy-making, much of it ostensibly in the interests of promoting public health but having failed to apply a fully systemic model to its harm prevention, costs and consequences.

Ultimately, this somewhat fractious spirit of international co-operation got adopted in 1948 within the World Health Organization, as an agency of the United Nations, to direct and co-ordinate intergovernmental health activities. The League of Nations, which preceded the UN, had been formed after the 1919 Treaty of

Versailles, which formalised European politics in the aftermath of the First World War. It is there that the beginnings of today's broad remit for the WHO lie. The League of Nations had created a Health Committee in 1920 and almost immediately began to consider the need for a focused international health organisation.[56] The case was championed there and outside, notably by epidemiologists. Although the 1919 influenza outbreak was in the process of globally killing more people than the First World War battlefields, the professions and the League itself cited cholera and typhus outbreaks rather than influenza as the trigger for international co-operation. By 1923 the case was being made strongly for the Health Committee to become a fully fledged organisation.[57] It was formally constituted the following year, with a Secretariat, an Epidemics Commission, and co-ordination of the Committee by a Council. The methods of work were specified as co-ordination not just of epidemiology (e.g. standardising national statistics) but of fact-finding missions to countries around the world to improve knowledge about public health services and the effectiveness of hygiene measures, specifically on malaria, TB, cancer, smallpox, leprosy, rabies, infant mortality and blindness. The drive to improve international professional knowledge of, and administrative responses to, these ailments meant the Health Organization spread its net wider than the 23-country membership of the League, and brought in the USSR (although post-Revolution), the USA (which had refused to join the League) and Mexico.[58]

The formation of the United Nations and institutions like the WHO, the United Nations Educational, Scientific and Cultural Organization (UNESCO) and others was an opportunity to start afresh, with greater support from the USA, which had had limited involvement with the League of Nations. The ecological thinkers of the time were enthusiastic. Julian Huxley (1887–1975), son of T.H. Huxley and a contributor to new evolutionary synthesis,[59] became the first director-general of UNESCO. In 1946 he wrote the organisation's founding documents, locating its mission squarely within the Enlightenment tradition, evolutionary biological and social theory and agnosticism towards all political and religious creeds.[60] His endorsement of such explicit progressivism may have contributed to his removal from the post, only two years into a six-year term. Nevertheless, some years later, his brother Aldous Huxley extolled the virtues and possibilities of such international structures as the 'beginning of ecological politics'. His summary is worth quoting at length:

> The beginnings of ecological politics are to be found in the special services of the United Nations Organization. UNESCO, the Food and Agriculture Organization, the World Health Organization, the various Technical Aid Services – all these are, partially or completely, concerned with the ecological problems of the human species. In a world where political problems are thought of and worked upon within a frame of reference whose coordinates are nationalism and military power, these ecology-oriented organizations are regarded as peripheral. If the problems of humanity could be thought about and acted upon within a frame of reference that has survival for the

species, the well-being of individuals, and the actualization of man's desirable potentialities as its coordinates, these peripheral organizations would become central. The subordinate politics of survival, happiness, and personal fulfilment would take the place now occupied by the politics of power, ideology, nationalistic idolatry, and unrelieved misery. In the process of reaching this kind of politics we shall find, no doubt, that we have done something, in President Wilson's prematurely optimistic words, 'to make the world safe for democracy'.[61]

This prescient passage links democracy with Ecological Public Health in the terms we mean it in this book. What occurred over the twentieth century was a process of widening the scope of public health beyond infectious disease (important though it still is, notably for many developing states) to an ever-broadening prospectus of involvement. In this later regard, international environmental law had, like law for infectious diseases, developed from collisions over shared borders or waterways. As with public health, the establishment of the League of Nations, the UN and its agencies was key to the development of international environmental law. However, two distinct branches of engagement emerged: international environmental law and the law of natural resources. While the former sought to protect nature and mitigate pollution, the latter endeavoured to protect developing countries. As new types of environmental problems emerged, internationalisation of law deepened. In the wake of decolonisation, newly independent countries were reluctant to be constrained from freely exploiting their own natural resources, arguing that they saw no reason to be restricted in the development process when the former colonial West had not been when it developed.[62] It is not surprising therefore that states embrace very different ways of looking at the environment and of codifying environmental considerations into law. In the USA, strongly advanced in some aspects of environmental law, although limited with regard to town planning, first the rail and then the road lobbies triumphed. Nevertheless, legal concepts were developed from within ecological thought (see Chapter 6).[63] Ecology in the USA centred on conservation and the protection of a 'balance of nature' rather than adopting a dynamic outlook.

Evolving governance: the range of actors and ideas

In part, the difficulties facing organisations and actors involved in health governance arise from changes in the economic and political order. Long gone are the days when magisterial public health doctors or their equivalent could pull levers of power. In truth that state of affairs rarely existed; as we have shown throughout this book, the tasks of public health have been endlessly fought over and redefined. The Democratic Transition, however, adds to the complexity of the public health project by changing the balance in the relationships of not just State and citizen but other authorities and the commercial sectors, as well as professions and other parties. In theory, too, the Democratic Transition is a process towards a situation where citizens are more equal. In fact, a more patchy situation often emerges, even as the process of democratisation continues.

Seen across the last century and a half, a big trend in public health has been the internationalisation of health governance and the sharing of, and much argument about, the right measures to adopt. If in the mid-nineteenth century the British State looked to the local level of government to resolve public health problems, exemplified by Chadwick's 1848 Public Health Act, elsewhere different levels of State structure were called upon. In the USA, many health powers were derived from Navy traditions, but the Federal Government was largely kept to the margins. The prime level for action was state government, with New York and Massachusetts being particularly progressive in their administrative or investigative arrangements. This was partly because they had to address the infectious diseases from ports, migration, urbanisation and industrialisation. In 1892, New York City opened a bacteriological laboratory headed by Hermann Biggs, which would become the first municipal laboratory in the world routinely to diagnose disease. That year, it would use its diagnostic tools to detect cholera on a ship of immigrants, enabling the City to take quick action to prevent another cholera epidemic.[64]

In Germany, Virchow (see Chapter 3) had argued for the establishment of an all-Germany ministry of health in the late 1840s, but German public health was mainly based at the local level, often co-ordinated by groups of medical practitioners. It eventually centralised with the growing Prussian hegemony later in the nineteenth century. One historian has argued that the German public health approach was innovative in its fusion of medicine and social science although less progressive for its authoritarianism, eugenicist resonances and coercive and unaccountable professions, ambivalences exploited by the Nazis in the 1930s.[65] In Canada, despite the British influence (as a colony), medical practitioners were wary of growing central administrative power over the professions, so tended to follow the USA.[66] Public health legislation in Australia and New Zealand, given the strong political and cultural links, followed the English, but it was poorly followed through. Until the 1890s, infant mortality rates were as high in Australian cities as in England.[67] The health of native Australians was dismal – no words could easily describe the rapid loss of their population – and was to remain so.

In the late twentieth century, general governance had stopped being so closely a function of government alone, if it ever truly was. Today, the world is more overtly multilevel: global to local. The dynamics of governance are not just of central to local state but also 'up' to the continental and global, far more, as well as across borders. Power and influence over the determinants of health have also broadened the range of actors. The private sector, commerce and civil society are important players in public health governance. Arguably, no company will ever be able to have the power that the East India Company had over India from the eighteenth century. It had its own armies, laws, systems of government, taxes and influences; it made and broke local fiefdoms, implemented health measures, canalised rivers, and so on. One of the longest sub-plots in the long history of British attempts to become more democratic and to define and democratise commercial power concerned the parliamentary and civil society attempts to rein back the East India Company's power. This culminated in the impeachment in 1787 of Warren Hastings, the all-powerful governor of India and head of the company before Parliament. He was ultimately acquitted in 1795, an eight-year-long trial process![68] The Company's reputation was diminished, as details emerged of how it had bought its legal influence and rights back in the parent country (the UK). It was there that its power had to be made accountable and redefined.[69]

Today's transnational corporations are immensely powerful, benefiting from, if not running, entire sub-continents, but there are more of them; thus compared to the East India Company their power is less hegemonic. That said, the sheer scale of twenty-first-century corporations is remarkable. The UN's Conference on Trade and Development (UNCTAD) calculates that there are around 63,000 significant multinational corporations (MNCs), with around 700,000 'branches' in different countries. They account for about a quarter of world economic output. In a much cited paper in 2000, Anderson and Cavanagh suggested that, of the 100 biggest 'economies' in the world, 51 were actually corporations and only 49 countries. This calculation was on the basis of comparing company sales data with country GDP.[70] Although this is not strictly measuring like for like, it gives an approximation of the economic weight of very large companies. One of the persistent criticisms of MNCs is that they can play tax regimes off against one another to their own advantage, thus flouting the Jeffersonian principle of 'no taxation without representation'. The top 200 corporations in the world, Anderson and Cavanagh suggested, had sales the equivalent of a quarter of global GDP, but employed only 0.78 per cent of the world's workforce. Of the top firms, 82 were US-based, with Japan the next largest with 41 of the top 200 MNCs.

In 1974, already conscious of emerging MNC influence and troubled by the critique that MNCs undermined developing countries' economic capacities, the UN created a Commission and Centre on Transnational Corporations. For nearly two decades, it became a funnel through which pressure was channelled for a Code of Conduct. The Code contained implied constraints on how MNCs could operate and was strongly resisted by MNCs and some governments. The Commission and Centre were 'dismantled' in 1993. Some of their work was transferred to UNCTAD, itself now marginalised by the World Trade Organization, which was created in 1994 by the General Agreement on Tariffs and Trade (GATT).[71] In place of the Code, what the world was offered by the dominant economic forces was a softer, voluntaristic Global Compact. This had little leverage when chaperoned into existence in 1990; de facto, it merely asked MNCs to be more honourable in their dealings with developing countries.[72]

The defeat of the campaign to get tougher regulation was connected to the emergence of intergovernmental efforts – heavily supported by commercial interests such as the International Chamber of Commerce and World Economic Forum. They strongly supported a new, more open set of world trade rules. The GATT had been launched at a 1948 London conference to create new trade rules and prevent the protectionism that some economists argued had accelerated the 1930s economic slump. Slowly, a system of ever stronger and wider trade rules emerged, signed on to by more nation states, through a series of negotiations known as rounds. In 1987 the most ambitious round was launched in Uruguay, culminating seven years later in the 1994 Marrakesh Treaty, which created the new World Trade Organization, as we noted above. As well as extending world trade rules into agriculture – the largest employment sector on the planet – it created the World Trade Organization as a fully fledged global organisation to promote liberalised trade rules. As the rapid expansion of MNC trade continued, the UN's 1999 Human Development Report, written by the UN Development Programme (UNDP), resuscitated the idea of a Code of Conduct to tame MNC power. This was part of its call to humanise the worst excesses of globalisation. This 'globalisation with a human face', as the UNDP report called it, and its appeal for the 'reinvention of the world government structure', never emerged. Tensions remained between the UN system and the Bretton Woods institutions set up at the end of the Second World War such as the World Bank, the International Monetary Fund and now the newer World Trade Organization which replaced the former GATT Secretariat. Global democratic institutions are further complicated by the emergence of ad hoc groups such as the powerful industrialised G7 and its counterpart the G77 grouping of developing nations.

In the twenty-first century, it has been suggested that globalisation has increased the need for new formalised frameworks for international health collaboration on matters of constantly expanding breadth, ranging across the safety of chemicals, pesticides, food and the disposal of hazardous wastes, environmentally damaging technologies as a source of biodiversity loss, marine pollution, ozone depletion, climate change and even human cloning. These matters bring together different realms of international law, such as intellectual property rights (patents), trade, human rights, environmental protection, defence and security. Health is a common thread across all of these policy issues.[73]

Legitimate drugs, products of the powerful pharmaceutical industry, illustrate why health governance is both complex and sensitive. The extraordinary sophistication and effectiveness of modern drugs mean that their supporters often hold the sector aloft as crucial for public health. Yet the history of pharmaceuticals is one of considerable risks and some (relatively rare) withdrawals of drugs, a notable case being thalidomide. In the late 1950s this drug was introduced as a sedative by Grünenthal, a German pharmaceutical company, and legalised. As the *British Medical Journal* later commented, 'clever marketing' that it had no side-effects led to it being sold in 46 countries.[74] Among other functions, it was found to be effective in reducing symptoms of morning sickness among pregnant women, which was its main marketing point, but it was withdrawn in 1961 following discovery of the causation of serious birth defects, after suspicions were explored by two doctors but suppressed. It was left to journalists to campaign doggedly for the full lessons to be learnt and for years of litigation and compensation to unfold.[75] One lesson was that side-effects were being noted by the parent company even before its sales took off. The tale is a classic of the genre, where a company lies, bribes, suppresses and distorts (to use the terms of the journalists' book) to keep opposing interpretations or facts at bay.

Thalidomide became a rallying cry for tougher testing procedures and new risk management processes for technical innovation. It had highlighted the different national cultures in regulatory procedures and processes. Some are more open; others occur behind closed doors. Some champion their own pharmaceutical companies; others follow rich-country guidance. The days of uncritical acceptance of scientific and technical advance are long gone. In 1955, Marver Bernstein first referred to the term and process of 'regulatory capture' to identify the process by which regulators come to serve the sector they were created to regulate.[76] Given thalidomide and problems with other drugs, the relations between regulatory bodies and the pharmaceutical industry have been much debated. The concerns raised are common to other industries and include: the power of lobbying; the 'revolving door', where personnel leave government to enter the private sector; 'agency capture' or 'regulatory capture', where over-close relations emerge between scientists who develop treatments and those who regulate the framing of research and safety; and the appointment procedures for membership of regulatory bodies.[77] Reliance on fixed procedures seems likely to be subject to such pressures.[78] For industries such as drugs, food and agrichemicals, common questions of governance are frequently raised, and how to create high-quality, high-standard systems of risk assessment, risk management and risk communication which warrant public respect and trust.[79] The response to this continual dilemma varies. The Washington Consensus (see Chapter 8) has favoured a trend to so-called 'light touch' systems and self-regulation, with government kept at arm's length, but in a crisis there is usually a shift to toughen up and to fund or (re)create more independent regulators.

The shift to 'new governance'

The story in this chapter has been of increasingly complex systems of governance being progressively applied across society, and of ebbs and flows in democratic scrutiny and intervention. Citizens take for granted today in any part of the developed world that – whether the issue is quality of goods in shops or the management of public utilities, schools and hospitals – all organisations and institutions necessarily should apply formal rules of governance and consistent operational procedures. In the case of the latter, sometimes private arrangements replace public systems. They might encompass regulations, staff guidance, supply chain management, risk management, methods of customer compliance and redress, ethics and more. Sometimes the privatisation of health governance is through the arrival of barely visible 'back office' arrangements. In other cases, it may be more visible, as with product labelling (see below). This web of governance illustrates the framework of often hidden rules to which John Searle was referring in the quotation in Chapter 1.

Bureaucracies, as is their nature, operate through rules. But the format and substance of such rules, and type of organisation which sets them are always historical outcomes. Nevertheless, in almost all independent types of organisation, once rules and standards are established they tend to proliferate, become codified through professional or industry good practice, spread from one place to another, and cross national boundaries. Many systems of standards are now global, such as through the International Organization for Standardization, but for some issues these are complicated owing to the coexistence of public and private standards. In food safety, for example, there are UN standards through the Codex Alimentarius Commission, but there is also a growing and powerful set of company standards through the international GlobalGAP system. Both pertain to setting good agricultural and food procedures, but the latter is hugely important within company supply chains because it is used within contracts and specifications.[80] In the past, owing to Britain's vast Empire, some British rules and standards covering such mundane matters as the measurement of energy or space (see Chapter 6) became adopted as the global standards and remain so. Energy is still measured by the British thermal unit (Btu). American economic hegemony is illustrated by its domination of computer engineering standards, for instance. The rise of the EU, which pools the standards of 27 countries, had become a counterweight to US power. GlobalGAP, for example, began in Europe as EurepGAP.[81]

Some neoliberals like to see standards as unnecessary intervention by governments, but such rule-making is not necessarily an imposition on business. Rather it is a means for creating a shared platform for business activity, the much-cited 'level playing field' or the conditions for interoperability. Nineteenth-century sanitarianism, it should be remembered, fought with private business but was utterly reliant on business at the same time. Civil servants do not construct drains, roads or railways. They rely on engineers and the ground rules of engineering, established in professional bodies and institutes, to create the infrastructure of health. Sir Edwin Chadwick, whose span of interest went far beyond public health, followed many of the ideas set out by his mentor Jeremy Bentham. He established a management formula based on the creation of expert-led executive bodies commissioning private companies. For him the issue was not 'who' but 'how', the watchwords being efficiency, accountability and minimisation of waste.[82] Not just in Britain but worldwide, the ensuing picture of urban infrastructure construction became a mixture of public and private (see Chapter 6).

Economists today make a distinction between private, public and mixed goods, but at no time until recently were these distinctions applied in any consistent form. In some countries, water utilities or electricity or gas suppliers were public, in others private. A similar tale could be told for healthcare provision or for that matter education, where even in societies committed to private solutions in health, like the USA, most education became public in its provision. Only later, in the 1980s, following political initiatives set in train by the British prime minister Margaret Thatcher and the US president Ronald Reagan was there a consistent effort to reduce the scope of the public sector and restructure the mode of its management. What was first termed 'denationalisation' in the UK, later called 'privatisation', was endorsed by international economic bodies such as the OECD and the International Monetary Fund.[83]

A consistent theme within twentieth-century debate about the Democratic Transition centres on the individual's freedom to choose within marketplaces. Citing inheritance from Adam Smith and the classical economists, the argument that consumer behaviour should be allowed to shape economies without an interfering State was championed most vociferously from the 1970s by the school of economists at Chicago University, most popularly by Milton Friedman. This drew on Middle Europeans such as Frederick Hayek (1899–1992) and his teacher Ludwig von Mises (1881–1973), the latter a friend of Max Weber (see Chapter 11). Their academic interests centred on money and how it conveys signals and value to consumers, through which market efficiencies can be communicated. For his work in this area, Hayek – by then based in Chicago – won the 1974 Nobel Prize for economics.

The central importance of the neoliberal argument put by these thinkers is that liberty is the most precious moral value within the democratic impulse. Efficiencies require unsullied and uncontaminated messages to pass between actors in economic systems, between producer, retailer and consumer. Within this picture, organised professional groups, like doctors, form a block against the proper operation of the market. There is no justification for licensing the medical profession, argued Milton Friedman; it results in inferior care and the establishment of medical cartels.[84] Friedman had a point about professional control resulting in monopolistic behaviours, although he and other US conservatives supported campaigns against the public organisation of US healthcare, which the US medical profession also opposed. Taken a stage further, the efficiencies of markets are so subtle and their signals and actors so diverse yet rational that society need not be encumbered by old systems of governance such as voting and parliaments when allocating resources. Markets can do this better. Thus, consumer 'votes' via purchasing decisions can replace electoral votes at the ballot box.[85] To market purists, this process is quicker in feedback and more efficient and has the added benefit of marginalising the State. It became a cornerstone argument of the New Right of Ronald Reagan and Margaret Thatcher, but was taken in a different direction by the ethical consumer movement championing fair trade,[86] and eco-health consumers supporting particular methods of food production. In 1970 Albert Hirschman diagnosed that economists like Friedman were avoiding the everyday realities of expressing one's views. In this conceptualisation, Friedman preferred 'exit' to 'voice'. In the case of schooling, to take one of Friedman's examples, this would mean that the neoliberal view was that, instead of campaigning for school improvement, parents should take the role of 'customers'. On the contrary, said Hirschman, expressing one's views, getting involved in the democratic deliberative process, was a better route to securing improvements and far better than retreating to the 'anonymity of the supermarket'.[87] Consumers only consume the world; citizens shape it.

Whichever route the consumerist argument takes – towards social justice and ethics reshaping markets or towards anti-statist and individual rights-driven economic systems – the role of information becomes a key policy issue. And it is here, in the issue of food labelling, that a heated public health argument has occurred for decades, championed first by consumer NGOs and latterly by public health bodies.

Better labelling had become a litmus test for the consumerist approach to democratic politics. Labels offer a tangible mechanism by which consumers can act responsibly in the marketplace. In a 1962 speech on consumer aspirations and rights to the US Congress, President John F. Kennedy outlined four rights: to safety, to be informed, to choose and to be heard.[88] Within a few decades, the four had been expanded by the UN-affiliated worldwide consumer movement (now called Consumers International) into eight, adding rights to satisfaction of basic needs, to redress, to education and to a healthy environment.[89] These rights all touch public health.

One might think that labelling would be a simple matter; far from it. What to declare on a label, whether to do so, the format chosen, the language, the size of print, whether the information is on the front or back of a package, whether opaque terms and claims can be made, and who adjudicates: all these issues and more litter the history of consumer movement pressure to provide the simple 'right' to be informed and educated, two of the eight rights. In the EU, for instance, following the decision to create a Single Market in the mid-1980s, all national food composition standards were abolished in 1987, deemed barriers to internal trade. Consumers were promised information on products to enable them to judge value for money.[90] Instead it took nearly two decades of wrangling before European consumers received labels where the contents were listed according to the quantitative ingredients declaration (QUID) system. And nutrient labelling was not resolved for another decade. This was an even more sensitive issue owing to rising population levels of obesity and the need to help consumers constrain calorific intake and tackle non-communicable diseases (see Chapter 9). Powerful sectors of the food processing industry were prepared to back a system which summarises for each packaged food its contribution to a notional guideline daily allowance, whereas consumer organisations preferred a 'traffic lights' system, which judged the food product as good (green), OK (amber) and less desirable (red) for nutritional health.[91]

Thus the theory of 'consumer votes' becomes in practice highly contested. Consumer aspirations are subject to a ceaseless barrage of information in the form of marketing and advertising, adding to information 'noise'.[92] Information is also systematically kept away from consumers, as has been the case for the labelling of genetically modified ingredients or for foods containing nanotechnology. The USA and EU had a long-running dispute over whether the EU, under WTO rules, had the right to refuse food products containing hormones, genetic modification and other process technologies on which consumers were sensitive. The demand for better sustainability or environmental labels has become another battleground, with information on residues or modes of production kept to a minimum, although there have been experiments with labels for embedded carbon and water.[93] From the public health perspective, far from resolving the issue of governance, food labelling and consumer rights become another site of democratic engagement and ongoing policy conflict.

Analysts of the 'new governance' that has emerged in the last quarter-century of globalised trade rules and measures suggest there has been a move to 'share power', to promote 'citizen autonomy' and civic engagement, to transform public administration and to promote new public–private arrangements. The new approach is a move away from what has been typified as hierarchical, 'command-and-control' methods of regulation to more transparent and flexible regulatory systems. Business regulation, in the new governance, is enjoined to take account of a range of economic, technical and social policy trends balancing needs of the market, current and future, with those of consumers and the public interest. Instead of governance being exercised directly through law and regulation, it is instead applied through expert-led processes of intelligence-gathering and decision-making which may make up soft rules or become formalised in law only in the last instance. Self-regulation is the preferred route. There may even be the deferment of regulation for company good behaviour. Companies are enjoined into corporate social responsibility, with government playing the role of the 'honest broker' between industry and civil society. An example is the UK government's promotion from 2010 of what it called 'Responsibility Deals' with industry. These were groups of business and non-threatening civil society bodies working together to come up with routes to consumer behaviour change. Everything is at the individual level, and there is a heavy reliance on social marketing and 'nudge' thinking (see Chapter 11).

There are other variants of the new soft governance thinking. They include: government-approved, private sector-led models, business-NGO initiatives, and multi-company and multi-NGO forums to try to get agreement. An example in Germany is the Plattform Ernährung und Bewegung (PEB), the Platform for Good Nutrition and Physical Exercise. This began in 2004, involving 100 organisations.[94] At the EU level another example is how the European Commission (EC) responded to pressure to 'do something' to tackle rising levels of obesity. The EC set up a public–private partnership (PPP) in the form of the European Platform for Action on Diet, Physical Activity and Health, established in March 2005.[95] This approach was backed by the WHO-organised European Conference on Obesity in 2006, which stated that it was 'essential to build partnerships between all stakeholders such as government, civil society, the private sector, professional networks, the media and international organisations, across all levels (national, sub-national and local)'.[96]

In these PPPs it is accepted that, while regulation may be part of the picture, business can play a role in easing the path to health improvement. It can reformulate its products on its own initiative. It can modify its marketing without the pressure of regulation. It can help shape healthier social norms. The question as to whether the measures achieve the sort of gains of earlier public–private parallel efforts, such as around the promotion of hygiene in the late nineteenth century, remains to be answered. Unlike those of the past, the conflicts of interest today are far more prominent. They are being formed in the open, subject to democratic scrutiny if not accountability always.

'Thin' and 'thick' democracy: civil society and capitalism

The role of the public health movement has a distinguished history within the Democratic Transition. It has promoted both primary standards of health and the notion that democracy is required. One interpretation of this role is that this is 'speaking truth to power', while we have presented it as a longer set of arguments and tensions. They include: the role of health in liberty versus authority; the deepening and sharing of improvements in quality of life; systems of accountability and responsibility; access to good data and information; and the assertion of collective needs. In this respect, the pursuit of the public health continues J.S. Mill's call for liberty to be the antidote to paternalism. That is why he called for worker co-operatives, seeing democracy as necessary not just in the political realm but also at work. Today, democratisation surely means more than just being conscious of the paternalism of the State. It surely includes, too, the role of powerful companies, ideologies, media and other vested interests. In a world where corporate responsibility is being offered as the route to better health, some caution is needed before public health proponents should rely upon that as the source of health improvement.

The picture we have painted is of the Democratic Transition as more than just a step from one status (e.g. serfdom) to another (e.g. mass suffrage). It is a long and continual process. Democracy can be weakened not just strengthened. Here we note an important distinction between 'thin' and 'thick' democracy. The US political theorist Robert A. Dahl (1915–) saw democratisation in three stages, the ultimate goal of which was what he termed 'polyarchy', a pluralist status in which power is spread not concentrated.[97] Dahl disagreed with the US sociologist C. Wright Mills (1916–62) and others who argued that power was concentrating.[98] Dahl's verdict on capitalism was that it has undemocratic tendencies but is the best philosophy so far. In practice, there are different types of capitalism, some which make broader arrangements of social welfare and hence are redistributive and others such as the so-called Anglo-American version which are less so.[99]

A central debate in the Democratic Transition concerns wealth not just power, inequality not just individual or collective liberties. A persistent argument for centuries has been that democracy must have a strong element of wealth-sharing for health gains to be collective, rather than accruing solely to an elite or special interest group. Dahl wrote, for example: 'unless we abandon the ideal of political equality . . . I do not see how we can live comfortably with the inequalities of power and political resources that we find around us'.[100] Wilkinson and Pickett's best-selling 2009 book *The Spirit Level* argued that unequal societies almost always perform worse than more equal societies across a wide range of indicators: crime, life expectancy, obesity, educational attainment, imprisonment, drug use and social mobility.[101] Although this work has been criticised for over-concentrating on psychological factors at the expense of material factors,[102] the authors return the project of public health to the material level of resources, too, arguing that the tradition of WHO's 1986 Ottawa Charter stressing health and well-being can come about only with a redistribution of wealth. This echoes the work of Sir Michael Marmot and his epidemiological colleagues and of the WHO Commission on Social Determinants of Health that the public health improvement requires a structural analysis and set of interventions.

An unanswered question, and one which is often ducked, is whether the public health can enhance democracy or whether it represents a form of disciplinary biopower, or governmentality, Michel Foucault's argument (see Chapters 1, 3 and 11).[103] Governmentality is not monolithic. It is itself up for grabs and may involve actors far beyond the national State, the rather limited site of Foucault's analysis. Even within states the outcome of any set of arguments about power cannot be predicted in advance – Foucault saw them as emergent – since a variety of tensions are at play. The form of governmentality and the content to which it is addressed change. Our argument is that the State, acting through professions or other forces, is often oppressive (as we have seen) and sometimes it is progressive (which we have also seen). Overall its contribution to liberal social democracies has undoubtedly been progressive, but in some states progressive features have yet to emerge. Another line of criticism, argued by a school of environmental theorists, is that, so far, democracy is not proving nimble enough to tackle environmental crises of resources, climate and other 'ecosystems services'. They raise a question of time scale. There is a huge gap between the evidence of the need to change and the Western consumerist models of behaviour so that the East can live and achieve well-being.[104] Instead, the world appears locked into a *danse macabre*, sliding inevitably to tragedy. Governments ultimately hold the circle of change but are paralysed by fear of confronting consumer aspirations and lifestyles. We prefer to believe that the gap is not inevitable. In some historical settings, states fail or are entirely co-opted by sectional interests.

The Democratic Transition is critical for public health. This has been inadequately discussed in the public literature yet infuses it. The pride of the public health movement is that it has generated better quality of life and expectancy yet, as we stated at the start of this book, public health suffers a certain invisibility. The account we have given here is of public health as active within the wider processes of the Democratic Transition. Our account has suggested that the Democratic Transition invokes all five models of public health given in Chapter 3. The Sanitary-Environmental model has promoted the strengthening of democratic processes. The Bio-Medical model was illustrated in the growth of international health law and institutions. The Techno-Economic model established the linkages between economic actors, the State and civil society. The Social-Behavioural model has become integrated into the information-giving mechanisms of both State and commercial products. And the Ecological Public Health model requires the construction of an integrated understanding of the web of health.

CONCLUSION TO PART II: AN OVERVIEW OF THE TRANSITIONS

The account of all the transitions we have presented in Part II is of the main dynamics shaping public health. The public health agenda has been informed by history, and we have recounted real events, pointing to live processes and continuing features. We have outlined key themes as the transitions emerged and were debated. We have given the transitions as persistent storylines which shape the world today. In Table P2.1, we summarise the transitions, giving their core ideas, some exponents and key features. This table is an aide-memoire, not a complete categorisation. It allows us to point to the contribution the transitions jointly make to the conceptualisation of public health.

In the Introduction to Part II, we quoted John Dewey's warnings of the limitations of thinking in compartments, and his principle of continuity. The account of the transitions we have presented surely justifies that statement. This is of public health addressing a continuous world in transition, whose dynamics can be understood and faced appropriately. In Part III and our final chapter, we explore more about the implications derived from this account of history, paying attention to how public health requires a special way of looking at and thinking about the world.

TABLE PII.1 The transitions summarised

Transition	Core idea	Exponents	Key dynamics for health	Contribution to public health thinking
Demographic	Over the last two centuries, Western societies have experienced rapidly reducing mortality and birth rates and extended longevity, leading to the rise of populations, a pattern repeated elsewhere.	T. Malthus, F. Notestein, A. Landry and K. Davies.	Industrialisation and modernisation improve living conditions and allow the birth rate to fall.	A map of progress in which a description of past experience is assumed to be a general prescription.
Epidemiological	Societies move from an age of pestilence and famine to one dominated by degenerative disease.	T. McKeown, A. Omran, J. Caldwell and R. Fogel.	Disease patterns follow the level of economic development and improved living standards.	The focus of public health switches from infectious to chronic diseases.
Urban	The move from rural to urban-based existence alters living conditions and modes of life.	L. Mumford, P. Geddes, D. Harvey, M. Davies and J. Jacobs.	Migration to cities concentrates populations and changes social dynamics.	The sanitation and social milieus are reshaped by growing towns and population intensification.
Energy	Cheaper and higher-output energy sources underpin societal and economic development.	S. Jevons, H. Haberl, M. Fischer-Kowalski, R. Fouquet and V. Smil.	The pursuit of cheap energy is shaped by the desire to replace human and animal labour.	Changes in energy sources transform heat, light and power, which underpin modern living.
Economic	There is a shift in modes of production, with higher inputs and outputs.	A. Smith, K. Marx, T. Veblen, W.W. Rostow and K. Boulding.	Progress is defined by the accumulation and distribution of wealth.	Economic development defines the scope of public health.
Nutrition	The shift from traditional to modern societies is characterised by changes in diet and physical activity.	H. Trowell, D. Burkitt, B. Popkin and R. Fogel.	Plentiful food transforms physiological growth and body size.	Public health has to address the mismatch of physiological requirements and dietary regime.

Biological and Ecological	Microbiological and natural ecological life are both being altered by human activity.	C. Darwin, A.R. Wallace, E. Haeckel, M. Curie, R. Koch, A. Tansley and A.J. McMichael.	Human activity is eroding biological and natural ecological processes on which civilisation depends.	Public health needs to respect human dependency on the natural world and biological processes.
Cultural	A shift from traditional society characterised by a fixed social location to modernity, which offers widened and displaced cultural possibilities for how to live.	G. Simmel, Frankfurt School, G.H. Mead, P. Bourdieu, D. Putnam and M. Foucault.	People's habits and everyday rules for living have enhanced health consequences.	Public health has to engage with how people think and conceive of themselves.
Democratic	Systems of governance in the commercial and public spheres become more accountable, rule-based and nominally democratic.	J.S. Mill, J. Dewey, J. Rawls and A. Sen.	Tensions emerge in and about the State over priorities and how health governance shapes health outcomes.	Public health has to take its place as a force for democracy, recognising the tensions between institutions and interventions expressed as functional systems of control and an alternative expression in which the citizenry is the guiding force and is where the fundamental ambitions of public health sit.

PART III

Reshaping the conditions for good health

13

THE IMPLICATIONS OF ECOLOGICAL PUBLIC HEALTH

It is part of human experience to learn how the past affects the present, how the moment for taking action can be gone in an instant, and how what is done today shapes the future, whether we like it or not. Among the fables credited to Aesop, the Greek slave and teller of tales, is the story of the ant and the grasshopper. In the fable the grasshopper has spent the summer months singing and enjoying the heat while the ant worked to store up food for winter. When that season arrives, the grasshopper finds itself short of food and hungry. Upon asking the ant for food the grasshopper is rebuked for its idleness. The moral of the tale is by way of warning about individual fecklessness: not being prepared or thinking ahead for when times may be hard. This and the other fables were first printed in English by William Caxton in 1484, one of the first books printed let alone printed in the newly settled English language. It has remained in print for over 500 years. J.S. Mill read it as a small child, in Greek. It has been told, retold, extended, turned into cartoons, even 'Disneyfied'. It gained new life with the near financial collapse of the Western economic model in the 2000s, when Martin Wolf, an economics writer on the *Financial Times*, retold the tale thus: the ants are the industrious societies (the Germans, Chinese and Japanese) who prosper, while the grasshoppers are the consumer societies (the American, British, Greek, Irish and Spanish) who are in trouble.[1]

Fables are timeless. They warn of the future. They are encapsulations of the human condition. Many offer sober accounts of how weak humans are, how fallible, how subject to external troubles. They are often moralist. They remind people: you reap what you sow, you have to work for gain, the future can creep up on you, and so on. Many great novelists are judged great because they capture wider eternal lessons. George Eliot (the nom de plume of Mary Ann Evans, 1819–80), the Victorian novelist, was a particularly acute observer of how the present becomes the future under our very noses. In *The Mill on the Floss*, published in 1860, a minor character, Mr Deane, says to young Tom Tulliver, a major character:[2]

'You see, Tom,' said Mr. Deane at last, throwing himself backward, 'the world goes on at a smarter pace now than it did when I was a young fellow. Why, sir, forty years ago, when I was much such a strapping youngster as you, a man expected to pull between the shafts the best part of his life, before he got the whip in his hand. The looms went slowish, and fashions didn't alter quite so fast; I'd a best suit that lasted me six years. Everything was on a lower scale, sir, – in point of expenditure, I mean. It's this steam, you see, that has made the difference; it drives on every wheel double pace, and the wheel of fortune along with 'em.'

Eliot was here capturing the coming of the Economic and Energy Transitions at the beginning of the nineteenth century, as we have described them; she was noting how culture and aspirations change as a result of economic change. Modern public health, instigated in the time when Eliot was a young woman, often looks, in terms of image at least, like a story drawn from the past. We have argued that it is a story also for the future, and one which needs a good grasp of the past and how it has shaped the present and thus the future which public health bodies must address.

Eliot's character, the keen observer Mr Deane quoted above, saw part of societal transition in terms of the Energy Transition. In 1923 J.B.S. Haldane, the biologist referred to in our account of the Biological Transition (Chapter 10), proposed that 'the power question in England' would be solved by 'rows of metallic windmills working electric motors which in their turn supply current at a very high voltage to great electric mains'.[3] Although known as a great synthesiser of evolutionary biological thinking, he was anticipating a return to the dominance of renewable forms of energy which had existed prior to the 1800s but been replaced by the Energy Transition to coal and steam admired by Mr Deane in Eliot's novel. How right he was (at least on this topic; he also referred to smoking as the hallmark of civilised comfort and eagerly predicted an era of synthetic food!).

Half a century later, in the midst of the oil era, the world went into economic shock in the first great energy crisis, in the early 1970s. This was analysed by the Club of Rome and many writers since, and has been a theme of political economics for decades now. It accelerated debate about security and continuity, and fuelled the debate about sustainable development. This new perspective in world politics was perhaps first fully articulated in the Report of the World Commission on Environment and Development, chaired by Gro Harlem Brundtland, who later became director general of the World Health Organization.[4] Right to today, the energy question dominates public and corporate policy, and there are now thousands of energy watchers and institutes, all pointing to a crisis for the twenty-first century. Yet, as we write, the direction being mostly supported at the national political level is of variants of 'business as usual', how to get the world back into what is agreed elsewhere is an unsustainable direction.[5]

The case emerging from our own account in Part II is not opposed to change; on the contrary, change is inevitable, a fact of life after Darwin, and one which frames how public health has to be understood. Further, we have shown how public health actions are often reactions to change in politics, economy and society, let alone in the natural world and environment. It may be that, as a movement or force for progress, those who champion the public health will inevitably be reactive, always responding to the outcome of other forces. Therein lies a strength of ecological thinking. It helps conceptualise public health appropriately because it assumes change is the nature of existence and that everything interacts. One reaction to ecological thinking – in the interactive sense – is that this makes everything so complex, inducing retreat: 'It's too complex. We cannot do anything about it.' Our view is that, if this is the nature of existence, then that complexity can be grasped sufficiently to be able to make a difference. We have offered our heuristic of the four dimensions of existence as a way to conceive of health. They provide a 'lens' for Ecological Public Health. Seeking out the juxtaposition of the material, biological, social and cultural dimensions of existence for any problem helps provide a template, a lens, a grid – choose your metaphor – through which one looks at public health. Issues which are seen as purely biological or material issues are enriched by the addition of the cultural and social dimension, and vice versa. Thus, for example, the nineteenth-century (and present) campaigns against dirt and squalor are about changing not just the material and biological worlds but also the cultural and social worlds.

In the rest of this chapter, we draw out some key implications from this analysis and the preceding chapters. The aim is to offer a pathway through the complexity in pursuit of better public health.

Implication 1: Use ecological thinking to address public health

In Chapter 3, we outlined five models of the public health. They were: Sanitary-Environmental, Social-Behavioural, Bio-Medical, Techno-Economic and Ecological Public Health. Each of these has been seen to have value, and to address elements of public health challenges. The Sanitary-Environmental model addresses a world of concentrated populations and burgeoning industrial and economic activity. The Social-Behavioural model addresses the world of belief and behaviour, appropriate for a world apparently resolving the Malthusian scarcity problem. The Bio-Medical model was ascendant in the twentieth century and offered workable interventions for newly understood microbiological problems. The Techno-Economic model draws from the alliance of scientific knowledge and capital to offer focused technical answers to mass public health problems. The Ecological Public Health model stresses the integration of different spheres of existence, suggesting interdisciplinary knowledge and a society-wide framework of intervention and action.

So why do we find this latter model so important and worthy of a higher profile? It is the title of our book. For us, the Ecological Public Health model is the most important, although currently most marginal, being mainly associated with the environment. Despite the other models having advantages and richness, this one has particular advantages. Firstly and crucially it is unifying. Ecological Public Health is 'ecological' in two senses. It both provides a way of looking at interactions – Darwin's entangled bank (see Part I) – and addresses divisions between human health and the 'health' and working of the natural environment. It reminds societies which have apparently bought the illusion that the environment can be endlessly raided, mined, treated badly or simply ignored that evolutionary and ecological forces underpin life. This model is also unifying in that it stresses links across the disciplinary boundaries. It helps in understanding the world as it is evolving. It points to continual transitions which influence health. In some people's language, this is the determinants of health. These transitions are the ground on which health is shaped. They are, in this book's subtitle's terms, the conditions which need to be reshaped for good health. The transitions themselves continuously interact, generating complexity. Ecological thinking assumes this state of affairs and provides an intellectual lens through which that complexity can be understood. Complexity does not need to be daunting; it is the inevitable reality.

A tricky issue that arises from Ecological Public Health thinking is actually another advantage: the allocation of responsibility for public health. If public health is multi-sectoral and complex, the fantasy evaporates that there is always a single 'lever', or even a group of 'levers', to pull – the dream of emulating Dr John Snow's mythical removal of the Broad Street water pump handle (see Chapter 1). Scientific superheroes and -heroines are rare beings and rarely acknowledged in their day. Edward Jenner, the originator of vaccination certainly was, but John Snow, the emblematic dogged investigator of environmental woes, was not. His status was only revived years after his death.[6] The complexity and multiple interactions which Ecological Public Health assumes mean that no one or few institutions, bodies or professions can resolve public health problems on their own. Public health is inevitably about teams, about the collectivity of actors, not the intrinsic superiority of one profession. Planners, for example, might be more important than physicians in enabling people to live and work in healthy environments. The relative imbalance of public or private provision of transport might be more important, although more silently so, than the provision of gyms to tackle physical inactivity. Key actors in public health promotion might be the public itself. Health, like ill-health, can be communicable: hence our focus on the social dynamics and importance of culture in the transitions described in Part II. But stressing the case for team thinking and work does not preclude simplicity of purpose or action. Sometimes the public health is improved by simple actions: the provision of clean water, toilets, uncontaminated food and life-building employment. These may appear 'simple' but can be very hard to achieve; their enactment requires a diversity of actors and forces.

Another advantage of the Ecological Public Health model is that it champions a rebalancing of what is meant by health activity, away from healthcare as the primary focus to prevention as the primary focus. For those people who like the 'stream' analogue of change, Ecological Public Health requires 'upstream' thinking and action to avoid 'downstream' problems. A political difficulty is that the public – not just politicians – is often happier to show commitment to hospitals and healthcare than to what seems long-term or diffuse in prevention work. Both forms of action – cure and prevention – are needed; like everyone else, we use them, rely on them and have been saved by them. Healthcare is visible; and its value is concentrated in the rich, developed world. Public health protection, however, tends to be invisible until you have eyes or the nose for it – seeing open sewers in slums, or not having the provision of piped water, or breathing foul air or suspecting factory pollution. Ecological Public Health emphasises prevention but does not pose a false dichotomy between prevention and cure. Our case is that more emphasis is always required in society to promote prevention; healthcare institutions always garner full support, but they too will be changed if an Ecological Public Health approach is the basis for health policy. As we saw, the effectiveness of antimicrobials and antibiotics has been undermined by over-reliance. More emphasis on prevention might have lengthened their utility. The same logic looks to be true for the explosion of diabetes; more attention on prevention makes sense, not least for treatment.

Our proposition is that Ecological Public Health integrates and overlaps the best of the other models set out in Part I. In the next implication, we apply our heuristic of the four dimensions of existence as a way of translating Ecological Public Health thinking into public health analysis.

Implication 2: Use the four dimensions to address complexity

In a complex world, inhabited by billions of people, in diverse circumstances, with different traditions and social structures, public health could easily become just another source of complexity. The case we set out early in this book is that it is helpful to look at public health through the lens of four dimensions:

- the *material*, which refers to the physical and energetic infrastructure of existence;
- the *biological*, which refers to the bio-physiological processes and elements, not just 'blood and bodies' but plants and all that grows;
- the *cultural*, which refers to the importance of how people think and to the formation of collective consciousness;
- the *social*, by which we mean interactions between people, and their mutual engagement as collectivities, in the form of the institutions through which societies operate.

These four dimensions are 'heuristics', our offering of a lens through which people working in public health can order and conceptualise their tasks and roles. The four dimensions help clarify what otherwise can become competing factors and forces. The history of public health is of tackling major problems and responding to processes which cross borders, cross categories, and override the intellectual fragments. These are not easy to pin down or sometimes even understand. Yet they must be tackled if the public health is to be protected and improved. Even in the nineteenth century, this was a daunting task: hence the furious battles about actions sketched in all histories of public health. In the twenty-first century, to an already complex mix of dynamics and factors is being added a welter of awesome tensions such as climate change, water stress, and energy and resources using technical advances. These issues require multilevel action.

An example of modern complexity is surely rising obesity and overweight. It is defying quick-fix responses, yet is widely agreed to be a major public health problem worldwide. Different interest groups compete to offer policy-makers their 'solutions': drugs, psychology, surgery, labels, product reformulation, gyms and more, amounting to what we have called elsewhere a policy cacophony, a wall of competing analyses and appeals. The evidence that there is a problem is not in doubt; it has been building for decades, first noted at WHO level in the 1980s, alarmingly so by the 2000s.[7] In the mid-twentieth century, if one had said that obesity would be a factor that ought to reshape the food system and that would raise questions about the implications of society escaping the Malthusian trap by being able to produce previously unimaginable amounts of cheap, nutrient-dense foods (see Chapter 9), few would have believed you. René Dubos was unusual in predicting a mismatch between human bodies and food supply systems; here was an Ecological Public Health theorist applying the model and predicting health worsening.[8]

Yet, by the early twenty-first century, the number of obese and overweight people on the planet had exceeded the number of the malnourished.[9] Even though the number of hungry people had risen alarmingly to nearly 1 billion – following the 2007–08 oil, commodity and speculation crisis[10] – the number of overweight people had already risen to 1.5 billion people. This was the figure of people aged 20 years and over with a body mass index of 25 and over, plus obese people with a body mass index of 30 and over. Of this 1.5 billion, over 200 million men and almost 300 million women were obese. These are not perfect measures, but they underscore the trend. The WHO estimated in 2011 that 65 per cent of the world's population live in countries where overweight and obesity kills more people than underweight. Nearly 43 million children under the age of five were overweight in 2010. All this is for an officially categorised disease that is preventable yet has more than doubled worldwide since 1980.[11]

As these figures and clinical concerns rose in the early 2000s, governments began to worry about the healthcare costs. Thus far, most attempts to tackle obesity and overweight had been health education: advice, labelling, information, media shows, some withdrawal of the supply of soft drinks in schools, and so on. Generally, these were 'soft' policy measures. Few regulations or fiscal measures and no serious bans had been introduced, with the exception of a few pioneering public health experiments such as New York's soft drink ban in schools, and restrictions on trans-fatty acids in Denmark. The food industry worldwide had fiercely resisted for years any attempts to impede the relationship between consumers and market choice. Politicians were also wary of being seen as 'nannies' or 'big brothers' (see Chapter 1).

The obesity problem began to appear intractable. Yet pressure rose mainly owing to anticipated healthcare costs ahead.

In England, for example, the pressure on public policy was first expressed not within public health but by the National Audit Office, the body charged to review and ensure efficient use of public money.[12] This was utilitarian thinking, and effective in that it was followed by the chief medical officer of England, in his annual report, labelling obesity as a 'timebomb'.[13] A parliamentary inquiry followed, producing a damning report on obesity's systemic nature.[14] To tackle rising weight required a society-wide change, yet there was no appetite for this, nor even did a magic bullet or single 'lever' or measure offer itself. Further delay happened when the chief scientist of England was asked to conduct an in-depth forecasting study.[15] This was effective. It produced a sobering account (in the Foresight report) of the structural nature of rising weight, including a celebrated systems map (see Figure 13.1). This map put at its centre the basic metabolic fact of overweight: if people consume more than their bodies expend in energy, human physiology (a legacy of evolution) will put on weight. Around this central 'engine of energy (im)balance' were modelled a vast number of factors. The Foresight report showed, much as we argue for Ecological Public Health, that these factors can be identified and are clustered (see Figure 13.1). The clusters

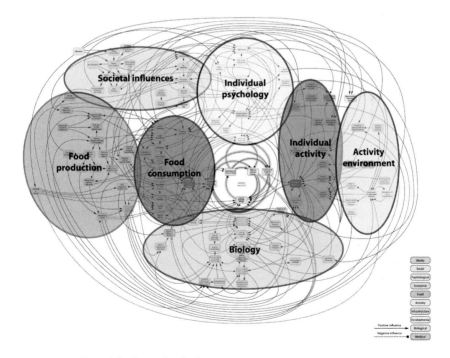

FIGURE 13.1   Foresight thematic obesity map

Note: The grey lines in the background, as reproduced here, are all interactions with varying degrees of strength more easily viewed in the full-size original.

included biological inheritance, societal influences, individual psychology, activity, environment and food production. It followed from this analysis that the Foresight report recommended cross-sectoral, 'multi-stakeholder', interdisciplinary actions. There was agreement by scientists, if not yet by the media, that obesity was the 'climate change of public health'.[16]

Within a few months, a three-ministry £0.3 billion programme was launched: Healthy Weight, Healthy Lives.[17] This was ostensibly to translate the systemic analysis into public policy, setting targets to slow the rise in obesity. The biggest single expenditure item of the £0.3 billion was in fact on a social marketing campaign, Change4Life (see Chapter 11). The Healthy Weight, Healthy Lives strategy appeared to follow on from the Foresight systems analysis, but in fact was shaped around the least controversial and feasible measures. Some trial health towns were set up with three years' funding. Pilot schemes for improving fruit and vegetable consumption from convenience stores in low-income areas were created. A healthy food code was drafted. Obesity climbed up the local public health agenda. All these actions were positive, but were they sufficient to make a difference? Meanwhile, there was a change of government; a year and a half later, the new government softened the approach still further, relied on 'nudge' thinking and merely made another 'call for action' in late 2011, a decade after that had already been done by the National Audit Office.[18] And did they really follow Foresight's systems analysis? We think not. In truth, the Foresight analysis and policy mix were incomplete. Obesity has taken decades to create. Decades of car-based planning have made it harder for people to build their lives around daily exercise. There are long distances between home, work, school and shops. The goal of building exercise and good food into daily life and culture have been systematically, not haphazardly, made hard. Cultural signals celebrate cheap, fatty, sugary foods. These are ubiquitous in their offer. Prices are low (historically) because cheap food policies have been pursued. Advertising and marketing bombard consumers with the messages 'Eat me, enjoy, now.' In short, obesity is a symptom of and coexistent with various transitions we have described in Part II: Energy, Nutrition, Culture and Economic Transitions. The four dimensions of Ecological Public Health are represented in the Foresight analysis, but where it fell down was in translating these into a robust policy mix. Transport, for example, was almost completely ignored: the car-based culture was untouchable.

What should happen if a society really wanted to tackle overweight and obesity? Short of an oil crisis which would cause the modern food system to collapse and force people to walk or bicycle to work, school or shop, what could an Ecological Public Health approach suggest? We have sketched such an account. Firstly, a long-term perspective is needed. Obesity did not emerge overnight but as a result of decades of actions and public and private policy choices, such as town and transport planning, consumerism, economic pricing, signals to the food industry, acceptance of sedentary lifestyles, and much more. To be serious about tackling obesity, these need to be in the analytic framework. No quick fix is likely, but changes are possible. These would need to be multi-sectoral, multilevel and multi-institutional.

Table 13.1 gives our view of the necessary kind of mix of thinking and action.[19] It makes a conventional policy distinction between actions which can be expedited by commercial activity (markets), government (the State) and the public (citizens). Taking those three foci for policy action, it then gives examples across the four dimensions we propose.

Our point in this implication is to show that public health analysis need not drown in complexity. It can analyse and confront it. It makes a virtue out of necessity, suggesting the case of teamwork and multi-sectoral action to reshape the conditions of health. It exposes, too, the immensity of changing the environment. This means nothing less than redirecting the legacy of the past. It is comparable to the vision of the nineteenth-century sanitarians daring to tackle urban squalor. If that is necessary, that is what must be done. Soft policy routes on their own are not just bound to fail; they are often part of the problem, obfuscating the task.

Implication 3: Address the transitions to face the future

Our case for spelling out the history of thinking about the transitions in Part II was that it is impossible to clarify public health, let alone which model of public health could be invoked most effectively, unless there is clarity about what the problem is, what drives public health, what it aspires to be and do, and what it is up against.

Like any compilation, the nine transitions presented above are an incomplete list. There are others perhaps that ought to be mapped or which the reader might wish to see included. We might perhaps have proposed that there had been a Habitat Transition, a transformation of housing and homes, where and how people live domestically, a major historical shift from transient homes to fixed roofs (even if plastic). Another candidate might have been physical security, from worlds of fear and insecurity to states where safety and protection are the norm (mostly). Both these transitions feature within the UN and WHO's public health strategies.[20] It could be argued, too, from a women's perspective, that there should be an Emancipation Transition, with a long-term shift from women as chattels to women as self-directing beings. One could characterise the Democratic and part of the Cultural Transitions as just that. We made our list of transitions, however, mindful that ecological thinking requires cross-cutting analysis. Others might champion different transitions or emphases than we have presented, but we remain convinced that the nine we have offered are essential for any understanding of public health. The list is not fixed, however.

What are the collective insights the transitions offer?

- *Understanding dynamics.* The transitions are reminders that public health has always been about understanding dynamics in order to confront and change them. In this sense, protection of the public health is, among other things, a task of constantly changing how and why the conditions of health need to be addressed. We showed how energy production, for example, influenced and

TABLE 13.1 Tackling obesity with the Ecological Public Health model

Focus of action		Altering the four dimensions of existence to reshape diet and physical activity			
		Material world	*Biological world*	*Cultural world*	*Social world*
	Making markets work for health by:	Linking profitability to healthier food ranges.	Changing price signals of food to favour fruit and vegetables.	Agreeing not to target children.	Promoting good, wholesome food to all, but especially to low-income social groups.
		Making food acquisition costs reflect environmental externalities.	Shopping more often for less to burn energy from food rather than fuel.	Supporting honest consumer information.	Aligning companies' success with consumer health.
		Reducing reliance on fossil fuels to encourage physical activity in daily life.	Promoting smaller portion sizes.	Promoting more flexible and diverse social role models.	Accepting restrictions on the commoditisation of relationships in food marketing.
		Ensuring health targets are built into wastage reduction targets.	Farmers producing less fat, sugar, meat and dairy products.		Promoting only self-regulation that works for health.
		Making environmental indicators meaningful for obesity policy.			
	Making governments work for health by:	Making it secure to walk or bicycle to work, school or leisure.	Setting incentives for better-quality food for all socio-economic groups and ethnic minorities.	Setting clear, long-term cultural goals.	Setting minimum income standards for a sustainably produced, wholesome diet.
		Aligning sustainable consumption targets with public health targets.	Focusing subsidies to promote healthier food ranges.	Helping educate 'taste' to be more discriminatory.	Ensuring all citizens have a requisite level of food choosing, sourcing and preparation, and general food literacy.

Making the public live healthily by:	Incorporating health into food industry sustainability strategy targets.	Using public procurement and other fiscal measures to manage demand.	Supporting the strengthening of social rituals when people bond through food.	Introducing fiscal measures such as aligning taxation of marketing expenditures with the health properties of food and drink.
	Using planning functions to build physical activity into daily life (school, work, local).	Setting and paying for high standards of public sector catering.		Providing more remedial support for overweight people.
	Demanding an extension of 'defensible' public space beyond home and protected malls, etc.	Ensuring local government fully reflects national obesity targets.	Accepting the need to eat less unless they engage in more physical activity.	Eating together, regular meal-times and breakfasts.
	Enabling children to play in streets and parks.	Altering the composition of their diets.	Being more health-discerning about when, how often and what to eat.	Using food as an affirmative social engagement.
	Getting out of their homes more to reclaim civic space.	Building exercise into daily life to promote energy balance.	Being prepared to redefine parental responsibility for long-term benefit rather than short-term family peace.	
	Accepting fewer parking spaces for cars.	Creating new cultures of daily activity, e.g. accepting less car use.		

continues to affect levels of pollution and environmental despoliation, as well as providing improvements to people's lives. The unleashing of stored carbon in the form of coal and coal gas, both for direct heating and to drive electricity generation, has vastly improved women's lives, enabling cooking, cleaning and the washing of clothes to be done in less time and with less direct physical harm. And yet such sources of energy are now widely agreed to be finite (a debate that began with Jevons in the mid-nineteenth century), requiring replacement by sustainable sources, and controls to limit CO_2 and climate change gas emissions. Nor can one have romance about more 'primitive' or traditional forms of energy – firewood, simple biomass, etc. – since they too cause harm to households and those who gather them via indoor pollution and environmental degradation.

- *Focusing on whole populations.* Populations have dynamics just as individuals do, but one cannot reduce the former to the latter. The health of the public can be affected without a mass of people necessarily individually knowing why. Outcomes can be indirect, as emerged in the discussion of the Epidemiological and Health Transition, for example. The public health is about population not just individual levels of action. This is not a new insight, of course. Whether the action is bodily intervention, such as vaccination or drugs, or the establishment of new habits, as we explored in the Cultural Transition, or the confrontation of power that we noted in the Democratic and Economic Transitions, the public health has been about challenging and altering mass behaviour, society-wide processes and the collective experience. Promoting the public health recognises that individuals operate and exist within social frameworks, mediated by groups, a point lost by laissez-faire or individualist approaches. One can address the public health, even at the minimalist level that the opponents of public health are prepared to accept (see Image 9 in Chapter 1), only if the societal and group dimensions of existence are in the frame. The health of the public cannot be built on an atomised perspective of society as a collection of individuals. People might think of themselves as individuals – which they are genetically – but for public health what matters is the communality, the shared genes, the shared experience, the shared worlds, and only then the variations. As we saw in previous chapters, the great cholera epidemics of the past took place through the emerging microbial unification of the world. That world, because of the rapid potential spread of new or resurgent infectious diseases and the reducing effectiveness of antibiotics defences (reminding ourselves of the self-defeating nature of war metaphors), may be approaching new, more troubling zones of risk.

- *Confronting normality.* Acting for the public health has often been a matter of confronting normality, by which we mean questioning the acceptance of harms as inevitable. The protection of the public health has required a combination of theorising, experimentation and practicality. In all the transitions, whether the examples are Bazalgette's re-engineering of London's River Thames and its tributaries to transport away human sewage or New York City's ordinances against spitting to contain TB, normality was being confronted. To protect public health one needs to change normality, because it has been changed by human activity.

- *Taking the long view.* The transitions collectively provide a long time sequence. In a world fixated on the short-term, the immediate and the instant, this is important. Nothing that happens today is unaffected by the past. In the Energy Transition (Chapter 7), we saw that the main technologies or forms of energy processing in use today were products of the nineteenth century. A sense of history and a long future is essential when setting priorities and tracking long-term effects. The past is not just in museums or libraries but in arguments, ways of seeing and thinking, formulae for action, social experiments, and attempts at improvements. Taking the long view forces people within public health to be reflective. A contemporary example might be the acceptance of a high level of meat and dairy consumption as normal and understandable aspirations within culture. As was noted in the Nutrition Transition, the case for lowering Western levels from their high consumption levels (an average 82 kilograms per head per year) is considerable.[21] This requires public health specialists and activists to dare to confront what is now considered almost a 'right' to eat enormous amounts of meat. Animal production now accounts for about a third of all usable productive land, not least owing to half of all the world's cereals being fed to animals. The net effect is that public health messages about reducing fat and calorie intake now have to confront what is deemed normal and a reasonable aspiration. The long view gives public health activists confidence that human health does not require high-level meat and dairy consumption and that the future is likely to require a change of food cultural direction. And, on the other hand, the long view is sensitive to the long aspiration from previous generations which saw rising meat consumption as an indicator of progress. The long view is important because it addresses the meanings and actions in daily life which are inherited, not necessarily 'hard-wired'. It also shapes the task ahead, which is to help shift from consumerism to citizenship.[22]

Another example of the value of viewing public health through the transitions is the case of vaccination, presented earlier within the Biological Transition (see Chapter 10). Even in that short account, it was clear that tensions associated with the Democratic and Cultural Transitions emerged. Vaccination was not and is not a Bio-Medical intervention alone. Questions bubbled over the rights and wrongs of vaccination, over its evidence base, over whether a superior power – doctor, government, law, local government – could impose the technology on to the people. It raised the distinction between authority, the securing of confidence in science and therefore public legitimacy, and authoritarianism, the illegitimate imposition of science. No single transition can encompass vaccination as its territory alone. It also raised questions with regard to the Economic Transition, about efficiency and the capacity of health populations being available for work. Vaccination can be offered up as a success factor in the Epidemiological Transition, and a method which enables Urban Transitions to succeed rather than fail, by keeping disease at bay when humans are massed together, facilitating disease spread. We noted, too, how the vaccination story has a strong cultural element, in that people's beliefs shaped their reactions and support for or resistance to it. This is still true in the early twenty-first century.

The transitions were presented in Part II singly, yet each one was really an investigation of one part of common public health territory. This is, we believe, a perspective previously not championed as overtly as we do here. The transitions, we submit, have to be taken together, because they inhabit a shared universe, not parallel universes. As we have shown, many stories within the transitions demonstrate how public health cannot be compartmentalised, yet all the time simplification has to be achieved. That is why this book began with existing images of health. For the twenty-first century, public health needs new simplification, and new images of and for itself within a world of ever-growing complexity. People working to improve public health need to reconnect with this bigger picture of the interplay of large-scale forces and trends. Better conceptualisation of public health should lead to better results from public health actions. Figure 13.2 repeats the simple model of the interplay between human health and eco-systems health introduced in Chapter 2. We further argued there that a useful way to address that dynamic is through the 'lens' of what we called the four dimensions of health – material, biological, social and cultural. Figure 13.3 aligns both together – looking at the core dynamic through the lens of the four dimensions. In Part II, we have shown how health and ill-health emerge from the dynamics of the transitions. Figure 13.4 graphically represents the transitions combining to create the conditions on which health emerges. These conditions are the terrain on which the dynamic of human and eco-systems health is played out. Figure 13.5 combines all these three images and places the core dynamic of human and eco-systems health within the conditions shaped by the transitions but then further

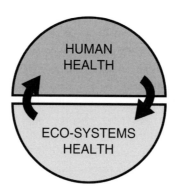

FIGURE 13.2   The dynamics of Ecological Public Health: a simple model

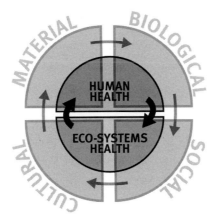

FIGURE 13.3   Aligning the four dimensions with the dynamics of Ecological Public Health

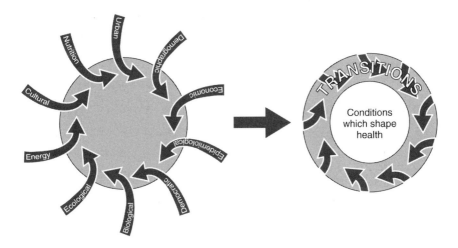

FIGURE 13.4   How the transitions create the conditions which shape Ecological Public Health

acted upon by events, time and human action and institutions – themes considered in this chapter. Figure 13.5 creates what we call here the complex model of Ecological Public Health. It pulls together the argument of this book. It represents how the flow of events can generate different health outcomes, here presented as either sustainable or unsustainable health futures. It posits the dynamics framing health as within not just the transitions but also the actions of social movements, the place of institutions and the passage of time. The rest of this chapter amplifies that interpretation of public health.

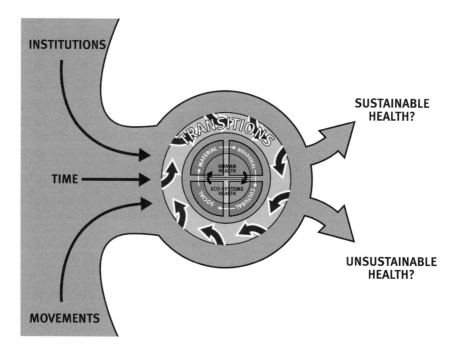

FIGURE 13.5 The complex model within the flow of events leading to different health outcomes

Implication 4: Invoke the public health imagination

An ingredient often absent from lists of public health capacities and skills is what we propose to call the public health imagination. Without it, public health, like so many army generals, is ready only for the last battle it won (or lost). Celebrating the public health imagination is one of the lessons from the transitions. By 'imagination', we do not mean fantasy or flying in the face of reality but being prepared to think beyond the situation. It is being sufficiently grounded to dare to think outside conventions. We are not abandoning tried-and-tested public health experience, although it is widely agreed that good practice always needs updating and revalidating. The public health imagination is daring to conceive of altering accepted reality and common sense. Public health thinking in this respect makes a cultural contribution. It can transform daily life, habits and expectations. It dares to imagine a world operating within different values, goals and norms.

Public health thinking needs to be constantly refreshed and updated. It needs the production of new hypotheses, a recommitment to meet the health needs of *all* the public, not just the exceptional 'healthy town' or marginalised at-risk groups. It engages abductive reasoning, the tentative and the expressive. It also needs to dare to think about confronting the widening of the health gap between rich and poor. That was the import of Geoffrey Rose's distinction between the population and the high-risk strategies (see Chapter 5). Thomas McKeown's challenge to the Bio-Medical model was that it alone could not provide the framework for public health advance. The imagination is about conceiving the possibility of taking the small social experiment – the healthy town – and writing it large, spreading it across all society. For us, a key feature of the public health imagination is critical thinking, what the ancient Greeks called 'scepticism'. It means imagining wholesale change and using opportunities when they come, as well as building change by steady incrementalism, if political circumstances dictate.

In 1987, a dreadful fire occurred in the London Underground at King's Cross station, caused most likely by a burning match or ash discarded by a traveller at the top of an escalator. Smoking was then allowed. This fallen match was thought to fall into the escalator where the running track underneath was dirty with grease and detritus, not having been cleaned since it was erected.[23] Smoking had been banned deep underground, on platforms and trains, two years earlier, following another fire on the Underground. For years, public health specialists had known that smoking in the confined space of underground railways gave people who did not smoke no choice (now known as passive smoking). The outcry and inquiry that followed the 1987 fire gave the opportunity to change behavioural norms – for workers, cleaners and passengers – for good. The case for seeing tobacco use in environmental terms had been established, as had the case for changing social norms. Eventually, broader measures on smoking in public places were introduced in all public settings. In so doing, the English contributed to a network of precedents and international experience at altering the boundaries of acceptable behaviour and the tacit rules for daily life. What was originally opposed by economic libertarians as impinging on individual liberties was more generally recognised and appreciated by the majority. Here, perhaps, was Jeremy Bentham's 'greatest happiness of the greatest number' principle in action.

The public health imagination dares to think of the possibility of the public good. It seeks opportunities for cultural shift. Imagination is required to see that factors, social groups and dimensions of existence (in our terms) might interact with each other. It means being prepared to think laterally and to change the categories which are measured. To refer to Geoffrey Rose again, it requires default thinking to shift away from seeing health risks as an amalgamation of individual risks (protecting oneself) to being able to grasp the dynamics of population risks (protecting everyone).[24] This is to move from personalised to systems failures, and therefore from personalised to systems change.

Discussion about achieving change within public health circles often dissolves into a debate about resources. Have we sufficient labour force or the right institutional location, influence or leadership? Of course, resources are needed to change the conditions for health. Investment in infrastructure, skills and material change is vitally needed in many parts of the world, from ensuring good water and sewerage to housing and safe work. But even there at the front line of global public health inequality, the public health imagination is needed. There might actually be sufficient resources but in the wrong hands, or corrupted, or working in inappropriate directions, or unacknowledged.[25] The problem is not resources but the politics of ownership. In the case of obesity, most of the marketing resources are in the hands of those who want to sell more inappropriate foods to more people. Even a large amount of money in public health hands is unlikely to be able to compete with the sheer weight of 'conventional' advertising, what we called earlier anti-social marketing (see Chapter 11). We note that the RAND Corporation, one of the oldest Western think tanks, funded by the Douglas Aircraft Corporation to advance military strategy in the 1940s but now with a far wider remit, has proposed that advertising and marketing should come under far more restrictive controls. Its researchers have suggested that they be licensed.[26] Within the neoliberal approach to economic governance, self-regulation is always preferred, and presented as the best route to corporate involvement with public health. Yet history also suggests that self-regulation can mean little or no change or symbolic change only, with sales and profits taking a higher priority. Even though corporations are powerful, the public health imagination dares to conceive of a world where they too have to conform to population measures. What is needed is to change the environment and to impede the routine and active reinforcement of anti-health behaviour.

The public health imagination, as we sketch it, is not a new perspective; we merely seek to polish and champion an old and honourable tradition for today. Chadwick's report which led to the 1848 Public Health Act in England and Shattuck's plans for Massachusetts in the USA a decade later were early attempts to change the parameters of health.[27] They staked a claim that a better public health is desirable and essential. Here we are restating a core argument that public health is not about whether or not there is a doctor, profession or institution with the words 'public health' in the title, but about transforming society, the economy and everyday culture to obtain the public health. When Chadwick or Shattuck spoke of public health in the mid-nineteenth century, they meant it either as a description of a condition of the population or as an aspiration to achieve a desirable status. Also for Chadwick, ever the analyser of costs versus benefits, public health had a prime cash value: hence his preparedness to change the ground rules in the interests of health.

Although at the start of this book we described the critique of public health as being bossy, interfering and controlling (Image 9 in Chapter 1), we nonetheless see the public health movement as firmly located within the Enlightenment. It believes in progress, but the debate is about for whom and how it may be achieved. One group of historians of US public health have noted that a century ago one of the acknowledged heroes of the public health movement, Hermann Biggs, once described public health as both 'autocratic' and 'radical' in nature.[28] Yet, even at its most 'bossy', the public health movement has been a proponent of progress, variously defined, but united in the sense of a better future and a controllable present. The ethos has been that 'things' (people, events, situations, environments) can be changed. The message has been that people may not like it or how it is done, but the assumption is that humanity does not need to wait for God-given or 'natural' events or even shocks (such as wars) to improve its lot in the reconstruction.

Destiny can be shaped; general risks can be minimised. Children do not need to die early. Parental suffering can be prevented. Ill-health is not inevitable. Circumstances can be improved. The criticism of being bossy or interfering sometimes levelled at public health has to be challenged. Fatalistic norms can be replaced by more optimistic norms.

Today, as we write, that optimism is cowed and in doubt. Financial turmoil, environmental threats, the rise of religious fundamentalism, and more are all proposed as reasons not to be positive about the future. Our argument is that these threats and this moment of cultural uncertainty offer the opportunity to reinvigorate and redefine progress. We need to confront the negatives of the age, just as the proponents of public health in the past have faced theirs. Today, the great ills are obvious: vast inequality and the excesses of a rampant minority which devalues and demeans humaneness and values vast wealth and conspicuous consumption over the sharing of wealth, time and possibility for all. This concern, expressed today across the public health field, is neither new nor original. It is shared with the most progressive trends of ecological thought. The most popular scientist of his own day, Alfred Russel Wallace, writing in 1898, referred to 'the perennial problem of wealth and poverty'. For Wallace, with Darwin the co-discoverer of natural selection, this issue assumed 'the greatest importance' over any other. 'In dealing with this question I have adduced a body of evidence showing that, accompanying our enormous increase of wealth, there has been a corresponding increase of poverty, of insanity, of suicide, and probably even of crime, together with other indications of moral and physical deterioration.'[29] If this argument remains as disputed today as then the causes and consequences of inequality are certainly more complicated. A better world requires better health, not more consumer goods or the creation of unrealisable fantasies that everyone can live a pop-star or football-idol lifestyle. There is much to be hugely grateful for about modern life: its openness, the need for power to prove its legitimacy, the holding of politicians to account, and some technical advances, particularly in medicine. But in the age of Twitter, Facebook and celebrity culture, public health figures lack 'street credibility' because they have not spoken for reform and progress.

To some extent, the vast investment in healthcare, and more material comforts that are associated with Westernisation have made public health a victim of its own success. A trip to the developing world or engagement with those societies characterised by brutal working lives, endless work and dire material existence reminds us how benign modern life for the developed world can be. Diseases have been pushed back. Preventive measures, such as vaccination, help populations ward off biological dangers. Hospitals and schools are available. Clean water flows from taps in houses. Electric light is reliable. Sewerage systems are deep underground, not seeping in streets. It is no wonder that immigrants to rich societies are so grateful for such infrastructure when so many in rich societies take it for granted. The immigrant might well know the drudgery let alone danger from a lack of such infrastructure. Appealing to that knowledge, the US Democratic Party chose its 1952 election slogan as 'You never had it so good', an appeal that was echoed in 1957 by the UK prime minister Harold Macmillan in a speech to his fellow Conservatives in the town of Bedford: 'let us be frank about it: most of our people have never had it so good'. That appeal to optimism and gratitude crossed political divides in the developed world, fresh from the Second World War. The process of development could be summed up in a political equation: 'wealth = health'. Often, the equation has substituted healthcare for health: one needs wealth to feed healthcare.

Aneurin Bevan (1897–1960), the British politician who steered the foundation of the British healthcare system (the National Health Service), articulated well how, if there is no healthcare or the arrangements are weak, the consequences fall on the individual or family when they are ill. And, when someone is ill, healthcare is wanted. Falling ill therefore is not simply a matter of physical incapacity but has profound economic and psychological consequences. It is no coincidence that Bevan titled his book giving his justifications for collective healthcare provision *In Place of Fear*.[30] He cited Jeremy Bentham, no less, to source the principle of the National Health Service, and yet he located its principal advantage in what it achieved for the relief of individual suffering.[31] 'Not even the apparently enlightened principle of the "greatest good for the greatest number" can excuse indifference to individual suffering. There is no test for progress other than its impact on the individual.'

By this he did not mean individualism as a social philosophy but rather how support for people (and their families) was capable of transforming their quality of life. As we showed in the discussion of the Epidemiological Transition, the contribution of healthcare to public health gain has been relatively recent. For the future, it may very well increase, although this causes deep anxiety to treasuries, which know that this can be paid for only by insurance or taxes, and are already frightened of the bills. Bevan thought that the combination of effective public health measures and the new NHS would result in the clearing up of the backlog of illness and disease. It was not that simple, as was seen in the discussion of the Epidemiological Transition (see Chapter 5). Some trends in medical development reduce treatment demand; others increase it. Increasing medical expenditure, an economist might say, results in declining marginal returns to health. But Bevan was right about prevention. It helps lessen the rising pace of medical demand due to the ageing of populations, but it will not remove it. Progress in health in this respect, at least from the financial point of view, will always be double-edged.

The public health imagination needs to be stretched for this century. One attempt is the argument that both public health and economics should be refocused around happiness.[32] For public health, this is not new; it is why the WHO and UN have championed 'well-being' for decades. It is embodied in the 1946 founding WHO goal of pursuing 'a state of complete physical, mental, and social well-being and not merely the absence of disease or infirmity'.[33] In the twenty-first century, when mental health problems loom very large on the public health agenda, this social-psychological dimension is deeply significant. It was also the centre of Bentham's thinking 200 years ago. It captured, too, the desire for a different world in post-Second World War social and economic reconstruction.

Another powerful contender for a reinvigorated public health imagination is through environmental, social and economic sustainability. In a world with shaky economic and financial structures, public health can and should contribute to a debate about what a good society is. The Western model of progress, now spread worldwide, has prioritised resource-hungry versions of economics.[34] It has fostered a values framework based on possessive individualism. Yet there is now growing recognition that there is a mismatch of aspirations and natural resources, between energy use and resources, and between human needs and consumerist demands. It is not surprising that there is revived interest in the connection between health and people's access to nature. People get healthier when their environment is greener.[35] Greener environments enable people to build exercise into their daily lives.[36] But what is required is society-wide change. Sustainable frameworks of living need to be articulated, designed and championed. This is a role, surely, for the public health imagination and advocates.

Implication 5: Shift from evidence to knowledge

What is evidence and what is knowledge? Here we address the difficulties that public health has over evidence. There is a modern mantra that all good policy is and should be evidence-based. This is championed in public health, but there are also serious debates about whether public health can operate solely on evidence-based criteria.[37] While we agree that public health must be literate about sound science, we are more reserved about whether everything in public health can be or should be reduced to only that which is already evidence-based. The application of an evidence-based perspective has been taken far beyond medicine and public health. It has been argued that 'evidence-based practice' should be applied across management, education, criminology and social work.[38] Many governments like to think that they exemplify 'evidence-based policy-making', an appeal championed in the 1990s.[39]

Our reasoning goes back to the early philosophy of science. Knowledge is reached when a sense of uncertainty is reduced sufficiently to take action. This view of knowledge, not only for science but also for common sense, was supported by the American scientist and philosopher Charles Sanders Peirce in the nineteenth century. Peirce's approach to science and knowledge, what became known as the pragmatic school of philosophy (see Chapter 11), came from his reading of European continental philosophy, in particular Kant and Hegel, but mixed with British empiricism, including Locke, Hume and J.S. Mill, together with the influence of his own practice as a working scientist. He thought empiricism was a significant advance over the forms of reasoning that had preceded it, but he also thought it too simplistic. Peirce concluded that humankind's search for knowledge and its battle against dogma occurred not only because humans are curious but because they need to act. Even so, all knowledge is intrinsically fallibilistic (from the Latin *fallibilis*, 'liable to error'). Absolute certainty is impossible. Empirical knowledge, and our theories, will always be subject to revision.[40] The acceptance of fallibilism does not imply the need to abandon the search for knowledge, nor do we need to have conclusive proof. Rather we accept when we do act that we do so on the basis that the knowledge we employ might later be proved false. Scientific knowledge, for Peirce, was the process by which knowledge was argued over, tussled over and tested. He described knowledge as driven by deduction, induction and, a new concept, abduction, a creative principle for forming hypotheses. Underlying the search for knowledge was the postulate that scientists might only agree in the long term, when actions need to occur in the short term (as all policy-makers know). Although Peirce thought that science was a special part of human activity, more concentrated, more specialist, he thought that the essential rules of knowledge and action applied to everyone.

T.H. Huxley, Darwin's friend and colleague, and probably the person who did most to establish a scientific culture in late Victorian Britain, knew how difficult it was to fix one's view when confronted with complex, often contradictory evidence. He too understood that evidence was part of knowledge but not its sum. It was by its nature fissiparous, pulling in different directions. In an editorial in *The Times* of London (attributed to him), he said:[41]

> To observe correctly, though commonly thought very easy, every man of science knows to be difficult. Our faculties are liable to report falsely from two opposite causes – the presence of hypothesis, and the absence of hypothesis. To the dangers arising from one or other of these, every observation we make is exposed; and between the two it hard to see any fact quite truly.

The basis of much public health thinking is based upon the appeal to evidence and science, but the question remains how much evidence and how much uncertainty over evidence. In the real world, pragmatism and urgency frequently force an answer; action has to happen. In his 1943 book on the history of epidemic disease, C.-E. Winslow quoted a passage from Chadwick's 1842 *Report on the Sanitary Condition* to the effect that the medical controversy around the causes of fever 'does not for practical purposes need be considered, except that its effect is prejudicial to diverting attention from the practical means for prevention'. To this, Winslow appended the remark: 'Blessed was the rugged common sense of the nineteenth century!' He went on to note that miasmatic theory while incomplete had enough truth in it to work. This was, he argued, the 'first generalization of epidemiology to be actually – and on a world-scale – justified by its fruits'.[42] As knowledge grows, the level of uncertainty seems to increase and the grounds for action in many cases narrow. Offering a level of acceptable proof on the likely causes of obesity, for example, would be a major – perhaps impossible – challenge. Look how hard it is to calculate the impact of food marketing on adult consumption. And yet the case for undertaking action to counteract it, as with tobacco advertising before it, seems powerful.

Our discussion of the impact of the transitions was interpretative. Evidence is always uncertain. It changes. It is fallible, as Peirce had observed. People are always trying to make sense of evidence. The evidence of today, moreover, will be replaced by the evidence of tomorrow, and so on. That is the progress of scientific knowledge. How then can evidence be used in making decisions, if it is such an accrual process? Accruing more evidence might take a long time and still not provide cast-iron certainty for strategy. Evidence grows by being tussled over; it is bounced and zig-zagged between reference points and questioners. It is contested all the time. Public health arguments have, over history, been constructed around contested evidence, ignored evidence, rediscovered evidence, right evidence with the wrong theory, wrong theory with the right evidence, evidence gathered without policy conse-quences or, perhaps the best kind, slow-burning evidence which leads to a radical change in knowledge. Our historical account of the transitions gave ample examples. We showed how difficult it is to make the translation between evidence and knowl-edge and onward from knowledge to policy and action. In fact the latter phase is at least as difficult as the first. Some policy analysts point to an ideal cycle of evidence-gathering within the process of policy and practice.[43] This is a virtuous circle of searching for evidence, testing hypotheses and translating the resulting evidence into policy, which then informs practice and which is in turn subjected to renewed scru-tiny and testing. This is the idealised framework championed for the public health world, but little in the world does operate in that way! Our view is not to fantasise about an unrealisable state of perfect synchronicity between evidence, policy and practice. Nor is it to slump into a cynical view that policy and practice can ignore evidence. The task is to produce knowledge which helps frame and guide policy and action through or over the gap between evidence and policy or practice.

Why has this debate taken such hold in public health? The impetus for the evidence-based perspective came from medicine. The approach was established by the Scottish doctor Archie Cochrane (1909–88), although the roots of evidence-based thinking in medicine are ancient. What is called the Cochrane Collaboration has been established alongside the term evidence-based medicine (EBM), which first appeared in the scientific literature in the 1990s. Its aim, and it is an honourable one, has been to raise the standard of knowledge in medicine by ridding it of poor science and poor practice through more rigorous review of evidence.[44] In particular the use of the randomised controlled trials (RCTs) or, better, the systematic review of multiple RCTs has become the 'gold standard' for judging whether a treatment does more good than harm.[45] EBM has been presented as one of the most impor-tant medical milestones of the last 160 years, in the same category as innovations such as antibiotics and anaesthesia.[46]

Although widely accepted – who can argue with the principle of toughly questioned evidence for surgery, for instance? – this approach remains contro-versial, for example when applied to the world of the chronically sick and the interplay between mind and body.[47] The plea has been made that the analytic knowledge provided by EBM review should sit alongside, but not replace, the accumulated experience and knowledge of the physician.[48] EBM calls for the scrupulous use of statistics and employs mathematical reasoning to test associa-tions. Certainly, removing subjectivism from the review of evidence might lead to more disinterested insights. However, as we saw in the Economic Transition (Chapter 8), the employment of mathematical reasoning can come with a cost. Judgement is frequently sacrificed on the altar of mathematical modelling and rule-based thinking. While statistical methods can help resolve some difficulties, they cannot replace the value of human scrutiny, argument and judgement.[49]

It is important to have an open mind about evidence. The pursuit of evidence is framed by assumptions, embedded in the questions and beliefs about what evidence is. Market-based neoclassical economics, for example, is the dominant framework through which much governance and commerce has operated for the last 40 years. But it, like all paradigms, eschews evidence that does not fit within its conceptual construction, that values can be translated into monetary value. In Chapter 8, we identified the incapacity of current dominant economic thinking to explain the financial crisis of the late 2000s onwards. This is a consistently identified failing of neoclassical thinking. Lord Keynes, who devised the world's economic architecture in the immediate aftermath of the Second World War, was lionised as a great economic and social theorist, but he maintained an open mind on the relationship of evidence to need and its place in economics. When criticised by a colleague that he had changed his mind on key aspects of monetary policy during the worst days of the Great Depression in the 1930s, he responded: 'When the facts change, I change my mind. What do you do, sir?'[50] His understanding of evidence was not only commendable but entirely realistic. As noted, evidence – 'the facts' – changes and so do the circumstances affecting fellow humanity. This too is evidence, even if hard to conduct an RCT on or to put through the EBM mill. To stretch the metaphor further, evidence-based policy-making might be a good approach for distinguishing between cogs in the mill but not for looking at whether to redesign the mill.

A more difficult question is why people do not change their perspective as new evidence comes to light. Why, for example, did economists fail to adjust their analyses in the light of the destabilisation of the financial world from 2008? Why do people continue gambling despite not winning? One of the arguments offered is that economists, like everyone, cannot cope with cognitive dissonance (evidence which undermines an entire outlook). When Semmelweis urged his Viennese colleagues to wash their hands before touching patients in the nineteenth century, for which he was derided at the time (see Chapter 3), it is likely his recommendations were greeted as an affront to his colleagues' dignity and thus rejected. This is cognitive dissonance on a group scale. An entirely different explanation (on which C.S. Peirce also commented) is that human assessments are often guided by habit. Once people have fixed a course in their minds, they no longer consider alternatives and instead go on to automatic response. This is not because people are lazy. It is merely the character of the human mind, and indeed an evolutionary advantage. Appeals to think or modify are beside the point; people normally do not think through every action they make. Different psychological dynamics operate. Civilisation advances by extending the number of operations which can be performed without thinking about them, to be conducted on a routine or automatic basis.

Where does this leave public health? If the twenty-first century requires different cultural reflexes and habits, as we have argued emerges from the transitions, the public health movement and professions must overtly champion and adopt changes of mindset. Culture needs different reflexes to be normalised. A.N. Whitehead, the philosopher, considered that operations of thought are like cavalry charges in a battle – they are strictly limited in number, require fresh horses, and must be made only at decisive moments.[51] In modern terms, public health must work by changing mass reflexes so that thought is *not* necessary. Culture must change without forcing every person on the planet to spend their entire days wrapped in calculations and rational choices and weighing up evidence. This can be threatening to Western democracies which celebrate individualism and personal choice.

Another difficulty for public health knowledge is that it has to take the long perspective. In the USA it has been suggested that the 1964 Report of the Advisory Committee to the Surgeon General on Smoking and Health provided 'a paradigm of evidence-based public health policy'.[52] In fact, it took decades of intense arguments and furious political fights against an immensely powerful industry for such evidence to be fully accepted and converted into policy. Moreover, it now transpires that the tobacco industry had the evidence that its products were harmful for a long time, but withheld it.[53] A similarly long time frame is already apparent with the issue of climate change. Decades ago, scientists and amateur observers began collecting and measuring climate data. This now enables the sober assessments of today to be made and built upon.

Such long perspectives have generated the argument that policy and practice may need to be changed before a perfect state of knowledge is achieved, i.e. without the full evidence desired by EBM or evidence-based policy proponents. This realism generated the view that a 'precautionary principle' should be adopted in policy and scientific discourse.[54] An illustration was the case of chlorofluorocarbons (CFCs), used by refrigerator manufacturers as a coolant. The role of CFCs became highly controversial when it was suggested that they were a part-cause of ozone loss in the earth's atmosphere – the discovery of which won Paul Crutzen, Mario Molina and Sherwood Rowland the Nobel Prize for chemistry in 1995. CFCs were not the sole cause of the decline in the thickness of the ozone layer from the 1950s to the 1990s, but their role was significant. Thus a technical advance – previously seen within public health, let alone domestic life worldwide, as a boon – had to be re-categorised as a threat to health. CFCs were banned in 1996, and it is estimated it will take a century or more for the ozone layer to recover.

A not dissimilar transition from wonder to risk has happened to agrichemicals. Heralded as almost miraculous modern farming aids in the mid-twentieth century, they had been found to be a cause of pollution, with residues in food and even breastmilk, by the end of the century. The problem raised by this tale is the issue of how to weigh up relative risks, not the evidence per se.[55] In that respect, contemporary science, often for practical reasons (ranging from the availability of funding to scientific fads and fashions) and for publication reasons, is preoccupied with what exists in the short term. It finds it harder to account for the longer term or for what is missing.[56] Gregory Bateson, the ecologist, argued that this is why ecological or systems-wide studies are needed. Good knowledge can emerge only if entire frameworks are subject to critical assessment. Even small changes in the balance between predator and predated can shift the entire picture and dimensions of an eco-system.[57] That is why systems thinking, notions of feedback, and the complex rebalancing of change are so integral to ecological thinking as we sketch it for Ecological Public Health. This underlines the case for not confining the incremental growth of knowledge to disciplinary compartments.

Being able to assess evidence and refresh conceptions of the world by scientific endeavour is of huge value, but the case we are making here is that the public health cannot rely on scientific *evidence* alone. The pursuit of evidence is obviously a good thing, but it can never be the sole basis for criticism in public health, not least since public health requires interdisciplinary thinking. It cannot be the responsibility of single-issue, expert-led professions. There must be access to a wide range of knowledge and the use of all the sciences not just the natural sciences. Epidemiology, the use of statistical modelling and other forms of advanced statistical reasoning are all part of that project, but the claim that epidemiology alone provides the science in public health should not be accepted.[58] Ecological Public Health requires interdisciplinary knowledge if it is to be able to examine the natural and human worlds critically and hopefully. Knowledge of value for Ecological Public Health is never reducible to one approach or epistemology. The sciences contribute to the Ecological Public Health as a project but cannot colonise it. In making this point we are not alone or new. It had been made by Sir Arthur Newsholme (1885–1935), the Englishman who had held at some time all of the most important posts in public health in England in the early twentieth century.[59] When speaking to the Massachusetts Board of Health in the USA in September 1919, on the occasion of the fifteenth anniversary of the administrative structure first proposed by Lemuel Shattuck, he gave the following opinion:[60]

> Let me in passing comment on the fact that neither Lemuel Shattuck in Boston nor Edwin Chadwick in London was a physician; but a perusal of their writings shows that they were men of sound judgment, of earnest zeal for their fellow men, with a wide and statesmanlike outlook, ready to search out, to accept and to apply the medical knowledge on which necessarily the prevention of disease is based. They illustrate once for all the need for partnership between all well-wishers of humanity in this work, and the importance of combined effort by the sociologist and the physician, as well as of experts in each branch of sanitation, if all attainable success is to be attained.

We propose that, just as Ecological Public Health needs a range of intellectual and experiential backgrounds to inform it in the twenty-first century, it also requires a range of evidence and cannot be purist or absolutist about evidence. The status of evidence is always provisional and subject to later revision. The difficulty with the purist position, championed by EBM as applied to the world beyond medicine, is that it assumes definitive evidence can be found, if only practitioners worked harder, got smarter, made a breakthrough or were better funded. A more realistic view, again to follow the philosopher C.S. Peirce, is to see all evidence and all theories as provisional, the best that one has at the moment, for practical purposes. In that sense, we are arguing that evidence is contingent on circumstances and dependent on what is available at any given moment to people in a situation. If evidence is always incomplete or provisional, then decisions have to be made on the basis of existing not ideal evidence. Judgement is inevitable and not to be shrouded in pseudo-evidence language. Public health action is a matter of judgement. It is better, we propose, to be open about the role of judgement. Failure to do so exacerbates the common difficulty of rogue studies being used by vested interests to dismiss all science. The contrarian line of reasoning emerges. 'They [scientists] cannot agree' becomes 'Do what you like; they cannot make up their minds', a default of tabloid journalism.

Ecological Public Health thus has to be open about the mix of judgement, best evidence, broad bases of knowledge and the necessity of constant critical reassessment. One approach to this new perspective is to be open about what are called the 'framing assumptions' in knowledge and policy-making. This perspective reviews what information is considered relevant and what is left out and how and why evidence is weighted. An example of such knowledge generation is the function of the new wave of public health observatories. These combine data-gathering, analysis and modelling of the future, offering composite foresight analysis to policy-makers and the public.

Our case here is not anti-science or robust evidence. On the contrary, we seek to reconnect the sciences with the public good. Ecological Public Health requires knowledge and also offers knowledge to society. We note the scepticism raised in 1923 by the British mathematician and philosopher Bertrand Russell (1872–1970) in his point that science 'has not given men more self-control, more kindliness, or more power of discounting their passions in deciding upon a course of action'.[61] Our desire is to forge more realistic links between the sciences and the public through public health: science for the public good. The Frankfurt School had argued that the hopes for a scientific enlightenment had been dashed by the Second World War and by the emergence of new means of manipulation and control, such as the marketing industries and the media. We, too, do not glorify science as outside society but as subject to its funding, controls and ideological framing assumptions – exposed as we noted in tobacco, and emerging over the food industry and the scandals of coexisting hunger and obesity in the world. On the contrary, the sciences reflect society in all its complexity, which is why we believe that the moves in recent years to include the public in scientific debate – about risks, new technologies, etc. – are right. The Ecological Public Health requires its adherents to face outwards. Inclusivity, we argue, counteracts fear and lack of knowledge.

Implication 6: Reinvigorate public health institutions and structures

We saw in Part I how public health emerged not just as a way of thinking but as competing arguments about reordering society. We also suggested that behind the everyday exchanges and interactions of daily life are located durable social rules or institutions. Such institutions, we saw, could be of many kinds and appear within society in numerous different ways, such as through language or visual communication with its rich use of metaphor, driving conventions setting the 'rules of the road', table manners, the means by which one blows one's nose in public, or for that matter the private accomplishment of bodily functions that all of us would prefer to keep discreet (although not in some other cultures and at some other times). Such institutions may have been built up over millennia; others, like the use of a handkerchief or toilet tissue, are relatively recent. Some have clear health consequences but in their performance may appear more as matters of manners or politeness. These common social institutions over time become habits or properties of mind, both enabling and constraining behaviour.

Institutions also emerged of a far more formal type. For public health to have a lasting impact, laws need to be established and propounded, organisations developed, funded and staffed, and skills, technologies and knowledge developed, debated, diffused and overseen, as we have just seen. The effectiveness of public health measures in terms of this form of institutional response to society's health needs is in part revealed in the quality of the match between the 'lived' social institutions which guide behaviour and the quality and effectiveness of formal institutions which produce yet another kind of societal response, be they expressed through law, organisational performance or professional task. It is to this realm of action that we now turn.

An implication of the case we have made for Ecological Public Health in this book, having reviewed the immensity of the transitions in Part II, is that the legacy of institutions and structures, inherited from the past two centuries, might need to be revalidated and reformed. New ways of formalising inter-agency processes are urgently needed if Ecological Public Health is to be pursued. In policy circles, this is called the challenge of 'cross-cutting agendas', the recognition that the real world requires collaboration. But this raises thorny issues about how to create collaborative effort and whether current institutions are able to tackle the existing distributions of power which frame public health. Our case is not that there is a lack of institutions – often there are many – but that there is insufficient unity of purpose and resolve to tackle the real conditions which frame public health. A process of better linking the four dimensions of existence mapped in this book – the material, biological, cultural and social – needs to be factored into all inter-agency work.

One particular issue is troubling. The modern world is now multilevel. There are global institutions, regional and continental ones, and national, sub-national and local ones. All these need to work in the same direction if Ecological Public

Health is to be achieved. Too often, fine words and declarations are made at the global level which are not translated at the local or national level. Equally, governments pronounce and make decisions which are hopelessly weak before commercial interests or, worse, are framed by fear of upsetting particular interests or the media. Such politicking is inevitable, of course, but we seek a renewed resolve by people within institutions and roles to work more effectively across agencies and professions. That requires them to have a better narrative about public health for the public. Building public support has to be part of the public health project.

We turn first to the global level. Is the UN adequately promoting Ecological Public Health, the better integration of environment, society, economy and development? As we noted, the Huxley brothers, Julian (head of UNESCO) and Aldous (the writer), hoped that the UN could adopt an ecological perspective collectively. In the succeeding half-century and more, the UN's record is patchy. Partly it is bound into single-issue compartments, laid down in its legal framework and agency remits, created in the post-Second World War reconstruction. And partly it does a decent job in constantly seeking to cross those imposed boundaries. Many of the landmark initiatives from the UN are in fact multi-agency actions, such as the UNCED Rio Declaration of 1992 and the Convention on Biodiversity, or the 2004 WHO–FAO strategy on combating non-communicable diseases.

The conventional map of modern global institutions of public health focuses on what the UN itself likes to call the UN 'family' – WHO, FAO, ILO, UNESCO, Unicef – and the many programmes and post-conference secretariats: UNCTAD, UNCED ('Rio' and 'Rio+20'), UN Habitat, etc. These all have regional or continental presence, but are strictly advisory. The UN is a talking body and only rarely a service deliverer. An exception is the World Food Programme, which distributes food aid in emergencies. In the main, political power over what the UN discusses and advises remains with national member states, a combination of elected governments and some governments accepted into the UN despite lack of democratic governance. In moral terms, the UN is a 'broad church', diverse and divergent.

The defence of the UN 'family' of institutions is that it is cheap. When we did a study for the WHO of how the world's top 25 food corporations were engaging with the WHO–FAO 2004 Global Strategy on Diet, Physical Activity and Health,[62] itself the result of decades of evidence-building,[63] one of the most startling facts that emerged for us was how the marketing budget of just one company, Coca-Cola, dwarfed the entire budget of the WHO for all its work, not just food. The soft drinks company had $2.2 billion for annual marketing, more than the WHO's budget for *two* years.[64] In 1949, the WHO's entire budget was a princely $5 million. Sixty years later, it was just under $5 billion for its two-year budget, but in 2010 that biennium budget was cut by 20 per cent to meet a $300 million shortfall, and in 2011 the total biennial budget was down to under $4 billion, i.e. $2 billion a year, with the Geneva workforce of 2,500 cut by hundreds. Only a quarter of the WHO's budget is core funding from governments; the rest is raised on an ad hoc project basis, and thus subject to donor power. The FAO's budget is larger, around $2 billion a year, with about half that coming from governments for its core functions, the rest from donations and projects. By contrast, UNEP, the UN family member for environmental action, is positively tiny. Its Environment Fund was approximately $200 million in 2009, with only 4 per cent given by member states, the rest from donations.[65]

Now contrast that to the might of the finance or transport sector. An overview by the OECD in 2007 – before the price bubble and crash – showed the hedge fund 'industry', which speculates on asset management, to be a $1.4 *trillion* market, with leverage (financial engagement power) over $5 trillion worth of asset funds.[66] (The OECD paper shows a dexterous way with words when defining hedge funds thus: 'lightly-regulated managers of private capital that use an active investment approach to play arbitrage opportunities that arise when mis-pricing of financial instruments emerge'.[67]) The derivatives industry, which stands accused of sparking the 2007 financial crisis,[68] was a market of $3.8 trillion. This is for funds which speculate. The automobile industry, which at least makes something, employs 5 per cent of the world's labour force, according to the ILO, and has a turnover (sales) which exceeds the gross domestic product of France. When car sales dropped by a fifth or more after the 2008 financial crisis, the European Investment Bank gave an €8.9 billion loan to the European car industry to tide it over.[69] For Ecological Public Health, the contradiction is stark: funds are accessible to support an industry which is unhealthy but has jobs which enable its workforce to live, yet those who control public funds continue to invest in modes of travel which fail the test of sustainability and add to the burden of overweight and obesity. For us, this is a failure both of institutions and of the public health imagination. Yet analyses do exist which could refocus public health. Ian Roberts, professor of public health at the London School of Hygiene, has produced such an analysis. In *The Energy Glut*, Roberts and Phil Edwards show how an Ecological Public Health perspective transforms but explains that situation.[70] It is a democratic failure to control institutions which cause ill-health.

What of the professions? Henry Sigerist (1891–1957), the French-born historian of public health, based at Johns Hopkins University in Baltimore, USA, argued that 'public health officers' always found themselves in situations which were 'the result of definite historical developments'. Hence they not only needed to be 'more than a technician' but required 'a philosophy' to guide their actions. If you know these things, he said, 'you are bound to act more intelligently'.[71] Public health began, we suggested, with a ready-made philosophical system, utilitarianism. This understanding of society easily incorporated a population-based perspective yet was always in tension with values-based approaches, more attuned to the aspirations of individuals or groups. Often what propelled events and change in the past was fear – of contagion, disorder and economic disruption. Today, we are suggesting, the public health would also benefit from a better mix of judgement, evidence and framing knowledge. In the previous implication about knowledge, we singled out processes such as the Foresight programmes and the public health observatories, but in truth they are purely advisory, when they need better institutional backing and translation. 'Advice' is easy to dismiss or park. Realistically, we think Ecological

Public Health is likely to be driven by a mixture of motives, part utilitarianism, part values, part fear and part foresight. They remain the essential co-ordinates of public health. The question now, as in the past, is their relative priority and backers.

The question of priorities always applies. Earlier chapters gave more attention to some societies than others. One country of focus was the USA, which followed the public health route set in the UK, in part because it too industrialised and urbanised. In the nineteenth century the UK was the dominant power on the globe; by the early twentieth century, the pre-eminent power was the USA, which began to exert more influence over the establishment and conduct of international arrangements, treaties and other organisations for public health (see Chapter 12). The USA was a major force in the establishment of the UN system, symbolised by its location in New York, moved from Geneva, where the League of Nations had been based. The name 'United Nations' was coined by President F.D. Roosevelt.

The historical narrative of public health as a Bio-Medical field of interventions is sometimes described as beginning with the 1915 US Welch–Rose Report, authored by William Welch, who a year later became founding dean of the now celebrated Johns Hopkins School of Public Health (now the Bloomberg School), and Wickliffe Rose of the Rockefeller Foundation. This combination of big corporate, now charitable, funding with disease prevention has been significant in appealing to the medicalisation and professionalisation of public health. By the end of the twentieth century, the USA had 29 schools of public health in universities. In fact, a better starting point for US public health history might be Lemuel Shattuck's proposals for Massachusetts in 1850, the US counterpart to Chadwick's efforts in England, Griscom's report on New York City and the efforts of people like Hermann Biggs in New York (see Chapters 2 and 3). C.-E. Winslow, as we saw, attempted to set out a framework for public health of multiple disciplines and backgrounds, citizens and experts. His vision was of public health as pursued by front-line people not just 'top people'. Winslow's vision was medical but also social, preventive and imaginative. His project was to 'sanitise' the environment but realise historic 'birthrights'.

This was a broad vision, but critics argue that it has been diffused and weakened by ceding authority to medicine and other professions. Our Ecological Public Health restores the vision of public health as about the condition of daily lives – housing, food, air, work. This vision, sketched by Shattuck, Winslow and others, has been marginalised, replaced by 'a science-based identity'.[72] This is all very well and utopian, one might think, but where are the budgets? Who has the power and responsibility for bringing it all about? Is the combination of 'public + health' to be addressed only at the population level? Is public health now solely about mass-scale interventions such as vaccines or drainage? Does its intellectual heartland lie in medicine or in social policy or politics? Or is it, as Winslow saw, in engineering, biology and medicine? In the USA, John Hanlon and others in the 1960s tried to restore a model of Ecological Public Health which aligned nature on one side and human organisation and behaviour on the other.[73] The goal today, as then, is to create institutions that could deliver a new conceptual settlement.

In the UK, parallel institutional debates and developments occurred to those in the USA. They happened much earlier but lacked the multidisciplinary and inclusive efforts of the American Public Health Association, which as we saw helped nurture a broader conception of public health than the British one. The combination of Empire and hygiene framed the UK's efforts. In both London and Liverpool, schools of hygiene and tropical medicine were created. The foundation of modern public health is often depicted as the 1848 Public Health Act.[74] This was driven by a civil servant who believed in a theory which was contentious in its day and was proven to be hopelessly wrong afterwards but which 'got the job done'.

What are the functions of public health? In Chapter 2 we looked at efforts to define public health. Summarising the work of the US Surgeon General (the head of US public health), the National Library of Medicine concluded in 2010 that in the last half of the twentieth century the notion of public health had 'not [been] fixed but has changed over time, and changed the practice of medicine, as well, to include areas such as human behavior and mental health'.[75] Note the assumption that public health *was* centrally based in medicine but is now being pulled more broadly! The analysis continued: 'That fact has broad implications for our understanding of health and risk, personal pleasure and social norms, science and moral standards, and individual freedoms and public policy.' The picture here is that public health has been modernised to address the new challenges such as AIDS, nutrition and mental health. This is, in the nicest of senses, a misunderstanding of public health history. Our contention is that public health has always been broad, and always since Shattuck in 1850 has been about personal not just population liberty, about both physiological and social-psychological well-being. But, whatever the past, today the definition and meaning of public health require re-evaluation and that institutional forms should follow from that. We see such a process.

In the UK, the Faculty of Public Health, the organisation representing many public health professionals, proposes that the public health means operating on three domains: health improvement (covering issues such as inequalities, education, housing, employment, lifestyles and disease monitoring), improving services (which includes efficiency, service planning and clinical effectiveness) and health protection (tackling infectious diseases, chemical pollution, etc.).[76] The UK Faculty states that the skills and tasks of its profession are shaped by core values, such as wishing to be equitable, evidence-based and effective. From this, a 'map' is derived for the promotion of nine key areas for public health activity and professional involvement, which include: surveillance and assessment of the population's health and well-being; assessing the evidence of effectiveness of health and healthcare interventions, programmes and services; policy and strategy development and implementation; strategic leadership and collaborative working for health; health improvement; health protection; health and social service quality; public health intelligence; and academic public health.

The Faculty used to represent public health doctors only, although their professional title has changed over the years, just as the Faculty itself has been renamed. The posts were and are based at the local level – first in local authorities, then in the health service and now back again in the local authority. The post title used to be 'social medicine' and was renamed 'community medicine' after government reorganisation in 1974. It is now called 'public health medicine', with a remit which views epidemiology and statistics as core skills and with some inclusion of economics, sociology, psychology and management skills.[77] Today, the Faculty operates on a welcome and even broader terrain, seeking to extend its membership beyond the medically qualified. It now incorporates an upstart movement of the 'new public health', established in the 1980s, the UK Public Health Association, started by people who thought the sweep of involvement should be broader and bolder.[78] Alongside these is one of the oldest organisations, the Royal Society for Public Health, founded in 1876, and today 'dedicated to the promotion and protection of collective human health and well-being'. The body representing the Chadwickian tradition is now called the Chartered Institute of Environmental Health, the most overtly pro-Ecological Public Health of all UK bodies. There are many other professional bodies, ranging from community nurses to pharmacists.

What can be learnt from this variety of public health bodies? In the UK, this fragmentation does not help generate a unified voice for public health. Is it any wonder that the emerging broad vision that we here articulate, and which others do too, has little impact across government and other institutions, let alone on civil society and all-powerful commercial interests? The potential for any model of public health, let alone Ecological Public Health, is dissipated. Ironically, this is not helped by a strong and divergent NGO and civil society sector, which adds greatly to the vibrancy of public health debate but not enough to the co-ordinated and focused injection of public health into the body politic. Many powerful NGOs are still primarily concerned with body parts − cancer, the heart, the brain. Each one competes in the public sphere for money, the public attention and awareness.

The American Public Health Association (APHA) offers an interesting difference to the UK's lead bodies in public health. The APHA is a multi-profession umbrella body. It has a greater emphasis on leadership; public health practitioners are openly encouraged to lead. It covers everything and holds massive conferences, where a dizzying breadth of papers are read and debated. The concern about US public health is not that it lacks focus or breadth but that its aspirations do not accord with the drive and trends of US society. Yet the APHA has been an umbrella under which many progressive forces shelter and through which a socially just voice about the more brutal attributes of US society has been continually expressed. It has contained thinkers who have reshaped the parameters of public health thinking. It is a prime example of a professional institution formed from the social movement that drove public health in the nineteenth century which has retained a continuity and moral purpose ever since. That it exists is wonderful, but from the perspective of Ecological Public Health it has to be concluded that it is not seemingly able to transform US political economy into an ecologically sound way of living. The failure to address obesity is glaring evidence of this.

Across the world, in both rich and less developed societies, it is sobering how many professional societies are now co-opted and subverted by commercial sponsorship, which underpins the large conferences that become the movement's notice boards. Too often, nutrition conferences are sponsored by large food companies whose business is selling sugary, fatty foods, or by sports organisations, themselves sponsored by soft drinks companies. To pay the travel of star speakers and to subsidise facilities, the professions have little alternative, argue the organisers. The intellectual distortion is further twisted by the presence of numerous commercial organisations promoting their own technical fixes. Our view is that the public health movement needs to strengthen its own governance procedures and ethical scrutiny or move into new ways of hosting conferences.

The positive case for the growth of the institutions and professions of public health is that only by getting organised and meeting in person can networks and personal commitments be strengthened. That, after all, was one of the great successes of medicine and social medicine, their professionalisation and exclusivity. Medicine has developed from marginality and 'quackery' to the pinnacle of social respectability. As we have sketched it, Ecological Public Health cannot go that route. It requires interdisciplinarity, focus and efficiency defined as meeting ecological principles, not the narrow cost–benefit approach to cost-effectiveness.

Where does this implication leave Ecological Public Health for the future? Political scientists see what has been described here as normal, and symptomatic of the messiness of modern governance. It is normal to have ineffective or marginalised institutions. Governments do not govern, in the sense that autocratic monarchs do or used to. Modern governance is multilevel, multi-sectoral and increasingly wrapped in the language of 'partnerships', 'co-responsibility' and 'stakeholders'. Consultation is continual, but some voices are listened to more than others, as new, more subtle power relations are forged. This is the world described by the notion of the 'hollowed-out state',[79] where institutions with nominal roles as arbiters of the public interest over particular sectors – industry, health, food, transport, local government, foreign policy, etc. – have few levers to pull, less influence than they might, and more deference across internal powers. In this new world – championed by the Washington Consensus and appeals for weaker government – which health ministry stands up to the ministry in charge of finance or business? This is the cry often made by departing ministers or senior civil servants in private, yet it continues.

Realistically, how could there be one organisation or one institution capable of capturing the diversity of what is required for Ecological Public Health? The answer lies not in wanting a new ministry of Ecological Public Health but in seeing that public health institutions are all over the place, in two senses. One needs to map, firstly, which institutions scattered over society drive the causes of ill-health and, secondly, which might have a positive impact. There is a plethora of institutions. The trouble, as we have spelt out for obesity earlier, is that they inhabit a world where there is policy cacophony: multiple solutions seeking to be heard. Ecological Public Health's promise is that it points to the need to weave together diverse organisations and arguments to confront the drivers of ill-health. That is the lesson of efforts to tackle climate change, where alliances of interest which a decade or so ago would have barely known of each other now strategise and campaign together. Greenpeace and environmental organisations now work alongside eminent professional bodies and work with the UN's success story here, the Intergovernmental Panel on Climate Change (IPCC). Together they are stronger and have helped push back resistance to acting on climate change, not enough of course, but at least they have begun.

We think public health institutions would benefit from reform and refocus. A debate is needed at national, international and local levels. Should the WHO be merged with environmental bodies such as UNEP and given a new Ecological Public Health remit? Or would the new agenda be better served by merely strengthening the environmental bodies by calling for their merger? Either way, what is needed is tougher cross-UN working, and the WHO urgently needs boosting. A parallel reinvigoration of institutions and professional bodies is needed at national and local levels. This book started with a discussion of public health's invisibility yet ubiquity. The Ecological Public Health needs to be articulated. That requires stronger institutions. This requires new narratives, better ways of communicating with daily lives. Single-issue NGOs have often been good at that, engaging with the constituencies. The task ahead is to weave the bigger picture.

Implication 7: Re-energise public health as a social movement

Our view is that public health has to be seen as a movement or it is nothing. This is because it is inevitably having both to react and to anticipate – hence our analysis of the issues of evidence and knowledge and of the institutions above. The modern move to improve public health began in Northern Europe and, in Britain at least, as a movement by the middle classes to clean up their towns. It was partly patronising, partly self-interested. To make towns more inhabitable and pleasant, they had to deal with the sources of disease. What began as the health of towns movement became the public health movement.[80] According to the microbiologist and ecologist René Dubos, this became the prototype of present-day voluntary health associations 'around the world'.[81] Pressure for administrative reform linked to 'public health agitation'.[82] It then became arguments and strategies for persuading the State to manage conditions better. It was taken up across the social classes, with powerful voices, like that of the remarkable Annie Besant, championing the interests of the working classes. There was endless dissent about how far this State action and the advancement of the public interest should go, for example over issues such as sexual health and birth control. Variations of this development of public health as societal reform occurred elsewhere. The early public health movement thus took a marginalised view – that life could be improved – and made it mainstream. It could do this partly because, with the spread and deepening of industrial capitalism, everything was being changed and challenged, not least by the growing working-class movements and the sciences. At its inception, by its nature, the public health movement was also an environmental movement. Therein lie the rudiments of the arguments explored in this book.

Edwin Chadwick in Britain, Lemuel Shattuck in Massachusetts, Rudolf Virchow in Germany, and Louis-René Villermé in France all recognised that unless movements infiltrated the State – easy in the case of Chadwick because he was already powerful within it! – they would never achieve resources or influence to effect change. But the Chadwicks are rare, raising the question: is it individuals who provoke change or movements? Individuals certainly matter in pushing for historical change. 'Great men' [sic], wrote the philosopher and psychologist William James in 1880, have an undoubted role in pushing the frontiers of change. Darwin thought 'spontaneous variations' would change the biological course of species, and so too could remarkable people set the pace of change for better or worse. 'Human beings, by changing the inner attitudes of their minds, can change the outer aspects of their lives', said James. For such distinctive individuals, he thought, 'The greatest use of life is to spend it for something that will outlast it.'[83] H.G. Wells, who had a profound influence on thinking about both history and the future, thought negatively about great men, holding a more jaundiced view after the First World War, when 'great men' led millions to slaughter on the fields of battle. James's main point was that, as with Darwinian theory, environments and individuals acted to shape each other reciprocally.

In public health, the role of motivated individuals and the greater movement is symbiotic. Where movements were not present, efforts failed, as in Shattuck's Boston. It is movements, often outside the upper echelons or dominant power elite in societies, which push for the change. As the Western world industrialised, and experienced the degradation first witnessed in the UK, others went through not dissimilar processes of argument, learning and strategy development. A whole succession of movements followed. Civil and professional societies positively exploded into life, transforming it. Some were no more than groups getting together in the name of civic pride. Some are embarrassing, such as the eugenics movement later in the nineteenth and early twentieth centuries, which spread across the Western world. Others continue to inspire: local sanitary and housing societies, for example. Some were patronising, some in the name of religion and saving people's souls not just their health. Some religious ones were radical, others punitive. Some were presented as an exercise in the 'medical policing' of infectious disease rather than for the benefit of the poor. 'If it had been proposed at that time to organize clinics for free treatment of disease among school children,' said C.-E. Winslow about the new Boston schools medical programme in 1894, 'the proposal would probably have been denounced as socialism of the most dangerous kind.'[84] Some were radical and political movements from below in society, others more wedded to the status quo, championing public health to control populations and to prevent dissent or destabilisation.

In New York there was the city parks movement, whose legacy is the beauty and grandeur of Central Park today (one of many designed by Frederick Law Olmsted, at one time head of the US Sanitary Commission). It has been argued that the creation of parks and urban planning were attempts by the social elites to manage the urban environment by managing the lower classes.[85] This was true, but the point of contrast might be the elites who provided no parks. Across Europe, there was a new town planning movement, which argued the drastic case of rebuilding cities on sanitarian lines, not just to improve the conditions of the poor. In Britain there was the formation of the National Trust in 1895, and before it the anti-adulteration food movement, which took from the 1820s to the 1890s to achieve decent legislation and food practices. Its goals are summarised, as the 1860 law first expressed it, as a requirement that food should be 'of the nature, quality and substance demanded'.[86] That requirement is still the cornerstone of UK food law, despite being superseded by EU food law from 2000. The pursuit of decent food, or the realisation that raw capitalism could not be relied upon to deliver what healthy bodies required, itself spawned the co-operative movement from the 1840s, now one of the biggest social movements in the world.[87]

The fate of the German public health movement is instructive. In Germany the orientation of health reform movements was 'hygiene', understood not only as cleanliness but 'as indications of political and social sickness which could be tackled by thorough democratisation of society'.[88] Established by the hygiene products industry in the early 1900s, and designed to spread an everyday culture of health, the German Hygiene Museum brought 5 million visitors to Dresden in 1911. But within a few decades it fell into the service of 'Nazi racist ideology', as the reborn Museum itself describes that phase today.[89] For public health, as with other largely progressive movements, the results of the trauma were tragic. Health thinking separated into rival Nazi and socialist camps, the latter to be destroyed – individually dispersed or put into concentration camps.[90]

Public health is about the condition of society, yet the reflex when talking about public health is often to think of medicine and technical support, as we have constantly stated. People experience public health through a set of services which provide the public health infrastructure – water, pavements, clean air, energy to houses – and through healthcare, via hospitals and doctors. The cause of women's health, for example, was tirelessly championed by movements on both sides of the Atlantic, in the UK by people like Elizabeth Garrett Anderson (1836–1917) and in both the UK and the USA by the Blackwell sisters (see Chapters 1 and 12). Such names represent large and active movements within which they worked, held meetings and corresponded. This process of pushing for reform, refusing to accept normality, appealing to fellow citizens, and confronting and cajoling power is what we mean by social movements. They have been critical in the aspiration to improve the conditions for public health.

Our conception of social movements sees the connections between campaigns for public parks or planting trees in towns with mothers campaigning for a pedestrian crossing for safe passage for their children or for play areas or safe bike or walk-to-school routes. As the public health world has professionalised, it has tended to fragment and formed hierarchies, partly for understandable reasons. But the effect is that campaigners for safe school routes do not conceive of themselves as public health actors but as acting for safety or neighbourhood or mothers' rights or themselves. Looking ahead in the twenty-first century, we suggest that the public health movement as it currently is must re-energise itself and reconnect with the local, the small and the unprofessional. Only then will it become a sufficiently broad movement to unify what is currently fragmented. We point to a two-way reconnection process, from the professions to civil society and back.

Although the Ecological Public Health is a complex approach, it has the great advantage of posing the challenge of democracy. Materialist and purely physiological approaches to health lend themselves to expert-led, 'top-down' solutions where technology rules. For us, democracy refers to the process of civic engagement, as discussed in the Democratic Transition (see Chapter 12). Political theorists have for decades taught that democracy comes in different packages, much like public health. For us, 'health democracy' is about a set of rules for public involvement and engagement in matters which affect society, and not simply a means for electing rulers or political representatives. This echoes the distinction between formal and substantive democracy, expressed by Max Weber. The more societies focus on organisational matters, the more they become dominated by formal rationality, he thought. Substantive issues get marginalised. Weber's position was ultimately pessimistic in that he argued that bureaucracy will always triumph and fossilise progress. We are more optimistic, because we see social movements as the brake on the worst tendencies of bureaucracy, and also as the defenders of the case for good bureaucracies which are the essential basis for consistent, equitable and effective public health services.

From within social science 'high' theory, there are two views of the role of social movements and civil society. Representing one, Michel Foucault, mentioned at various points in this book, argued that the modern State is not a work of social progress (as presented in some accounts of public health) but merely a sideways extension of existing authority. The growth of professions, endorsed by the State, ends up giving professionals power and control over human bodies and minds. Professions shape what bodies do, how they exist and how they are interpreted. For Foucault, this was a theory of 'governmentality', the internalisation of external governance over individual behaviour.[91] Although critical of the State, Foucault had a notion of power in public health that went beyond being simply a notion of State control. He saw this as illustrative of the modern condition where autonomy is fiction. Foucault has a major point. Power in health is not just a lever stemming from economic power. In *Discipline and Punish*, he presented an image of someone being hung, drawn and quartered as the expression of surplus, unnecessary 'old' power. For Foucault, power can infuse both mind and matter, body and brain.[92] His image of 'modern' power was Jeremy Bentham's panopticon, a jail in which people are watched from above and afar by all-seeing jailors. Bentham, of course, was the mentor of Edwin Chadwick. For Foucault, civil society and therefore social movements are a sham. They are part of, rather than distant from, lines of power.

The other tradition of high theory about social movements begins with the autonomous development of civil society. In this tradition, people combine to comment on the world. They fight for the right to act, desiring change, conceiving of a better society. This is a world of social movements that began with the anti-slavery societies which confronted the State, conventional morality and entrenched economic interests. This, as Charles Taylor has argued, provided a social formula 'which has been repeated continually, through the US abolitionist crusade, countless temperance movements, to the great American civil rights movement of the 1960s and beyond'.[93] It is social movements as expressed by South Africa's and the world's anti-apartheid movement. Key founders of the US public health movement were stalwart anti-slavers. What was formed in 1839 as the British and Foreign Anti-Slavery Society is now Anti-Slavery International, an organisation which continues to identify slavery worldwide in terms of forced labour, bonded labour, child labour, people trafficking and slavery.[94] The movement still exists because slavery still exists.

This is the version of social movements as a progressive improving force which was seen in the health of towns movement in Britain, referred to above, and countless general amelioration societies across Europe and the world as it industrialised. They derive from a world where discussion often began in coffee shops or parlours, which champions the free press, and debates the present and future. This is the world which Habermas described as the early cultural phase of modern capitalism,[95] and which the Enlightenment fired from the eighteenth century. It is there that the public health movement in all its elements begins.

Although fractured by class, the early public health movement advanced the idea of public space, open to all. With this rich history and perspective, public health in the twenty-first century will have to address the question of public space itself and the right and capacity to speak. The erosion of public space comes in new forms. One manifestation is the shift from public streets to private shopping malls, with private police forces. Another is media and communications ownership, increasingly being narrowed and global, which shapes debate about health. Another is the infection of commercial involvement in public health campaigns. Sometimes this is mild or even positive, but sometimes too it disguises conflicts of interest and skews public interest towards private benefit. Another is the rise of intellectual property rights, which is arguably the second enclosure movement, mimicking a past era when common land, owned by no one and everyone, was ceded to powerful individuals. The ownership of genes, of ideas, of techniques and of cultures is being extended in order to be traded and controlled. These are new forms of power which are reshaping the conditions within which public health can either flourish or be divided.

On the surface, it could be claimed that public health has little to do with power, that it is all about scientific, objective and neutral knowledge. As we have shown, that position is alive and well within public health, but our argument is that the public health has to be involved in democratising power. Power defines its duties, its possibilities, its roles and its funding. Historically, public health has been most effective when being rolled out at the local level, often by a centralising State. The critics of public health say it is about the exercise of power by the State, the institutions and even capital on the individual and over the individual body. From this discourse, we propose that public health has countervailing tendencies with regard to power. At different times and in different settings, it has to be both pro and anti, pro the State and anti it, pro and anti business, pro and anti existing popular movements. In some settings, the public health system can work effectively if left alone by politicians. In other settings, the public health services needs to be challenged and transformed. Sometimes public health movements can harness business; sometimes they need to be confronted and reshaped. In today's world of multilevel governance where power and institutions move between and across levels – local, subnational, national, regional, continental and global – the public health movements need to operate on and change the conditions for public health on all levels.

The history of public health has tended to be piecemeal, working on the 'inside', accommodating to the State. In the twenty-first century, when power has shifted to corporations, that accommodation needs to be reviewed. It requires the public health world to think carefully about who its allies are and where the compromises are. Does this mean working with the horticulture industry, for example, to increase fruit and vegetable output to promote consumption? On the other hand, does it mean being financially supported by large soft drink companies which assure people that they are now ethical, committed to improving their products, and have corporate responsibility reports to 'prove' it?

A touchstone for how serious public health movements are is surely the issue of inequalities. The twenty-first century is deeply fissured by health inequalities within and between societies. Many reports and commissions show this to be the case. Surely this has to be confronted. History comes to our aid. Previous generations have had to tackle such inequalities, and learnt to build movements – of diverse political hues – to rein back the disproportionate economic disparities unleashed in the name of neoliberalism or authoritarian paternalisation (see Chapter 8). Public health has to use the full range of economic measures, not restrict itself to 'soft' measures, if it wants to reduce inequalities in health. The argument for tackling inequalities is both self-interested – a better society is nicer for all – and values-based in that it promotes a citizenry where people are accorded dignity and respect whatever their origins or differences. This is a society which builds trust not social capital (see Chapter 11). It overtly proclaims the virtues of democratic life and strives to create conditions which allow people room to live decent lives, improve themselves and be free as far as possible from the fear of ill-health.

The challenge for the public health movement today and in this century lies in incorporating many elements and clarifying many complex processes. Public health, as the editorial of one health journal announced in 2004, 'is no longer the domain of any one bounded discipline'.[96] The truth is that it never was; at some points diversity ruled, and at other points one profession, usually medically based, was in the ascendant. In the current period there is a fear too that some in medical care have become disengaged. Public health has always, in the modern period, been the domain of movements. Sometimes it has been organised and powerful; at other times it has been weak, dissipated or in thrall to bureaucratic, technological, professional and in recent times commercialising impulses. The case for Ecological Public Health is that it engages many professions and people who have no nominal health affiliation. In the future, as the conditions of health steadily shift from complacency to threat this same movement will have to create engaging narratives which link what otherwise appears technical or one-off. The twenty-first-century health movements need to refine their narratives and to connect matters which countervailing interests prefer to leave disconnected.

Implication 8: Unify natural and human sustainability

'How can humans live sustainably on the planet and do so in a way that manages to preserve some biodiversity?' That was the question asked by the American journal *Science* in 2005 under the rhetorical title 'Will Malthus Continue to Be Wrong?'[97] The same journal, a century before, had witnessed a ferocious debate, not unusual between academic disciplines, over who owns good ideas. Some argued that ecology, then a newly fashionable term, was a biological concept. Others said that its true meaning and focus lay in botany. The journal was now reviving a much older and more important debate, one forever indelibly associated with the name of the Reverend Dr Thomas Malthus. Was nature – for Malthus the tension between agriculture and population growth – the inevitable fate of humankind? If so, would this tension be resolved by disease or social disorder? How could it be that someone judged so definitely wrong over two centuries can still be part of debate in the twenty-first century?

The vitality of Malthus's perspective – there is much to be buried and forgotten within it – is that it exposes the dangers for humankind in its relationship with nature. If nature is despoiled, or if agriculture (or the sea, or water or energy systems, or biology and more) fails to produce 'goods' for economic consumption sustainably, to put the debate in a more modern language and context, in the final instance it is humankind which will be the loser. There is now a possibility of humans being if not eradicated (as were the dinosaurs) then definitely curtailed and brought back to live within environmental limits and ecological processes.

The conflict between humans and nature has often been missed because the appeal from the modern environmental movement has been that the natural environment needs to be protected rather than humankind from itself and its pretensions to live unecologically. The conservation movement champions the natural environment, protected from humanity rather than living with it. The journal *Science* suggested that agriculture was under increasing pressure to provide food for ever-rising populations but with less environmental damage. This theme is now widely accepted. Scientists are under pressure to provide answers to the question of how far eco-systems are being degraded and if resilience thresholds have been breached. Social scientists are under pressure to investigate housing and urbanisation and the impact of urban existence on issues as fundamental as energy use, drinking water and foodways. Most scientific judgement is that 'The world clearly can't support 10 billion people living like Americans do today.' The word 'sustainability' is now used to carry all this! It actually implies a radical transformation of societies, aspirations and all that pertains to public health.

There were numerous responses to the article in *Science*. In one eloquent response, Theodore C. Okeahialam, a professor of paediatrics in Nigeria, who had researched malnutrition among Nigerian children during that country's civil war,[98] noted that the true picture was not entirely dismal. The world had witnessed the increasing adoption of democratic principles and rapid scientific advances. But he noted the persistence of global, social and economic inequalities and, while agriculture required close attention, eco-system degradation, global warming, and pollution in developing countries like his own were also being contributed to by the multinational companies of industrial countries. What was desperately needed in the developing world, he said, was responsible, selfless democratic leadership with political commitment, accountability, and good governance devoid of corruption. It was critical that female education and female empowerment for employment were promoted, not only because they limited the number of children in the average family but for their own sake; indeed no programme of change 'including population control' could be meaningful in the lives of the people without it.

He was right. The cause of sustainability, a term which must be central to all public health thinking, from the avoidance of microbial feedback to health that empowers not just manipulates, must centrally focus on improving the quality of people's lives and not, as in the original Malthusian formulation, become a reason for one social class's impoverishment. Sustainability is the single greatest challenge to the Enlightenment tradition of progress. It is also its inheritor. The eighteenth-century Enlightenment was based on a belief in the possibility of improving the quality of life for all, by reorganising society and technology to uplift the public and the individual. In the twenty-first century, a new Enlightenment is needed.

The convention of sustainable development, ever since the 1987 Brundtland report, is to see sustainability as about balancing environment, society and economy. The picture we have painted in this book suggests that health sits at the heart of any notion of sustainability. Human bodies live off the natural environment, and without that environment they could not exist. Darwin's entangled bank of ecological relationships needs to have a social dimension to it. Humans have become the predator that is altering the bank, and our (financial) banks are funding that process.

The Ecological Public Health model offers the four dimensions of existence as a lens through which to look at the huge trends or transitions that have been described in this book. The public health world and movements now need to engage with the overriding question: how can progress be pursued in an economy based on ecological principles? To answer that question requires a society which takes all the people's health, globally, more seriously. This will not happen in a world driven by consumerism, where ceaseless pursuit of material goods is a substitute for well-being, and now the basis for economic activity. Some fundamental questions need to be debated. Our argument is that the public health movements are a key location for this debate. The public health movement is well placed to both lead and participate.

We end with our offering of a new definition of public health for the twenty-first century. The tradition to seek perfect health was first fully articulated by Shattuck in the 1850s. Then it was re-honed in the WHO's founding statement in 1946. Since then, it has been given more operational definitions as a series of tasks and methods. We think these inadequate to the challenge of Ecological Public Health ahead. Our own definition is this:

> In the twenty-first century, the pursuit of public health requires the analysis of the composite interactions between the material, biological, social and cultural dimensions of existence. This demands a new mix of interventions and actions to alter and ameliorate the determinants of health; the better framing of public and private choices to achieve sustainable planetary, economic, societal and human health; and the active participation of movements to that end. Ecological Public Health is about shaping the conditions for good health for all.

NOTES

1 Introducing the notion of Ecological Public Health

1 K. Grahame, *Wind in the Willows* (London: Methuen & Co., 1908), ch. 8.
2 J. Hicks and G. Allen, *A Century of Change: Trends in UK Statistics since 1900*, Research Paper 99/111 (London: House of Commons Library, 1999).
3 I. Roberts and P. Edwards, *The Energy Glut: The Politics of Fatness in an Overheating World* (London: Zed Press, 2010).
4 WHO, *Global Status Report on Road Safety 2009* (Geneva: World Health Organization, 2009).
5 J.R. Searle, *The Construction of Social Reality* (New York: Free Press, 1995), p. 3.
6 D. Hemenway, Why We Don't Spend Enough on Public Health (*New England Journal of Medicine* 2010, 362, 18: 1657–1658).
7 R.H. Shryock, The Early American Public Health Movement (*American Journal of Public Health* 1937, 27, 10: 965–971).
8 L. Shattuck, N.P. Banks, Jr and J. Abbott, *Report of a General Plan for the Promotion of Public and Personal Health* (Boston, MA: Dutton and Wentworth, 1850).
9 G. Rosen, *A History of Public Health* (Baltimore, MD: Johns Hopkins University Press, 1993).
10 J.R. Walkowitz, *Prostitution and Victorian Society: Women, Class, and the State* (Cambridge: Cambridge University Press, 1982).
11 C. Quétel, *History of Syphilis* (Baltimore, MD: Johns Hopkins University Press, 1990).
12 J. D'Emilio and E.B. Freedman, *Intimate Matters: A History of Sexuality in America* (Chicago: University of Chicago Press, 1998), p. 205.
13 J.H. Jones, *Bad Blood* (New York: Free Press, 1993).
14 J.W. Leavitt, *Typhoid Mary: Captive to the Public's Health* (New York: Beacon Press, 1996).
15 J.S. Mill, *Autobiography* (Philadelphia: Pennsylvania State University, 2004 [1873]).
16 J.S. Mill, *On Liberty* (Kitchener, Ontario: Batoche Books, 2001 [1859]), p. 14.
17 E. Chadwick, *Report to Her Majesty's Principal Secretary of State for the Home Department from the Poor Law Commissioners on an Inquiry into the Sanitary Condition of the Labouring Population of Great Britain, with Appendices* (London: HMSO, 1842).
18 S.E. Finer, *The Life and Times of Sir Edwin Chadwick* (London: Taylor & Francis, 1952).
19 Commission on Macroeconomics and Health, *Macroeconomics and Health: Investing in*

Health for Economic Development (Geneva: Harvard University/Center for International Development/World Health Organization, 2002), p. 8.

20 H. Waitzkin, Report of the WHO Commission on Macroeconomics and Health: A Summary and Critique (*Lancet* 2003, 361: 523–526).

21 F. Engels, *The Condition of the Working Class in England* (New York: Panther, 1969 [1845]), p. 24.

22 R. Labonte, M. Polanyi, N. Muhajarine, T. McIntosh and A. Williams, Beyond the Divides: Towards Critical Population Health Research (*Critical Public Health* 2005, 15, 1: 5–17).

23 H. Heinonen-Tanski, S. Pradhan and P. Karinen, Sustainable Sanitation: A Cost-Effective Tool to Improve Plant Yields and the Environment (*Sustainability* 2010, 2, 1: 341–353).

24 P. Bennett, S. Murphy and D. Carroll, Paper One: Social Cognition Models as a Framework for Health Promotion: Necessary, but Not Sufficient (*Health Care Analysis* 1995, 3, 1: 15–22).

25 IRIS, *Health Perceptions around the Globe* (Adligenswil, Switzerland: International Research Institutes, 2004).

26 M. Brodie, D. Altman, C. Deane, S. Buscho and E. Hamel, Liking the Pieces, Not the Package: Contradictions in Public Opinion during Health Reform (*Health Affairs (Millwood)* 2010, 29, 6: 1125–1130).

27 R. Blendon and M. Kim, When It Comes to Health Policy, Americans Are Not British (*Harvard Health Policy Review* 2001, 2, 1: 72–75).

28 Manning Selvage & Lee, *Three out of Four Americans View Health as Their Personal Symbol of Success* (New York: Manning Selvage & Lee, 2008).

29 CDC, Public Opinion about Public Health – United States, 1999 (*Morbidity and Mortality Weekly Report* 2000, 49, 12: 258–260).

30 R.J. Blendon, J.M. Benson, G.K. SteelFisher and J.M. Connolly, Americans' Conflicting Views about the Public Health System, and How to Shore Up Support (*Health Affairs (Millwood)* 2010, 29, 11: 2033–2040).

31 M. Bury, Health Promotion and Lay Epidemiology: A Sociological View (*Health Care Analysis* 1994, 2, 1: 23–30).

32 J.C. Fell and R.B. Voas, Mothers against Drunk Driving (MADD): The First 25 Years (*Traffic Injury Prevention* 2006, 7, 3: 195–212).

33 W.G. Smillie, *Public Health: Its Promise for the Future* (New York: Macmillan, 1955), p. 470.

34 C. Julia and A.-J. Valleron, Louis-René Villermé (1782–1863), a Pioneer in Social Epidemiology: Re-analysis of His Data on Comparative Mortality in Paris in the Early 19th Century (*Journal of Epidemiology and Community Health* 2011, 65, 8 (August): 666–670).

35 A.F. La Berge, *Mission and Method: The Early Nineteenth-Century French Public Health Movement* (Cambridge: Cambridge University Press, 1992).

36 W.G. Smillie, The Great Pioneers of Public Health in America 1610–1925 (*American Journal of Public Health* 1953, 43, 9: 1077–1084).

37 H. Morris, *Portrait of a Chef: The Life of Alexis Soyer* (Oxford: Oxford University Press, 1980).

38 D. Porter, Changing Definitions of the History of Public Health (*History of Public Health: Current Themes and Approaches* 1999, 1, 1: 9–21).

39 A.M. Stern and H. Markel, The Public Health Service and Film Noir: A Look Back at Elia Kazan's Panic in the Streets (1950) (*Public Health Reports* 2003, 118, 3: 178–183).

40 Rosen, *History of Public Health*, p. 200.

41 G. Kearns, Cholera, Nuisances and Environmental Management in Islington, 1830–55 (*Medical History Supplement* 1991, 11).

42 Department of Health, Public Health, Web definition, http://www.dh.gov.uk/en/Publichealth/DH_081652 [accessed 21 March 2010] (London: Department of Health, 2010).

43 G.L. Armstrong, L.A. Conn and R.W. Pinner, Trends in Infectious Disease Mortality in the United States during the 20th Century (*Journal of the American Medical Association* 1999, 281, 1: 61–66).

44 P. Alcabes, *Dread: How Fear and Fantasy Have Fueled Epidemics from the Black Death to Avian Flu* (New York: PublicAffairs, 2010).

45 B.P. Zietz and H. Dunkelberg, The History of the Plague and the Research on the Causative Agent Yersinia Pestis (*International Journal of Hygiene and Environmental Health* 2004, 207, 2: 165–178).

46 M. Healy, Defoe's Journal and the English Plague Writing Tradition (*Literature and Medicine* 2003, 22, 1: 25–44).

47 W.B. Schwartz, *Life without Disease: The Pursuit of Medical Utopia* (Berkeley: University of California Press, 1998), p. 8.

48 D.J. Rothman, *Beginnings Count: The Technological Imperative in American Health Care* (New York: Oxford University Press, 1997).

49 OECD, *OECD Health Data 2011: How Does the United States Compare* (Paris: Organisation for Economic Co-operation and Development, 2011).

50 R.W. Fogel, *Forecasting the Cost of U.S. Health Care in 2040*, NBER Working Paper No. 14361 (Washington, DC: National Bureau of Economic Research, 2008).

51 World Health Organization, *The World Health Report 2000 – Health Systems: Improving Performance* (Geneva: World Health Organization, 2000).

52 OECD, *OECD Health Data 2011: How Does the United Kingdom Compare* (Paris: Organisation for Economic Co-operation and Development, 2011).

53 M. Millman, *The Unkindest Cut: Life in the Backrooms of Medicine* (New York: William Morrow, 1977).

54 St Augustine, *The City of God* (introduction by Sir Ernest Barker) (London: J. M. Dent & Sons, 1957 [426]).

55 S. Shapin, *The Scientific Revolution* (Chicago: University of Chicago Press, 1996).

56 G. Saliba, *Islamic Science and the Making of the European Renaissance* (Cambridge, MA: MIT Press, 2007).

57 R. Collingwood, *The Idea of Nature* (Oxford: Oxford University Press, 1966), p. 97.

58 U. Bronfenbrenner, *The Ecology of Human Development* (Cambridge, MA: Harvard University Press, 1979).

59 F. Baum, *The New Public Health: An Australian Perspective*, 2nd edn (Melbourne: Oxford University Press, 2002).

60 A.H. Dolan, M. Taylor, B. Neis, R. Ommer, J. Eyles, D. Schneider *et al.*, Restructuring and Health in Canadian Coastal Communities (*EcoHealth* 2005, 2, 3: 195–208).

61 P. Martens and J. Rotmans, Transitions in a Globalising World (*Futures* 2005, 37: 1133–1144).

62 World Bank, *NGO World Bank Collaboration*, http://wbln0018.worldbank.org/essd/essd.nsf/d3f59aa3a570f67a852567cf00695688/ce6b105aaa19360f85256966006c74e3?OpenDocument (Washington, DC: World Bank, 2011).

63 Union of International Associations, *Comparison of Yearbook of International Organizations*, www.uia.be/node/328022 (Brussels: Union of International Associations, 2011).

64 G. Palmer, *The Politics of Breastfeeding* (London: Pandora, 1988).

65 Alcabes, *Dread.*

66 G. Orwell, *Nineteen Eighty-Four: A Novel* (London: Secker & Warburg, 1949).

67 R.A. Epstein, *In Defense of the 'Old' Public Health: The Legal Framework for the Regulation of Public Health*, John M. Olin Law and Economics Working Paper (Chicago: University of Chicago, 2002).

68 R. Nozick, *Anarchy, State, and Utopia* (New York: Basic Books, 1974).

69 A. Rand, Introducing Objectivism (*Objectivist Newsletter* 1962: 35).

70 M. Foucault, *Power/Knowledge: Selected Interviews and Other Writings, 1972–1977*, ed. C. Gordon (New York: Pantheon Books, 1980).

71 G.B. Shaw, *Everybody's Political What's What?* (London: Constable & Co., 1944).

72 J. Sullum, *For Your Own Good: The Anti-Smoking Crusade and the Tyranny of Public Health* (New York: Free Press, 1998).

73 C. Petrini, Theoretical Models and Operational Frameworks in Public Health Ethics (*International Journal of Environmental Research and Public Health* 2010, 7: 189–202).

74 Mill, *On Liberty*.

75 J.F. Childress, R.R. Faden, R.D. Gaare, L.O. Gostin, J. Kahn, R.J. Bonnie *et al.*, Public Health Ethics: Mapping the Terrain (*Journal of Law and Medical Ethics* 2002, 30, 2: 170–178).

76 T.R.V. Nys, Paternalism in Public Health Care (*Public Health Ethics* 2008, 1, 1: 64–72).

2 Defining public health

1 L. Nordenfelt, *On the Nature of Health: An Action-Theoretic Approach* (Amsterdam: Kluwer, 1995).

2 J. Piaget, *Genetic Epistemology* (New York: Columbia University Press, 1970).

3 J.J. Spielvogel, *Western Civilization: Since 1300*, 8th edn (Boston, MA: Cengage Learning, 2011), p. 516.

4 S.D. Snobelen, Encyclopedia of the Enlightenment, in *Isaac Newton (1642–1727): Natural Philosopher, Biblical Scholar and Civil Servant*, ed. A.C. Kors (Oxford: Oxford University Press, 2003).

5 W. Heisenberg, *The Physicist's Conception of Nature* (London: Hutchinson, 1958), p. 29.

6 D. Porter, Changing Definitions of the History of Public Health (*History of Public Health: Current Themes and Approaches* 1999, 1, 1: 9–21).

7 M.P.J. Dillon, The Ecology of the Greek Sanctuary (*Zeitschrift für Papyrologie und Epigraphik* 1997, 118: 113–127).

8 R. Collingwood, *The Idea of Nature* (Oxford: Oxford University Press, 1966), p. 43.

9 M. Perry, M. Chase, J.R. Jacob, M.C. Jacob and T.H. Von Laue, *Western Civilization: Ideas, Politics and Society – From 1600* (Florence, KY: Cengage Learning, 2008).

10 D.A. Franco and C.E. Williams, 'Airs, Waters, Places' and Other Hippocratic Writings: Inferences for Control of Foodborne and Waterborne Disease (*Journal of Environmental Health* 2000, 62: 9–14).

11 G. Miller, 'Airs, Waters, and Places' in History (*Journal of the History of Medicine and Allied Sciences* 1962, XVII, 1: 129–140).

12 L.I. Conrad, M. Neve, V. Nutton, R. Porter and A. Wear (eds), *The Western Medical Tradition: 800 BC to AD 1800*, vol. 1 (Cambridge: Cambridge University Press, 1995), p. 20.

13 R.D. Lasker, *Medicine and Public Health: The Power of Collaboration* (New York: New York Academy of Medicine, 1997), p. 12.

14 A. Newsholme, *Public Health and Insurance: American Addresses* (Baltimore, MD: Johns Hopkins University Press, 1920), p. 3.

15 J.G. Freymann, Medicine's Great Schism: Prevention vs. Cure: An Historical Interpretation (*Medical Care* 1975, 13, 7: 525–536).

16 A.M. Brandt and M. Gardner, Antagonism and Accommodation: Interpreting the Relationship between Public Health and Medicine in the United States during the 20th Century (*American Journal of Public Health* 2000, 90, 5: 707–715).

17 W.G. Smillie, The Great Pioneers of Public Health in America 1610–1925 (*American Journal of Public Health* 1953, 43, 9: 1077–1084).

18 Editorial, Lemuel Shattuck (1793–1859): Prophet of American Public Health (*American Journal of Public Health* 1959, 49, 5: 676–677).

19 W. Winkelstein, Jr, The Development of American Public Health, a Commentary: Three Documents that Made an Impact (*Journal of Public Health Policy* 2009, 30, 1: 40–48).

20 M. Bloom, Editorial, Primary Prevention and Public Health: An Historical Note on Dr. John Hoskins Griscom (*Journal of Primary Prevention* 2001, 21, 3: 305–308).

21 J.H. Griscom, *The Sanitary Condition of the Laboring Population of New York, with Suggestions for Its Improvement: A Discourse* (New York: Harper and Brothers, 1845), p. 23.

22 W.G. Smillie, *Public Health: Its Promise for the Future* (New York: Macmillan, 1955), p. 256.

23 L. Shattuck, N.P. Banks, Jr and J. Abbott, *Report of a General Plan for the Promotion of Public and Personal Health* (Boston, MA: Dutton and Wentworth, 1850), p. 248.

24 Griscom, *Sanitary Condition of the Laboring Population of New York*, p. 4.

25 Shattuck, Banks and Abbott, *Report of a General Plan for the Promotion of Public and Personal Health*, p. 9.

26 Ibid., p. 10.

27 C.-E.A. Winslow, The Untilled Fields of Public Health (*Science* 1920, 51 (New Series), 1306: 23–33).

28 A. Yankauer, The American Journal of Public Health, 1911–85 (*American Journal of Public Health* 1986, 76, 7: 809–815).

29 D. Acheson, *Public Health in England: The Report of the Committee of the Enquiry into the Future Development of the Public Health Function* (London: HMSO, 1988).

30 D.J. Hunter, L. Marks and K. Smith, *The Public Health System in England: A Scoping Study* (Durham: Centre for Public Policy and Health, 2007).

31 M. Verweij and A. Dawson, The Meaning of 'Public' in 'Public Health', in *Ethics, Prevention, and Public Health*, ed. A. Dawson and M. Verweij (Oxford: Clarendon Press, 2007), pp. 13–29.

32 Committee for the Study of the Future of Public Health, Division of Health Care Services, Institute of Medicine, *The Future of Public Health* (Washington, DC: National Academies Press, 1988), p. 1.

33 Ibid., pp. 40–41.

34 R. Riegelman, *Public Health 101: Healthy People – Healthy Populations* (Sudbury, MA: Jones and Bartlett, 2010), p. 4.

35 C.-E.A. Winslow, *The Conquest of Epidemic Disease: A Chapter in the History of Ideas* (Princeton, NJ: Princeton University Press, 1943), p. 28.

36 J. Duffy, *The Sanitarians: A History of American Public Health* (Champaign: University of Illinois Press, 1992), p. 199.

37 A.J. Viseltear, C.-E.A. Winslow and the Early Years of Public Health at Yale, 1915–1925 (*Yale Journal of Biology and Medicine* 1982, 55: 137–151).

38 A.J. Viseltear, Milton C. Winternitz and the Yale Institute of Human Relations: A Brief Chapter in the History of Social Medicine (*Yale Journal of Biology and Medicine* 1984, 57: 32–58).

39 C. Boorse, On the Distinction between Disease and Illness (*Philosophy and Public Affairs* 1975, 5: 49–68).

40 K.C. Carter, *The Rise of Causal Theories of Disease* (Aldershot and Burlington, VT: Ashgate, 2003).

41 R. Nesse, On the Difficulty of Defining Disease: A Darwinian Perspective (*Medicine, Health Care and Philosophy* 2001, 4, 1: 37–46).

42 G.W. Brown, Social Factors and Disease: The Sociological Perspective (*BMJ* 1987, 294: 1026–1028).

43 S. DeVito, On the Value-Neutrality of the Concepts of Health and Disease: Unto the Breach Again (*Journal of Medicine and Philosophy* 2000, 25, 5: 539–567).

44 WHO, Preamble to the Constitution of the World Health Organization as Adopted by the International Health Conference, New York, 19 June – 22 July 1946; Signed on 22 July 1946 by the Representatives of 61 States, in *Official Records of the World Health Organization*, no. 2 (Geneva: World Health Organization, 1946), p. 100.

45 R.M. Titmuss, *Commitment to Welfare* (London: Unwin University Books, 1968).

46 R.J. Dubos, *Mirage of Health: Utopias, Progress and Biological Change* (New York: Rutgers University Press, 1987 [1959]).

47 O. Wilde, *The Soul of Man under Socialism* (Charleston, SC: Forgotten Books, 2008 [1891]), p. 18.

48 J.S. Larson, The World Health Organization's Definition of Health: Social versus Spiritual Health (*Social Indicators Research* 1996, 38, 2: 181–192).

49 R. Saracci, The World Health Organization Needs to Reconsider Its Definition of Health (*BMJ* 1997, 314, 7091: 1409).

50 A.R. Jadad and L. O'Grady, How Should Health Be Defined? (*BMJ* 2008, 337 (10 December): a2900).

51 J. Kovács, Concepts of Health and Disease (*Journal of Medicine and Philosophy* 1989, 14, 3: 261–267).

52 M. Fine, J.W. Peters and R.S. Lawrence, *The Nature of Health: How America Lost, and Can Regain, a Basic Human Value* (Oxford: Radcliffe, 2007), p. 136.

53 Anon., Declaration of Alma-Ata, in *International Conference on Primary Health Care* (Alma-Ata: World Health Organization, 1978).

54 L. Breslow, Origins and Development of the International Epidemiological Association (*International Journal of Epidemiology* 2005, 34, 4: 725–729).

55 R. Costanza, Towards an Operational Definition of Ecosystem Health, in *Ecosystem Health: New Goals for Environmental Management*, ed. R. Costanza, B.G. Norton and B.D. Haskell (Washington, DC: Island Press, 1992: 239–256).

56 A.C. Gatrell, Complexity Theory and Geographies of Health: A Critical Assessment (*Social Science and Medicine* 2005, 60: 2661–2671).

57 M. Gell-Mann, *The Quark and the Jaguar: Adventures in the Simple and the Complex* (New York: Henry Holt, 1995).

58 M.C. Taylor, *The Moment of Complexity: Emerging Network Culture* (Chicago: University of Chicago Press, 2001).

59 J. Habermas, Modernity: An Unfinished Project, in *Habermas and the Unfinished Project of Modernity: Critical Essays on The Philosophical Discourse of Modernity*, ed. M.P. d'Entrèves and S. Benhabib (Cambridge, MA: MIT Press, 1997: 38–55).

60 P. Philippe and O. Mansi, Nonlinearity in the Epidemiology of Complex Health and Disease Processes (*Theoretical Medicine and Bioethics* 1998, 19, 6).

61 S. Galea, M. Riddle and G.A. Kaplan, Causal Thinking and Complex System Approaches in Epidemiology (*International Journal of Epidemiology* 2010, 39, 1: 97–106).

62 J.C. Riley, *Rising Life Expectancy: A Global History* (Cambridge: Cambridge University Press, 2001), p. xi.

63 D.H. Crawford, *Deadly Companions: How Microbes Shaped Our History* (Oxford: Oxford University Press, 2009), p. 189.

64 E.R. Choffnes, D.A. Relman and A. Mack, *Antibiotic Resistance: Implications for Global Health and Novel Intervention Strategies: Workshop Summary* (Washington, DC: Institute of Medicine (US) Forum on Microbial Threats, 2010). J. Davies, Everything Depends on Everything Else (*Clinical Microbiology and Infection* 2009, 15, 1: 1–4). K. Outterson, The Vanishing Public Domain: Antibiotic Resistance, Pharmaceutical Innovation and Global Public Health (*University of Pittsburgh Law Review* 2005, 67: 67–123).

65 J. Komlos, *On the Biological Standard of Living of Eighteenth-Century Americans: Taller, Richer, Healthier*, Munich Discussion Papers 2003-9 (Munich: University of Munich, Department of Economics, 2003).

66 Shattuck, Banks and Abbott, *Report of a General Plan for the Promotion of Public and Personal Health*.

67 K. Marx, *Writings of the Young Marx on Philosophy and Society*, ed. L.D. Easton and K.H. Guddat (Indianapolis, IN: Hackett, 1997), p. 381.

68 Dubos, *Mirage of Health*, p. 52.

69 S.L. Syme, Historical Perspective: The Social Determinants of Disease – Some Roots of the Movement (*Epidemiologic Perspectives and Innovations* 2005, 2, 1: 2).

70 R. Labonte, Healthy Public Policy and the World Trade Organization: A Proposal for an International Health Presence in Future World Trade/Investment Talks (*Health Promotion International* 1998, 13, 3: 245–256). D. Dollar, Is Globalization Good for

Your Health? (*Bulletin of the World Health Organization* 2001, 79: 827–833). T. Lang, The New Globalisation, Food and Health: Is Public Health Receiving Its Due Emphasis? (*Journal of Epidemiology and Community Health* 1998, 52, 9: 538–539). G. Rayner, C. Hawkes, T. Lang and W. Bello, Trade Liberalisation and the Diet Transition: A Public Health Response (*Health Promotion International* 2006, 21 (Supplement 1): 67–74). R. Beaglehole and D. Yach, Globalisation and the Prevention and Control of Non-Communicable Disease: The Neglected Chronic Diseases of Adults (*Lancet* 2003, 362 (13 September): 903–908). D.W. Bettcher, D. Yach and G.E. Guindon, Global Trade and Health: Key Linkages and Future Challenges (*Bulletin of the World Health Organization* 2000, 78: 521–534).

71 D. Held, *Global Transformations: Politics, Economics and Culture* (Cambridge: Polity Press, 1999), pp. xxiii, 515.

72 N. Robins, *The Corporation that Changed the World: How the East India Company Shaped the Modern Multinational* (London: Pluto, 2006).

73 S.W. Mintz, *Sweetness and Power: The Place of Sugar in Modern History* (Harmondsworth: Penguin Books, 1985). R. Blackburn, *The Overthrow of Colonial Slavery 1776–1848* (London: Verso, 2007).

74 World Health Assembly, *Preventing Violence: A Public Health Priority*, Resolution WHA 49.25 (Geneva: World Health Organization, 1996). World Health Organization, *World Report on Violence and Health* (Geneva: World Health Organization, 2002).

75 A. Sen, *Poverty and Famines: An Essay on Entitlement and Deprivation* (Oxford: Oxford University Press, 1982).

76 P. Guyer (ed.), Kant, Immanuel, in *Routledge Encyclopedia of Philosophy*, ed. E. Craig (London: Routledge, 2004).

77 S. Johnson and J. Kwak, *13 Bankers: The Wall Street Takeover and the Next Financial Meltdown* (New York: Random House, 2011).

78 C. Darwin, *On the Origin of Species by Natural Selection* (London: John Murray, 1859).

79 Ibid., ch. 14.

80 E. Haeckel, *Generelle Morphologie der Organismen* (Berlin: Georg Reimer, 1866).

81 C.H. Smith, Alfred Russel Wallace, Societal Planning and Environmental Agenda (*Environmental Conservation* 2003, 30, 3: 215–218).

82 C. Darwin, *The Descent of Man, and Selection in Relation to Sex* (London: John Murray, 1871), p. 115.

3 The received wisdom of public health

1 L. Garrett, *The Coming Plague: Newly Emerging Diseases in a World out of Balance* (London: Penguin Books, 1995); *The Betrayal of Trust: The Collapse of Global Public Health* (Oxford: Oxford University Press, 2001); The Challenge of Global Health (*Foreign Affairs* 2007 (January/February)).

2 L. Mumford, *The City in History: Its Origins, Its Transformations and Its Prospects* (London: Secker & Warburg, 1961), p. 239.

3 E.D.G. Fraser and A. Rimas, *Empires of Food: Feast, Famine and the Rise and Fall of Civilizations* (London: Random House, 2010).

4 I. Milne, Sir John Pringle's Observations on the Diseases of the Army: An Early Scientific Account of Epidemiology and the Prevention of Cross Infection (*Journal of Epidemiology and Community Health* 2005, 59, 11: 966).

5 Anon., Life, Death and Health in the Navy, www.nelsonsnavy.co.uk/broadside2.html (*Broadside* [accessed 15 March 2011], 2011).

6 R. Walter, *Anson's Voyage round the World* (London, 1901).

7 H. Zinsser, *Rats, Lice and History* (New Brunswick, NJ: Transaction Publishers, 2008 [1935]).

8 J. Lind, *A Treatise of the Scurvy, Containing an Inquiry into the Nature, Causes and Cure, of That Disease, together with a Critical and Chronological View of What Has Been Published*

on the Subject (3 volumes) (Edinburgh: printed by Sands, Murray and Cochran for A. Kincaid and A. Donaldson, 1753).

9 E. Martini, Treatment for Scurvy Not Discovered by Lind (*Lancet* 2004, 364, 9452: 2180).

10 J.H. Baron, Sailors' Scurvy before and after James Lind: A Reassessment (*Nutrition Reviews* 2009, 67, 6: 315–332). D.E. Hammerschmidt, 250 Years of Controlled Clinical Trials: Where It All Began (*Journal of Laboratory and Clinical Medicine* 2004, 143, 1: 68–69).

11 F. Nightingale, *Notes on Nursing: What It Is, and What It Is Not* (London: Harrison, 1859).

12 G. Hastings, M. Stead, L. Macdermott, A. Forsyth, A.M. Mackintosh, M. Rayner *et al.*, *Review of Research on the Effects of Food Promotion to Children*, Final Report to the Food Standards Agency by the Centre for Social Marketing, University of Strathclyde (London: Food Standards Agency, 2004). WHO, *Marketing of Food and Non-Alcoholic Beverages to Children*, Report of a WHO Forum and Technical Meeting, Oslo, 2–5 May 2006 (Geneva: World Health Organization, 2006).

13 C. Hamlin, *Public Health and Social Justice in the Age of Chadwick: Britain, 1800–1854* (Cambridge: Cambridge University Press, 1998), p. 16.

14 J. Hanley, Edwin Chadwick and the Poverty of Statistics (*Medical History* 2002, 46: 21–40).

15 B. Harrison, *Drink and the Victorians: The Temperance Question in England 1815–1872* (London: Faber and Faber, 1971).

16 J. Stuart, *A Counter-Blaste to Tobacco* (London: R.B., 1604).

17 N. Elias, *The Civilizing Process*, vol. I: *The History of Manners* (Oxford: Blackwell, 1969); vol. II: *State Formation and Civilization* (Oxford: Blackwell, 1982).

18 H.P. Young, Social Norms, Department of Economics Discussion Paper 307 (Oxford University, Oxford, 2007).

19 R. Porter, *The Enlightenment* (London: Palgrave Macmillan, 2001).

20 M. Potts and M. Campbell, History of Contraception, in *Gynecology and Obstetrics CD-ROM*, ed. J.J. Sciarra (Philadelphia, PA: Lippincott Williams & Wilkins, 2003).

21 M. Sanger, Opening Address for Birth Control Clinical Research Bureau Dinner (Margaret Sanger Papers, Sophia Smith Collection, Smith College, Margaret Sanger Microfilm S71:153, 1929).

22 P. Weindling, Public Health in Germany, in *The History of Public Health and the Modern State*, ed. D. Porter (Amsterdam and Atlanta, GA: Editions Rodopi, 1994: 119–131).

23 J. Sivulka, *Stronger than Dirt: A Cultural History of Advertising: Personal Hygiene in America 1875–1940* (New York: Humanity Books, 2001).

24 J. Mokyr, *The Gifts of Athena: Historical Origins of the Knowledge Economy* (Princeton, NJ: Princeton University Press, 2002).

25 R. Ashcraft, John Stuart Mill and the Theoretical Foundations of Democratic Socialism, in *Mill and the Moral Character of Liberalism*, ed. E.J. Eisenach (University Park: Pennsylvania State University Press, 1999: 169–190).

26 C.-E.A. Winslow, The Untilled Fields of Public Health (*Science* 1920, 51, 1306: 23–33).

27 R. Thaler and C. Sunstein, *Nudge: Improving Decisions about Health, Wealth, and Happiness* (New Haven, CT: Yale University Press, 2008).

28 J.C. Caldwell, Education as a Factor in Mortality Decline: An Examination of Nigerian Data (*Population Studies* 1979, 33: 395–413).

29 K.D. Brownell and J.P. Koplan, Front-of-Package Nutrition Labeling: An Abuse of Trust by the Food Industry? (*New England Journal of Medicine* 2011, 364, 25: 2373–2375).

30 M.E. Porter and M.R. Kramer, The Big Idea: Creating Shared Value (*Harvard Business Review* 2011 (January/February): 62–77).

31 I.S. Kickbusch, Health Literacy: Addressing the Health and Education Divide (*Health Promotion International* 2001, 16, 3: 289–297).

32 K.R. McLeroy, D. Bibeau, A. Steckler and K. Glanz, An Ecological Perspective on Health Promotion Programs (*Health Education Quarterly* 1988, 15, 4: 351–377).

33 M. Rothschild, Carrots, Sticks and Promises: A Conceptual Framework for the Management of Public Health and Social Issues Behaviors (*Journal of Marketing* 1999, 63 (October): 24–37).

34 A.R. Andreasen, *Marketing Social Change: Changing Behaviour to Promote Health, Social Development and the Environment* (San Francisco, CA: Jossey-Bass, 1995).

35 M. Horkheimer and T. Adorno, *The Dialectic of Enlightenment* (New York: Herder and Herder, 1997 [1947]).

36 U. Bronfenbrenner, *The Ecology of Human Development: Experiments by Nature and Design* (Cambridge, MA: Harvard University Press, 1979).

37 M. Fishbein and I. Ajzen, *Belief, Attitude, Intention, and Behavior: An Introduction to Theory and Research* (Reading, MA: Addison-Wesley, 1975), p. 511.

38 I. Ajzen and M. Fishbein, *Understanding Attitudes and Predicting Social Behavior* (Englewood Cliffs, NJ: Prentice-Hall, 1980).

39 Bronfenbrenner, *Ecology of Human Development*.

40 A.H. Hawley, *Human Ecology: A Theory of Community Structure* (New York: Ronald Press, 1950).

41 McLeroy *et al.*, Ecological Perspective on Health Promotion Programs.

42 D. Stokols, Social Ecology and Behavioral Medicine: Implications for Training, Practice, and Policy (*Behavioral Medicine* 2000, 26, 3: 129–138). D. Stokols, J.G. Grzywacz, S. McMahan and K. Phillips, Increasing the Health Promotive Capacity of Human Environments (*American Journal of Health Promotion* 2003, 18, 1: 4–13). D. Stokols, S. Misra, M.G. Runnerstrom and J.A. Hipp, Psychology in an Age of Ecological Crisis: From Personal Angst to Collective Action (*American Psychologist* 2009, 64, 3: 181–193).

43 Stokols *et al.*, Psychology in an Age of Ecological Crisis.

44 E.G. Krug, L.L. Dahlberg, J.A. Mercy, A.B. Zwi and R. Lozano (eds), *World Report on Violence and Health* (Geneva: World Health Organization, 2002).

45 G. Jones, *Social Hygiene in Twentieth Century Britain* (London: Croom Helm, 1986).

46 J.A. Bargh and T.L. Chartrand, The Unbearable Automaticity of Being (*American Psychologist* 1999, 54, 7: 462–479).

47 M. Foucault, What Is Enlightenment?, in *The Foucault Reader*, ed. P. Rabinow (New York: Pantheon Books, 1984: 32–50).

48 M. Foucault, *Power/Knowledge: Selected Interviews and Other Writings, 1972–1977*, ed. C. Gordon (New York: Pantheon Books, 1980).

49 R. Cockett, *Thinking the Unthinkable: Think-Tanks and the Economic Counter-Revolution, 1931–1983* (London: HarperCollins, 1994).

50 D. Harsanyi, *Nanny State: How Food Fascists, Teetotaling Do-Gooders, Priggish Moralists, and Other Boneheaded Bureaucrats Are Turning America into a Nation of Children* (New York: Random House, 2007).

51 Thaler and Sunstein, *Nudge*, p. 248.

52 O. Lobel and O. Amir, Stumble, Predict, Nudge: How Behavioral Economics Informs Law and Policy (*Columbia Law Review* 2009, 108, 8: 2098–2138).

53 Quoted in G. Rosen, Approaches to a Concept of Social Medicine: A Historical Survey (*Milbank Memorial Fund Quarterly* 1948, 26, 1: 7–21).

54 T. McKeown, *The Modern Rise of Population* (London: Edward Arnold, 1976).

55 F. Macfarlane Burnet, *Biological Aspects of Infectious Disease* (New York: Macmillan, 1940).

56 F. Macfarlane Burnet and D.O. White, *Natural History of Infectious Disease*, 4th edn (Cambridge: Cambridge University Press Archive, 1972), p. 186.

57 I. Illich, *Medical Nemesis* (London: Calder & Boyars, 1974).

58 H. Selye, *The Stress of Life* (New York: McGraw-Hill, 1956).

59 F. Borrell-Carrió, A.L. Suchman and R.M. Epstein, The Biopsychosocial Model 25 Years Later: Principles, Practice, and Scientific Inquiry (*Annals of Family Medicine* 2004, 6: 576–582).

60 H. Zinsser, *Rats, Lice and History* (New Brunswick, NJ: Transaction Publishers, 2008 [1935]), p. 168.

61 J. Diamond, *Guns, Germs and Steel: A Short History of Everybody for the Last 13,000 Years* (London: Chatto & Windus, 1997).

62 R. Porter, *The Greatest Benefit to Mankind: A Medical History of Humanity* (London: HarperCollins, 1997).

63 Winslow, The Untilled Fields of Public Health.

64 S. Marble, Why the Military Makes Public Health a Priority (*Newsletter of the Foreign Policy Research Institute* 2010, 15, 4).

65 E.R. Brown, *Rockefeller Medicine Men: Medicine and Capitalism in America* (Berkeley and London: University of California Press, 1979).

66 D. Wilsford, The Cohesion and Fragmentation of Organized Medicine in France and the United States (*Journal of Health Politics, Policy and Law* 1987, 12, 3: 481–503).

67 Porter, *The Greatest Benefit to Mankind*.

68 D. Wootton, *Bad Medicine: Doctors Doing Harm since Hippocrates* (Oxford: Oxford University Press, 2006).

69 P.Q. Hirst, *Durkheim, Bernard and Epistemology* (London: Routledge, 1975).

70 Cochrane Collaboration, About the Cochrane Collaboration, www.cochrane.org (Oxford: Cochrane Collaboration, 2008).

71 J.C. Venter, M.D. Adams, E.W. Myers, P.W. Li, R.J. Mural, G.G. Sutton *et al.*, The Sequence of the Human Genome (*Science* 2001, 291, 5507: 1304–1351).

72 E. Hood and K. Jenkins, Evolutionary Medicine: A Powerful Tool for Improving Human Health (*Evolution: Education and Outreach* 2008, 1, 2: 114–120). S.C. Stearns, R.M. Nesse, D.R. Govindaraju and P.T. Ellison, Evolutionary Perspectives on Health and Medicine (*Proceedings of the National Academy of Sciences* 2010, 107 (Supplement 1): 1691–1695).

73 S. Sondheim and L. Bernstein, Gee, Officer Krupke, in *West Side Story* (New York: Leonard Bernstein Publishing Company/Boosey & Hawkes, 1956).

74 B.J. Foster, *The 'Public Health' Approach to Gun Control*, http://www.mcrgo.org/mcrgo/doc_pdf/politics_public_health.pdf [accessed 26 February 2011] (Michigan: Michigan Coalition for Responsible Gun Owners, n.d.).

75 M. Stagnitti, *Anti-Depressant Use in the US Civilian Non-Institutionalised Population 2002*, Statistical Brief (Rockville, MD: Medical Expenditure Panel of the Agency for Health-care Research and Quality, 2005).

76 J. Moncrieff, Psychiatric Drug Promotion and the Politics of Neoliberalism (*British Journal of Psychiatry* 2006, 188, 4: 301–302).

77 McKeown, *Modern Rise of Population*; *Medicine in Modern Society* (London: Allen & Unwin, 1965); *The Origins of Human Disease* (London: Blackwell, 1988).

78 T. McKeown, Medical Issues in Historical Demography, in *Modern Methods in the History of Medicine*, ed. E. Clarke (London: Athlone Press, 1971: 57–74).

79 Ibid.

80 L.G. Wilson, Commentary: Medicine, Population, and Tuberculosis (*International Journal of Epidemiology* 2005, 34, 3: 521–524). S. Szreter, Rethinking McKeown: The Relationship between Public Health and Social Change (*American Journal of Public Health* 2002, 92, 5: 722–725).

81 Szreter, Rethinking McKeown.

82 Mokyr, *Gifts of Athena*.

83 E. Beinhocker, *The Origin of Wealth: Evolution, Complexity, and the Radical Remaking of Economics* (Boston, MA: Harvard Business Press, 2006), p. 259.

84 W.W. Rostow, *Stages of Economic Growth: A Non-Communist Manifesto* (Cambridge: Cambridge University Press, 1971).

85 J. Williamson, What Washington Means by Policy Reform, in *Latin American Read-justment: How Much Has Happened?*, ed. J. Williamson (Washington, DC: Institute for International Economics, 1989: 5–20).

86 D. Dollar, Is Globalization Good for Your Health? (*Bulletin of the World Health*

Organization 2001, 79: 827–833). D. Dollar and A. Kraay, Growth Is Good for the Poor (*Journal of Economic Growth* 2002, 7: 195–225).

87 WBCSD, *Sustainable Consumption Facts and Trends* (Conches, Geneva: World Business Council for Sustainable Development, 2008).

88 R.J. Dubos, *Mirage of Health: Utopias, Progress and Biological Change* (New York: Rutgers University Press, 1987 [1959]), p. 266.

89 Hippocrates, *Hippocratic Writings*, trans. J. Chadwick, W.N. Mann, I.M. Lonie and E.T. Withington (London: Penguin Classics, 2005).

90 C. Darwin, *On the Origin of Species by Natural Selection* (London: John Murray, 1859).

91 S.B. Eaton, M. Konner and M. Shostak, Stone Agers in the Fast Lane: Chronic Degenerative Diseases in Evolutionary Perspective (*American Journal of Medicine* 1988, 84, 4: 739–749). T.B. Gage, Are Modern Environments Really Bad for Us? Revisiting the Demographic and Epidemiologic Transitions (*American Journal of Physical Anthropology* 2005 (Supplement 41): 96–117).

92 P. Draper, *Health through Public Policy: Greening of Public Health* (London: Green Print, 1991).

93 J. Naydler, *Goethe on Science* (Edinburgh: Floris Books, 2000).

94 N. Rupke, *Alexander von Humboldt: A Metabiography* (Chicago: University of Chicago Press, 2008).

95 T.H. Huxley, Darwin and Haeckel (*Popular Science Monthly* 1875: 592–598).

96 A.G. Tansley, The Use and Abuse of Vegetational Concepts and Terms (*Ecology* 1935, 16, 3: 284–307).

97 H. Odum and E.C. Odum, *A Prosperous Way Down* (Boulder: University Press of Colorado, 2001).

98 T.G. Randolph, *Human Ecology and Susceptibility to the Chemical Environment* (Springfield, IL: Charles C. Thomas, 1962).

99 A.J. McMichael, *Human Frontiers, Environment and Disease* (Cambridge: Cambridge University Press, 2001).

100 P.A. Kropotkin, *Mutual Aid: A Factor of Evolution*, rev. and cheaper edn (London: Heinemann, 1904).

101 D. Lowenthal, *George Perkins Marsh, Prophet of Conservation* (Seattle: University of Washington Press, 2000).

102 B. Mollison, *Permaculture: A Designer's Manual* (Sisters Creek, Tasmania: Tagari Publications, 1988).

103 J.S. Mill, *Principles of Political Economy* (London, 1848), book IV, ch. 6.

104 C. Darwin, *The Formation of Vegetable Mould through the Action of Worms with Observations on Their Habits* (London: John Murray, 1881).

105 R.E. Park, E.W. Burgess and R.D. McKenzie, *The City* (Chicago: University of Chicago Press, 1967).

106 E.H.P.A. Haeckel and E.R. Lankester, *The History of Creation: Or, The Development of the Earth and Its Inhabitants by the Action of Natural Causes. A Popular Exposition of the Doctrine of Evolution in General, and of That of Darwin, Goethe and Lamarck in Particular*, 2nd edn (London: Henry S. King & Co., 1876).

107 R.J. Richards, *The Tragic Sense of Life: Ernst Haeckel and the Struggle over Evolutionary Thought* (Chicago: University of Chicago Press, 2008).

108 E. Haeckel, Ueber Entwickelungsgang und Aufgabe der Zoologie, *Gesammelte populare Vortrage aus dem Gebiete der Entwickelungslehre*, Heft 2 (Bonn: Strauss, 1879 [1869]).

109 D.R. Keller and F.B. Golley, *The Philosophy of Ecology: From Science to Synthesis* (Athens: University of Georgia Press, 2000).

110 D.P. Todes, *Darwin without Malthus: The Struggle for Existence in Russian Evolutionary Thought* (Oxford: Oxford University Press, 1989).

111 T.R. Malthus, *An Essay on the Principle of Population, as It Affects the Future Improvement of Society with Remarks on the Speculations of Mr. Godwin, M. Condorcet and Other Writers* (London: printed for J. Johnson, 1798).

112 M. Davis, *Late Victorian Holocausts: El Nino Famines and the Making of the Third World* (London: Verso, 2002).

113 S. Dresner, *The Principles of Sustainability* (London: Earthscan, 2008).

114 J.R. Richards, *Human Nature after Darwin: A Philosophical Introduction* (London: Routledge, 2000); Ernst Haeckel's Alleged Anti-Semitism and Contributions to Nazi Biology (*Biological Theory* 2007, 2, 1: 97–103).

115 H. Rose and S. Rose (eds), *Alas, Poor Darwin: Arguments against Evolutionary Psychology* (London: Jonathan Cape, 2000).

116 P.M. Vitousek, H.A. Mooney, J. Lubchenco and J.M. Melillo, Human Domination of Earth's Ecosystems (*Science* 1997, 277, 5325: 494–499).

117 IPCC, Climate Change 2001: Synthesis Report and Summary for Policymakers (approved at the IPCC Plenary XVIII, Wembley, 24–29 September 2001) (Geneva: Intergovernmental Panel on Climate Change Secretariat, 2001). A. McMichael, R. Woodruff and S. Hales, Climate Change and Human Health: Present and Future Risks (*Lancet* 2006, 367, 9513: 859–869).

118 Millennium Ecosystem Assessment, *Ecosystems and Human Well-Being: Synthesis* (Washington, DC: Island Press, 2005).

119 United Nations Environment Programme, *GEO4: Global Environmental Outlook* (Stevenage: EarthPrint, 2007).

120 H.E. Daly, J.B. Cobb and C.W. Cobb, *For the Common Good: Redirecting the Economy toward Community, the Environment, and a Sustainable Future* (London: Green Print, 1990). T. Jackson, *Prosperity without Growth: Economics for a Finite Planet* (London: Earthscan, 2009).

121 E. Mayr, Darwin's Influence on Modern Thought (Lecture delivered in Stockholm on receiving the Craford Prize from the Royal Swedish Academy of Science, 1999).

122 R.B. Laughlin and D. Pines, The Theory of Everything (*Proceedings of the National Academy of Sciences of the United States of America* 2000, 97, 1: 28–31).

123 E. Mayr, *One Long Argument: Charles Darwin's Influence on Evolutionary Thought* (Cambridge, MA: Harvard University Press, 1991), ch. 7.

124 M. Gross, Human Geography and Ecological Sociology: The Unfolding of a Human Ecology, 1890 to 1930 – and Beyond (*Social Science History* 2004, 28, 4: 575–605).

125 G. Rayner and T. Lang, Obesity: Using the Ecologic Public Health Approach to Overcome Policy Cacophony, in *Clinical Obesity in Adults and Children*, 3rd edn, ed. P.G. Kopelman, I.D. Caterson and W.H. Dietz (Oxford: John Wiley & Sons, 2009: 452–470).

126 L. McLaren and P. Hawe, Ecological Perspectives in Health Research, *Journal of Epidemiology and Community Health* 2005, 59, 1: 6–14.

127 H.L. Mencken, *The Divine Afflatus: A Mencken Chrestomathy* (New York: Vintage, 1982 [1949]), p. 449.

128 Commission on Social Determinants of Health, *Closing the Gap in a Generation: Health Equity through Action on the Social Determinants of Health*, Final report of the Commission on Social Determinants of Health, http://www.who.int/social_determinants/final_report/en/index.html (Geneva: World Health Organization, 2008).

129 G.C.M. M'Gonigle and J. Kirby, *Poverty and Public Health*, Left Book Club edn (London: Victor Gollancz, 1936).

130 L. Kartman, Human Ecology and Public Health (*American Journal of Public Health* 1967, 57, 5: 737–750).

131 J.J. Hanlon, An Ecologic View of Public Health (*American Journal of Public Health* 1969, 59, 1: 4–11).

132 Committee on Assuring the Health of the Public in the 21st Century, *The Future of the Public's Health in the 21st Century* (Washington, DC: National Academies Press, 2002). Institute of Medicine of the National Academies, *Preventing Childhood Obesity: Health in the Balance* (Washington, DC: Institute of Medicine of the National Academies, 2004).

133 Commission on the Social Determinants of Health, *Towards a Conceptual Framework for*

Analysis and Action on the Social Determinants of Health (Geneva: World Health Organization, 2005).

134 McMichael, *Human Frontiers, Environment and Disease*. N. Krieger, Theories for Social Epidemiology in the 21st Century: An Eco-Social Perspective (*International Journal of Epidemiology* 2001, 30: 668–677); Historical Roots of Social Epidemiology: Socioeconomic Gradients in Health and Contextual Analysis (*International Journal of Epidemiology* 2001, 30, 4: 899–900). N. Pearce and F. Merletti, Complexity, Simplicity, and Epidemiology (*International Journal of Epidemiology* 2006, 35, 3: 515–519). M. Susser and E. Susser, Choosing a Future for Epidemiology: I. Eras and Paradigms (*American Journal of Public Health* 1996, 86, 5: 668–673).

135 J.M. Last, *Public Health and Human Ecology* (Stamford, CT: Appleton & Lange, 1997), p. ix.

136 I. Kickbush, Approaches to an Ecological Base for Public Health (*Health Promotion* 1989, 4: 265–268).

137 M.J. Douglas, S.J. Watkins, D.R. Gorman and M. Higgins, Are Cars the New Tobacco? (*Journal of Public Health* 2011, 33, 2: 160–169).

138 J.L. Aron and J.A. Patz (eds), *Ecosystem Change and Public Health: A Global Perspective* (Baltimore, MD: Johns Hopkins University Press, 2001).

Introduction to Part II

1 J. Dewey, *The Influence of Darwin on Philosophy* (New York: Henry Holt, 1910).

2 J.A. Popp, *Evolution's First Philosopher: John Dewey and the Continuity of Nature* (Albany: State University of New York, 2007), p. 83.

3 R.J. Dubos, *Mirage of Health: Utopias, Progress and Biological Change* (New York: Rutgers University Press, 1987 [1959]), p. 1.

4 J. Dewey, *Art as Experience*, vol. 23 (New York: Perigee Books, 1980 [1934]).

5 M. Gell-Mann, *The Quark and the Jaguar: Adventures in the Simple and the Complex* (New York: Henry Holt, 1995).

6 M. Gell-Mann, Transformations of the Twenty-First Century: Transitions to Greater Sustainability, in *Global Sustainability: A Nobel Cause*, ed. H.J. Schellnhuber, M. Molina, N. Stern, V. Huber and S. Kadner (Cambridge: Cambridge University Press, 2010), pp. 1–7.

4 Demographic Transition

1 A. Landry, Adolphe Landry on the Demographic Revolution (*Population and Development Review* 1987, 13, 4: 731–740).

2 A. Landry, *La révolution démographique: Études et essais sur les problèmes de la population* (Paris: Institut National d'Études Demographiques/Presses Universitaires de France, 1934).

3 F.W. Notestein, Population: The Long View, in *Food for the World*, ed. T.W. Schultz (Chicago: University of Chicago Press, 1945), pp. 36–57.

4 J.-C. Chesnais, *The Demographic Transition: Stages, Patterns, and Economic Implications: A Longitudinal Study of Sixty-Seven Countries Covering the Period 1720–1984* (Oxford: Oxford University Press, 1992), ch. 1.

5 J.C. Caldwell, Demographers and the Study of Mortality: Scope, Perspectives, and Theory (*Annals of the New York Academy of Sciences* 2001, 954: 19–34).

6 A. Smith, *An Inquiry into the Nature and Causes of the Wealth of Nations* (Charleston, SC: Forgotten Books, 2008 [1776]), p. 55.

7 G. Mooney, Infectious Diseases and Epidemiologic Transition in Victorian Britain? Definitely (*Social History of Medicine* 2007, 20, 3: 595–606).

8 A. Macfarlane, *The Savage Wars of Peace: England, Japan and the Malthusian Trap* (Oxford: Blackwell, 1997).

9 S. Szreter, The Population Health Approach in Historical Perspective (*American Journal of Public Health* 2003, 93, 3: 421–431).

10 A. Maddison, *The World Economy: A Millennial Perspective* (Paris: Organisation for Economic Co-operation and Development, 2001).

11 T.R. Malthus, *An Essay on the Principle of Population, as It Affects the Future Improvement of Society with Remarks on the Speculations of Mr. Godwin, M. Condorcet and Other Writers* (London: printed for J. Johnson, 1798).

12 B. Dolan, Malthus' Political Economy of Health: The Critique of Scandinavia in the Essay on Population, in *Malthus, Medicine and Morality: Malthusianism after 1798*, ed. B. Dolan (Amsterdam: Editions Rodopi, 2000: 9–32).

13 Chesnais, *The Demographic Transition*, p. 1.

14 T.R. Malthus, *The Grounds of an Opinion on the Policy of Restricting the Importation of Foreign Corn: Intended as an Appendix to 'Observations on the Corn Law'* (London: John Murray and J. Johnson and Co., 1815).

15 K. Marx and F. Engels, *Collected Works*, vol. 3: *1843–44* (London: Lawrence & Wishart, 1975).

16 O. Galor and D.N. Weil, Population, Technology, and Growth: From Malthusian Stagnation to the Demographic Transition and Beyond (*American Economic Review* 2000, 90, 4: 806–828).

17 V.L. Bullough (ed.), *Encyclopedia of Birth Control* (Santa Barbara, CA: ABC-CLIO, 2001), p. 147.

18 J.S. Mill, *Autobiography* (Philadelphia: Pennsylvania State University, 2004 [1873]), p. 61.

19 R. Ledbetter, *A History of the Malthusian League, 1877–1927* (Columbus: Ohio State University, 1976).

20 R. Jütte, *Contraception: A History* (London: Polity Press, 2008).

21 R. Pearl and L.J. Reed, On the Rate of Growth of the Population of the United States since 1790 and Its Mathematical Representation (*Proceedings of the National Academy of Sciences* 1920, 6, 6: 175–288).

22 W.S. Thompson, *Population: A Study in Malthusianism* (New York: Columbia University, 1915).

23 W.S. Thompson, Population (*American Journal of Sociology* 1929, 34, 6: 959–975).

24 F.W. Notestein, Population: The Long View, in *Food for the World*, ed. T.W. Schultz (Chicago: Chicago University Press, 1945: 36–57).

25 S.R.S. Szreter, The Idea of Demographic Transition: A Critical Intellectual History (*Population and Development Review* 1993, 19, 4: 659–701).

26 J.C. Caldwell and B. Caldwell, *Demographic Transition Theory* (Dordrecht: Springer, 2006).

27 D. Kirk, Demographic Transition Theory (*Population Studies* 1986, 50: 361–387).

28 Chesnais, *The Demographic Transition*, p. 17.

29 J. Cleland, S. Bernstein, A. Ezeh, A. Faundes, A. Glasier and J. Innis, Family Planning: The Unfinished Agenda (*Lancet* 2006, 368: 1810–1827).

30 P.R. Ehrlich, *The Population Bomb* (New York: Ballantine, 1968).

31 UN Population Division, *World Population Prospects: The 2010 Revision* (New York: UN Population Division, Department of Economic and Social Affairs, 2011).

32 P.R. Ehrlich and A.H. Ehrlich, The Population Bomb Revisited (*Electronic Journal of Sustainable Development* 2009, 1, 3: 63–71).

5 Epidemiological and Health Transition

1 J.C. Riley, *Rising Life Expectancy: A Global History* (Cambridge: Cambridge University Press, 2001), p. 7.

2 A.R. Omran, The Epidemiologic Transition Theory: A Preliminary Update (*Journal of Tropical Pediatrics* 1983, 29: 305–316).

3 R. Lewontin, Death of TB (*New York Review of Books* 1979, 25, 21/22).

4 C.-E.A. Winslow, Preventive Medicine and Health Promotion: Ideals or Realities? (*Yale Journal of Biology and Medicine* 1942, 14, 5: 443–452).

5 J. Pemberton, Origins and Early History of the Society for Social Medicine in the UK and Ireland (*Journal of Epidemiology and Community Health* 2002, 56, 5: 342–346).

6 T. McKeown, Medicine and World Population (*Journal of Chronic Diseases* 1965, 18: 1067–1077); *Medicine in Modern Society* (London: Allen & Unwin, 1965); A Sociological Approach to the History of Medicine (*Medical History* 1970, 14, 4: 342–351); Medical Issues in Historical Demography, in *Modern Methods in the History of Medicine*, ed. E. Clarke (London: Athlone Press, 1971: 57–74); *The Modern Rise of Population* (London: Edward Arnold, 1976); Fertility, Mortality and Causes of Death: An Examination of Issues Related to the Modern Rise of Population (*Population Studies* 1978, 32, 3: 535–542); *The Role of Medicine: Dream, Mirage, or Nemesis?* (Princeton, NJ: Princeton University Press, 1979); *The Origins of Human Disease* (London: Basil Blackwell, 1988).

7 J. Vernon, *Hunger: A Modern History* (Cambridge, MA: Harvard University Press, 2007).

8 C. Alvarez-Dardet and M.T. Ruiz, Thomas McKeown and Archibald Cochrane: A Journey through the Diffusion of Their Ideas (*BMJ* 1993, 306, 6887: 1252–1254).

9 S. Glouberman and J. Millar, Evolution of the Determinants of Health, Health Policy, and Health Information Systems in Canada (*American Journal of Public Health* 2003, 93, 3: 388–392).

10 B.D. Smedley and S.L. Syme (eds), Committee on Capitalizing on Social Science and Behavioral Research to Improve the Public's Health, Division of Health Promotion and Disease Prevention, *Promoting Health: Intervention Strategies from Social and Behavioral Research* (Washington, DC: National Academies Press, 2000).

11 L.G. Wilson, Commentary: Medicine, Population, and Tuberculosis (*International Journal of Epidemiology* 2005, 34, 3: 521–524).

12 S. Szreter, Rethinking McKeown: The Relationship between Public Health and Social Change (*American Journal of Public Health* 2002, 92, 5: 722–725). J.F. Hutchinson, Historical Method and the Social History of Medicine (*Medical History* 1973, 17, 4: 423–431). E.A. Wrigley and R.S. Schofield, *The Population History of England, 1541–1871: A Reconstruction* (London: Edward Arnold, 1981). B. Bynum, The McKeown Thesis (*Lancet* 2008, 371, 9613: 644–645). S. Szreter, Szreter Responds (*American Journal of Public Health* 2003, 93, 7: 1032–1033).

13 S.R. Johansson, Commentary: The Pitfalls of Policy History – Writing the Past to Change the Present (*International Journal of Epidemiology* 2005, 34, 3: 526–529).

14 D.R. Hopkins, *The Greatest Killer: Smallpox in History* (with a new introduction) (Chicago: University of Chicago Press, 1983), p. 94.

15 S. Guha, The Importance of Social Intervention in England's Mortality Decline: The Evidence Reviewed (*Social History of Medicine* 1994, 7, 1: 89–113.

16 R.W. Fogel, *The Global Struggle to Escape from Chronic Malnutrition since 1700*, Proceedings of the World Food Programme/United Nations University (Rome: United Nations Food and Agriculture Organization, 1997).

17 G.A. Condran, Commentary: History in the Search of Policy (*International Journal of Epidemiology* 2005, 34, 3: 525–526).

18 R.G. Evans, Thomas McKeown, Meet Fidel Castro: Physicians, Population Health and the Cuban Paradox (*Healthcare Policy/Politiques de Santé* 2008, 3, 4: 21–32).

19 D. Acemoglu, S. Johnson and J. Robinson, Disease and Development in Historical Perspective (*Journal of the European Economic Association* 2003, 1, 2–3: 397–405).

20 G. Rayner, C. Hawkes, T. Lang and W. Bello, Trade Liberalisation and the Diet and Nutrition Transition: A Public Health Response (*Health Promotion International* 2006, 21 (Supplement 1): 67–74).

21 C. Mathers, G. Stevens and M. Mascarenhas, *Global Health Risks: Mortality and Burden of Disease Attributable to Selected Major Risks* (Geneva: World Health Organization, 2009).

22 S.J. Olshansky and A.B. Ault, The Fourth Stage of the Epidemiologic Transition: The Age of Delayed Degenerative Diseases (*Milbank Quarterly* 1986, 64, 3: 355–391).

23 OECD, *OECD Health Data 2011: How Does Japan Compare?* (Paris: Organisation for Economic Co-operation and Development, 2011).

24 W. Lutz, B.C. O'Neill and S. Scherbov, Europe's Population at a Turning Point (*Science* 2003, 299, 5615: 1991–1992).

25 S. Agyei-Mensah and A. de-Graft Aikins, Epidemiological Transition and the Double Burden of Disease in Accra, Ghana (*Journal of Urban Health* 2001, 87, 5: 879–897).

26 K.N. Dancause, C. Dehuff, L.E. Soloway, M. Vilar, C. Chan, M. Wilson *et al.*, Behavioral Changes Associated with Economic Development in the South Pacific: Health Transition in Vanuatu (*American Journal of Human Biology* 2011, 23, 3: 366–376).

27 J. Coreil, J.S. Levin and E.G. Jaco, Life Style: An Emergent Concept in the Sociomedical Sciences (*Culture, Medicine and Psychiatry* 1985, 9, 4: 423–437).

28 M. Ezzati, S. Vander Hoorn, C.M.M. Lawes, R. Leach, W.P.T. James, A.D. Lopez *et al.*, Rethinking the 'Diseases of Affluence' Paradigm: Global Patterns of Nutritional Risks in Relation to Economic Development (*PLoS Medicine* 2005, 2, 5: e133).

29 D. Phillips, Urbanization and Human Health (*Parasitology* 1993, 106 (Supplement): S93–107).

30 G. Rose, Sick Individuals and Sick Populations (*International Journal of Epidemiology* 2001, 30, 3: 427–432).

31 R.W. Fogel, *Nutrition, Physiological Capital, and Economic Growth* (Washington, DC: Pan American Health Organization, 2002).

32 B.G. Chariton, A Critique of Geoffrey Rose's 'Population Strategy' for Preventive Medicine (*Journal of the Royal Society of Medicine* 1995, 88: 607–610).

33 N. Krieger, *Epidemiology and the People's Health: Theory and Context* (New York: Oxford University Press, 2011).

34 S. Galea, M. Riddle and G.A. Kaplan, Causal Thinking and Complex System Approaches in Epidemiology (*International Journal of Epidemiology* 2010, 39, 1: 97–106).

35 J.M. Cohen, M.L. Wilson and A.E. Aiello, Analysis of Social Epidemiology Research on Infectious Diseases: Historical Patterns and Future Opportunities (*Journal of Epidemiology and Community Health* 2007, 61: 1021–1027).

36 M. Susser, The Logic in Ecological: I. The Logic of Analysis (*American Journal of Public Health* 1994, 84, 5: 825–829).

37 A.J. McMichael, Prisoners of the Proximate: Loosening the Constraints on Epidemiology in an Age of Change (*American Journal of Epidemiology* 1999, 149, 10: 887–897).

38 K. Popper, Natural Selection and the Emergence of Mind (*Dialectica* 1978, 32, 3–4: 339–355).

39 M. Marmot, *The Social Determinants of Health* (Oxford: Oxford University Press, 1999); *Status Syndrome: How Your Social Standing Directly Affects Your Health* (London: Bloomsbury, 2005).

40 R.G. Wilkinson and K. Pickett, *The Spirit Level: Why More Equal Societies Almost Always Do Better* (London: Allen Lane, 2009).

41 E. Durkheim, *Suicide: A Study in Sociology* (London: Routledge, 2002 [1912]).

42 J.W. Lynch, G. Davey-Smith, G.A. Kaplan and J.S. House, Income Inequality and Mortality: Importance to Health of Individual Income, Psychosocial Environment, or Material Conditions (*British Medical Journal* 2000, 320, 7243: 1200–1204).

43 C. Muntaner, J. Lynch and G. Davey-Smith, Social Capital, Disorganized Communities, and the Third Way: Understanding the Retreat from Structural Inequalities in Epidemiology and Public Health (*International Journal of Health Services* 2001, 31, 2: 213–237).

6 Urban Transition

1 UN Habitat, *State of the World's Cities 2010/2011 – Cities for All: Bridging the Urban Divide* (London: Earthscan, 2010), p. 5.

2 Ibid.

3 R.C. Allen, *The British Industrial Revolution in Global Perspective: How Commerce*

Created the Industrial Revolution and Modern Economic Growth (Oxford: Oxford University, Department of Economics and Nuffield College, 2006).

4 C. Tilly and A.L. Stinchcombe, *Roads from Past to Future* (Lanham, MD: Rowman & Littlefield, 1997).

5 F. Tönnies, *Gemeinschaft und Gesellschaft* (Leipzig: Fues Verlag, 1887).

6 M. Brown, From Foetid Air to Filth: The Cultural Transformation of British Epidemiological Thought, ca. 1780–1848 (*Bulletin of the History of Medicine* 2008, 82, 3: 515–544).

7 K. Ringen, Edwin Chadwick, the Market Ideology, and Sanitary Reform: On the Nature of the 19th-Century Public Health Movement (*International Journal of Health Services* 1979, 9, 1: 107–120).

8 Brown, From Foetid Air to Filth.

9 J.H. Cassedy, Hygeia: A Mid-Victorian Dream of a City of Health (*Journal of the History of Medicine and Allied Sciences* 1962, XVII, 2: 217–228).

10 G.C. Cook, Thomas Southwood Smith FRCP (1788–1861): Leading Exponent of Diseases of Poverty and Pioneer of Sanitary Reform in the Mid-Nineteenth Century (*Journal of Medical Biography* 2002, 10, 4: 194–205).

11 F. Engels, *The Condition of the Working Class in England in 1844* (London: Penguin Classics, 1987 [1845/1892]).

12 L.A. Baker, *The Water Environment of Cities* (New York: Springer, 2009), p. 6.

13 N. Howard-Jones, Robert Koch and the Cholera Vibrio: A Centenary (*British Medical Journal* 1984, 288: 379–381).

14 J.M. Eyler, The Changing Assessments of John Snow's and William Farr's Cholera Studies (*Sozial- und Präventivmedizin* 2001, 46, 4: 225–232).

15 R.A. Easterlin, *The Reluctant Economist: Perspectives on Economics, Economic History and Demography* (Cambridge: Cambridge University Press, 2004), p. 93.

16 P.D. Groote, J.P. Elhorst and P.G. Tassenaar, Standard of Living Effects Due to Infrastructure Improvements in the 19th Century (*Social Science Computer Review* 2009, 27, 3: 380–389).

17 S. Johnson, *The Ghost Map: A Street, a City, an Epidemic and the Hidden Power of Urban Networks* (London: Penguin Books, 2006).

18 D. Cutler and G. Miller, The Role of Public Health Improvements in Health Advances: The Twentieth Century United States (*Demography* 2005, 42, 1: 1–22).

19 M. Kalfus, *Frederick Law Olmsted: The Passion of a Public Artist* (New York: New York University Press, 1990), p. 291.

20 P. Thane, Government and Society in England and Wales, 1750–1914, in *The Cambridge Social History of Britain 1750–1950: Social Agencies and Institutions*, ed. F.M.L. Thompson (Cambridge: Cambridge University Press, 1993: 1–62), p. 18.

21 S. Sheard, Profit Is a Dirty Word: The Development of Public Baths and Wash-Houses in Britain 1847–1915 (*Social History of Medicine* 2000, 13, 1: 63–86).

22 P. Geddes, *Cities in Evolution: An Introduction to the Town Planning Movement and to the Study of Civics* (London: Williams and Norgate, 1915).

23 L. Mumford, The Natural History of Urbanization, in *Man's Role in Changing the Face of the Earth*, ed. W.L. Thomas, Jr (Chicago: University of Chicago Press, 1956).

24 L. Mumford, *The City in History: Its Origins, Its Transformations and Its Prospects* (London: Secker & Warburg, 1961).

25 Mumford, Natural History of Urbanization.

26 Ibid.

27 P.A. Kropotkin, *Fields, Factories and Workshops: Or Industry Combined with Agriculture and Brain Work with Manual Work*, new edn (London: S. Sonnenschein, 1901).

28 R.H. Kargon and A.P. Molella, *Invented Edens: Techno-Cities of the Twentieth Century* (Cambridge, MA: MIT Press, 2008).

29 L. Mumford, *The Highway and the City* (New York: New American Library, 1964).

30 A. Linklater, *Measuring America: How the United States Was Shaped by the Greatest Land Sale in History* (New York: HarperCollins, 2002).

31 A. Schiff, *The Father of Baseball: A Biography of Henry Chadwick* (Jefferson, NC: McFarland Publishing, 2008).

32 J.H. Kay, *Asphalt Nation: How the Automobile Took Over America, and How We Can Take It Back* (Berkeley and London: University of California Press, 1998).

33 International Energy Agency and OECD, *Transport, Energy and CO_2: Moving towards Sustainability – How the World Can Achieve Deep CO_2 Reductions in Transport by 2050* (Paris: International Energy Agency, 2009).

34 Ibid.

35 C. Kennedy, J. Steinberger, B. Gasson, Y. Hansen, T. Hillman, M. Havránek *et al.*, Greenhouse Gas Emissions from Global Cities (*Environmental Science and Technology* 2009, 43, 19: 7297–7302).

36 W. Zelinsky, The Hypothesis of the Mobility Transition (*Geographical Review* 1971, 61, 2: 219–249).

37 J. Jacobs, *The Death and Life of Great American Cities* (New York: Random House, 1961).

38 M. Davis, *Ecology of Fear: Los Angeles and the Imagination of Disaster* (New York: Vintage Books, 1999).

39 D. Harvey, *The Limits to Capital* (London: Verso, 2006).

40 D. Harvey, *Possible Urban Worlds: Megacities Lecture 4* (Amersfoort: Twynstra Gudde Management Consultants, 2000).

41 J.O. Abiodun, Urban Growth and Problems in Metropolitan Lagos (*Urban Studies* 1974, 11, 3: 341–347).

42 E. Cossou, Lagos Aims to Be Africa's Model Megacity, Africa Business Report, *BBC World News*, http://news.bbc.co.uk/1/hi/business/8473001.stm (London: BBC, 2010).

43 UN Habitat, *State of African Cities 2010: Governance, Inequalities and Urban Land Market* (Nairobi: UN Habitat, 2010).

44 Ibid.

45 R. Kipper and M. Fischer (eds), *Cairo's Informal Areas: Between Urban Challenges and Hidden Potentials. Facts. Voices. Visions* (Cairo: German Technical Cooperation, 2009), p. 32.

46 E. Van de Poela, O. O'Donnell and E. Van Doorslae, *The Health Penalty of China's Rapid Urbanization*, Tinbergen Institute Discussion Paper (Amsterdam: Tinbergen Institute, 2009).

47 B.W. Richardson, *Hygeia, a City of Health* (Gloucester: Dodo Press, 2008 [1876]).

48 Cassedy, Hygeia.

49 M. Davis and D.B. Monk, *Evil Paradises: Dreamworlds of Neoliberalism* (New York: New Press, 2007).

50 R. Dobbs, S. Smit, J. Remes, J. Manyika, C. Roxburgh and A. Restrepo, *Urban World: Mapping the Economic Power of Cities* (McKinsey Global Institute, 2011). B. Cohen, Urban Growth in Developing Countries: A Review of Current Trends and a Caution Regarding Existing Forecasts (*World Development* 2004, 32, 1: 23–51).

51 W. Easterly, *The White Man's Burden: Why the West's Efforts to Aid the Rest Have Done So Much Ill and So Little Good* (New York: Penguin, 2006).

52 Van de Poela, O'Donnell and Van Doorslae, *Health Penalty of China's Rapid Urbanization*.

53 UN Habitat, *Global Report on Human Settlements 2011: Cities and Climate Change* (New York: UN Habitat, 2011).

54 UN Population Fund, *International Conference on Population and Development: Summary of the Programme of Action*, Cairo, 5–13 September 1994, http://www.un.org/ecosocdev/geninfo/populatin/icpd.htm (New York: UN Population Fund, 1994).

55 UN Habitat, History, http://www.unhabitat.org/content.asp?typeid=19&catid=10&cid=927 [accessed 31 May 2011] (Nairobi: UN Habitat, 2011).

56 E.J. Kasowski, R.J. Garten and C.B. Bridges, Influenza Pandemic Epidemiologic and Virologic Diversity: Reminding Ourselves of the Possibilities (*Clinical Infectious Diseases* 2011, 52 (Supplement 1): S44–S49). N.M. Scalera and S.B. Mossad, The First

Pandemic of the 21st Century: A Review of the 2009 Pandemic Variant Influenza A (H1N1) Virus (*Postgraduate Medicine* 2009, 121, 5: 43–47).

57 R.E. Park and E.W. Burgess, *The City* (Chicago: University of Chicago Press, 1925).

58 H. Frumkin, J. Hess and S. Vindigni, Energy and Public Health: The Challenge of Peak Petroleum (*Public Health Reports* 2009, 124: 5–19).

59 P. Rode and R. Burdett (eds), *Towards a Green Economy: Pathways to Sustainable Development and Poverty Eradication* (New York: United Nations Environment Programme, 2011).

7 Energy Transition

1 T.B. Haugland, O. Helge and K. Roland, *Energy Structures and Environmental Futures* (Oxford: Oxford University Press, 1998).

2 G.H. Mead, *On the Influence of Darwin's Origin of Species* (Chicago: Chicago University, 1909).

3 A. Grubler, *Technology and Global Change* (Cambridge: Cambridge University Press, 1998); Transitions in Energy Use (*Encyclopedia of Energy* 2004, 6: 163–177).

4 H. Haberl, M. Fischer-Kowalski, F. Krausmann, J. Martinez-Alier and V. Winiwarter, A Socio-Metabolic Transition towards Sustainability? Challenges for Another Great Transformation (*Sustainable Development* 2009, 19, 1: 1–14).

5 J.C.J.M. van den Bergh and F.H. Oosterhuis, An Evolutionary Economic Analysis of Energy Transitions (45th Congress of the European Regional Science Association, 2005).

6 V. Smil, *Creating the Twentieth Century: Technical Innovations of 1867–1914 and Their Lasting Impact* (New York: Oxford University Press, 2005).

7 A.H. Lockwood, K. Welker-Hood, M. Rauch and B. Gottlieb, *Coal's Assault on Human Health* (Washington, DC: Physicians for Social Responsibility, 2009).

8 K. Mellanby (ed.), *Air Pollution, Acid Rain, and the Environment* (Barking: Springer, 1998).

9 E.A. Finkelstein and K.L. Strombotne, The Economics of Obesity (*American Journal of Clinical Nutrition* 2010, 91, 5: 1520S–1524).

10 S.H. Jacobson and L.A. McLay, The Economic Impact of Obesity on Automobile Fuel Consumption (*Engineering Economist: A Journal Devoted to the Problems of Capital Investment* 2006, 51, 4: 307–323). I. Roberts and P. Edwards, *The Energy Glut: The Politics of Fatness in an Overheating World* (London: Zed Press, 2010).

11 W. Steffen, P.J. Crutzen and J.R. McNeill, The Anthropocene: Are Humans Now Overwhelming the Great Forces of Nature? (*AMBIO: A Journal of the Human Environment* 2009, 36, 8: 614–621).

12 F. Pearce, *The Climate Files: The Battle for the Truth about Global Warming* (London: Guardian Books, 2010).

13 S. Kinzer, *All the Shah's Men: An American Coup and the Roots of Middle East Terror* (Hoboken, NJ: John Wiley, 2003).

14 N. Georgescu-Roegen, Energy and Economic Myths (*Southern Economic Journal* 1975, 41, 3: 347–381).

15 Ibid.

16 A. Maddison, Evidence Submitted to the Select Committee on Economic Affairs, House of Lords, London, for the Inquiry into Economics of Climate Change, *Economics of Climate Change: 2nd Report of Session 2005–06*, HL Paper 12-I (London: House of Lords, 2005).

17 A. Williams and G.H. Martin (eds), *Domesday Book (1186)* (London: Penguin Books, 1992).

18 J. Getzler, *A History of Water Rights at Common Law* (Oxford: Oxford University Press, 2004).

19 J. Hatcher, *The History of the British Coal Industry before 1700* (Oxford: Oxford University Press, 1993).

20 R.P. Sieferle, *The Subterranean Forest Energy Systems and the Industrial Revolution* (Cambridge: White Horse Press, 2001).

21 R.C. Allen, *The British Industrial Revolution in Global Perspective: How Commerce Created the Industrial Revolution and Modern Economic Growth* (Oxford: Oxford University, Department of Economics and Nuffield College, 2006).

22 T. Balderston, The Economics of Abundance: Coal and Cotton in Lancashire and the World (*Economic History Review* 2010, 63, 3: 569–590).

23 R. Fouquet, *The Slow Search for Solutions: Lessons from Historical Energy Transitions by Sector and Service*, BC3 Working Paper Series 2010-05 (Bilbao: Basque Centre for Climate Change, 2010).

24 S. Jevons, *The Coal Question* (London: Macmillan, 1865).

25 J. Hicks and G. Allen, *A Century of Change: Trends in UK Statistics since 1900*, Research Paper 99/111 (London: House of Commons Library, 1999).

26 D. Briggs, Environmental Pollution and the Global Burden of Disease (*British Medical Bulletin* 2003, 68, 1: 1–24).

27 R.A. Smith, *Air and Rain: The Beginning of Chemical Climatology* (London: Longmans, Green and Co., 1872).

28 W.H. TeBrake, Air Pollution and Fuel Crises in Preindustrial London, 1250–1650 (*Technological Culture* 1975, 16: 337–359).

29 C. Garwood, Green Crusaders or Captives of Industry? The British Alkali Inspectorate and the Ethics of Environmental Decision Making, 1864–95 (*Annals of Science* 2004, 61, 1: 99–117).

30 A. Gibson and W.V. Farrar, Robert Angus Smith, FRS, and 'Sanitary Science' (*Notes and Records of the Royal Society of London* 1974, 28, 2: 241–262).

31 C. Flick, The Movement for Smoke Abatement in Nineteenth-Century Britain (*Technology and Culture* 1980, 21, 1: 29–50).

32 B. Luckin, Pollution in the City, in *The Cambridge Urban History of Britain: 1840–1950*, ed. M.J. Daunton (Cambridge: Cambridge University Press, 2000: 207–228).

33 P. Brimblecombe, *The Big Smoke: A History of Air Pollution in London since Medieval Times* (London: Methuen, 1987). M.L. Bell, D.L. Davis and T. Fletcher, A Retrospective Assessment of Mortality from the London Smog Episode of 1952: The Role of Influenza and Pollution (*Environmental Health Perspectives* 2004, 112, 1: 6–8).

34 Briggs, Environmental Pollution.

35 B. Freese, *Coal: A Human History* (London: Penguin, 2004).

36 H. Haberl, H. Weisz, C. Amann, A. Bondeau, N. Eisenmenger, K.-H. Erb *et al.*, The Energetic Metabolism of the European Union and the United States: Decadal Energy Input Time-Series with an Emphasis on Biomass (*Journal of Industrial Ecology* 2006, 10, 4: 151–172).

37 FAO, *State of Food and Agriculture 2008: Biofuels – Prospects, Risks and Opportunities* (Rome: Food and Agriculture Organization, 2008).

38 J. Goodell, *Big Coal: The Dirty Secret behind America's Energy Future* (Boston, MA: Houghton Mifflin, 2006).

39 E. Crooks, Clouds Gather over US Coal-Fired Plants (*Financial Times* 2011 (29 August)).

40 BP, *BP Statistical Review of World Energy* (London: BP, 2009).

41 W. Bank, *Cost of Pollution in China: Economic Estimates of Physical Damages* (Washington, DC: World Bank, 2007). V. Smil, *China's Past, China's Future: Energy, Food, Environment*, Critical Asian Scholarship (New York: London: RoutledgeCurzon, 2004).

42 Smil, China's Past, China's Future. D.G. Streets, J. Hao, Y. Wu, J. Jiang, M. Chan, H. Tian *et al.*, Anthropogenic Mercury Emissions in China (*Atmospheric Environment* 2005, 39, 40: 7789–7806). F.X. Han, Y. Su, D.L. Monts, M.J. Plodinec, A. Banin and G.E. Triplett, Assessment of Global Industrial-Age Anthropogenic Arsenic Contamination (*Naturwissenschaften* 2003, 90, 9: 395–401). H.E. Belkin, B. Zheng, D. Zhou and R.B.

Finkelman, Chronic Arsenic Poisoning from Domestic Combustion of Coal in Rural China: A Case Study of the Relationship between Earth Materials and Human Health, in *Environmental Geochemistry: Site Characterization, Data Analysis and Case Histories*, ed. B. De Vivo, H.E. Belkin and A. Lima (Amsterdam: Elsevier, 2008: 401–420).

43 A. Grubler, Doing More with Less: Improving the Environment through Green Engineering (*Environment* 2006, 48, 2: 22–37).

44 K.R. Smith, S. Mehta and M. Maeusezahl-Feuz, Indoor Air-Pollution from Solid Fuel Use, in *Comparative Quantification of Health Risks: Global and Regional Burden of Disease Attributable to Selected Major Risk Factors*, ed. M. Ezzati, A.D. Lopez, A. Rodgers and C.J.L. Murray (Geneva: World Health Organization, 2004: 1435–1493).

45 T.V. Ramachandra, Y. Loerincik and B.V. Shruthi, Intra and Inter Country Energy Intensity Trends (*Journal of Energy and Development* 2006, 31, 1: 43–84).

46 P. Winch and R. Stepnitz, Peak Oil and Health in Low- and Middle-Income Countries: Impacts and Potential Responses (*American Journal of Public Health* 2011, 101, 9: 1607–1614). B.S. Schwartz, C.L. Parker, J. Hess and H. Frumkin, Public Health and Medicine in an Age of Energy Scarcity: The Case of Petroleum (*American Journal of Public Health* 2011, 101, 9: 1560–1567).

47 D.G. Fullerton, N. Bruce and S.B. Gordon, Indoor Air Pollution from Biomass Fuel Smoke Is a Major Health Concern in the Developing World (*Transactions of the Royal Society of Tropical Medicine and Hygiene* 2008, 102, 9: 843–851). O.P. Kurmi, S. Semple, P. Simkhada, W.C.S. Smith and J.G. Ayres, COPD and Chronic Bronchitis Risk of Indoor Air Pollution from Solid Fuel: A Systematic Review and Meta-Analysis (*Thorax* 2010, 65, 3: 221–228). E.A. Rehfuess, L. Tzala, N. Best, D.J. Briggs and M. Joffe, Solid Fuel Use and Cooking Practices as a Major Risk Factor for ALRI Mortality among African Children (*Journal of Epidemiology and Community Health* 2009, 63, 11: 887–892).

48 WHO, *Indoor Air Pollution and Health*, Factsheet (Geneva: World Health Organization, 2005).

49 Briggs, Environmental Pollution.

50 N. Stern, *The Economics of Climate Change: The Stern Review* (Cambridge: Cambridge University Press, 2007).

51 Ibid. N. Stern and S.-L. Garbett-Shiels, Towards a Global Deal on Climate Change, in *Global Sustainability: A Nobel Cause*, ed. H.J. Schellnhuber, M. Molina, N. Stern, V. Huber and S. Kadner (Cambridge: Cambridge University Press, 2010: 82–98).

52 US Energy Information Administration, *International Energy Outlook 2010* (Washington, DC: US Energy Information Administration, 2010).

53 Maddison, Evidence Submitted to the Select Committee on Economic Affairs.

54 US Energy Information Administration, *International Energy Outlook 2010*.

55 Fouquet, *Slow Search for Solutions*.

56 Haberl *et al.*, Energetic Metabolism.

57 J.D. Hughes, *An Environmental History of the World: Humankind's Changing Role in the Community of Life* (London: Routledge, 2001), p. 18. J. Goudsblom, *Fire and Civilization* (London: Allen Lane/Penguin, 1993).

58 V. Smil, Eating Meat: Evolution, Patterns, and Consequences (*Population and Development Review* 2002, 28, 4: 599–639).

59 Steffen, Crutzen and McNeill, Anthropocene.

60 H. Spencer, *The Principles of Sociology* (London: Williams and Norgate, 1876).

61 P.A. Corning, Thermoeconomics: Beyond the Second Law (*Journal of Bioeconomics* 2002, 4, 1: 57–88).

62 A.J. Lotka, Natural Selection as Physical Principle (*Proceedings of the National Academy of Sciences* 1922, 8: 151–154).

63 L.A. White, Energy and the Evolution of Culture (*American Anthropologist* 1943, 45, 3: 335–356).

64 L.A. White, *The Evolution of Culture: The Development of Civilization to the Fall of Rome* (New York: McGraw-Hill, 1959).

65 W.J. Peace, *Leslie A. White: Evolution and Revolution in Anthropology* (Lincoln: University of Nebraska Press, 2004).

66 J.W. Bennett, *The Ecological Transition: Cultural Anthropology and Human Adaptation* (Edison, NJ: Transaction Publishers, 2005).

67 J. Gowdy and S. Mesner, The Evolution of Georgescu-Roegen's Bioeconomics (*Review of Social Economy* 1998, LVI, 2: 136–156). K. Mayumi, *The Origins of Ecological Economics: The Bioeconomics of Georgescu-Roegen* (London: Routledge, 2001).

68 Corning, Thermoeconomics.

69 H.E. Daly, Uneconomic Growth in Theory and in Fact (First Annual Feasta Lecture, Trinity College, Dublin, 1999).

70 H.T. Odum and E.C. Odum, *A Prosperous Way Down* (Boulder: University Press of Colorado, 2001). J.J. Kay and H. Regier, Uncertainty, Complexity, and Ecological Integrity: Insights from an Ecosystem Approach, in *Implementing Ecological Integrity: Restoring Regional and Global Environmental and Human Health*, ed. P. Crabbé, A. Holland, L. Ryszkowski and L. Westra (Dordrecht: Kluwer, NATO Science Series, 2000). T. Jackson, *Prosperity without Growth: Economics for a Finite Planet* (London: Earthscan, 2009).

8 Economic Transition

1 B.D. Smith, *The Emergence of Agriculture* (New York: Scientific American Library/W.H. Freeman, 1995). C. Tudge, *Neanderthals, Bandits and Farmers: How Agriculture Really Began* (London: Weidenfeld & Nicolson, 1998).

2 J. Mokyr, *The Gifts of Athena: Historical Origins of the Knowledge Economy* (Princeton, NJ: Princeton University Press, 2002).

3 D. Dollar and A. Kraay, Growth Is Good for the Poor (*Journal of Economic Growth* 2002, 7: 195–225). L. Pritchett and LH. Summers, Wealthier Is Healthier (*Journal of Human Resources* 1996, 31, 4: 842–868).

4 M. Marmot, *The Social Determinants of Health* (Oxford: Oxford University Press, 1999). J.E. Stiglitz, *Globalization and Its Discontents*, 1st edn (New York: W.W. Norton, 2002).

5 A. Smith, *An Inquiry into the Nature and Causes of the Wealth of Nations* (Charleston, SC: Forgotten Books, 2008 [1776]), p. 584.

6 M. Schabas, *The Natural Origins of Economics* (Chicago: University of Chicago Press, 2005).

7 J.M. Keynes, *The General Theory of Employment, Interest, and Money* (London: Macmillan, 1936).

8 E. Beinhocker, *The Origin of Wealth: Evolution, Complexity, and the Radical Remaking of Economics* (Boston, MA: Harvard Business Press, 2006), p. 26

9 W. Grampp, What Did Smith Mean by the Invisible Hand? (*Journal of Political Economy* 2000, 108, 3: 441–465).

10 H. Peukert, Adam Smith's Invisible Hands, in *Economic Policy in an Orderly Framework: Liber Amicorum For Gerrit Meijer*, ed. J. Backhaus *et al.* (Münster: Lit Verlag, 2003: 344–360).

11 J.E. Alvey, Adam Smith's View of History: Consistent or Paradoxical? (*History of the Human Sciences* 2003, 16, 2: 1–25).

12 D. Winch, Adam Smith's 'Enduring Particular Result': A Political and Cosmopolitan Perspective, in *Wealth and Virtue: The Shaping of Political Economy in the Scottish Enlightenment*, ed. I. Hont and M. Ignatieff (Cambridge: Cambridge University Press, 1983: 253–270).

13 T.R. Malthus, *An Essay on the Principle of Population, as It Affects the Future Improvement of Society with Remarks on the Speculations of Mr. Godwin, M. Condorcet and Other Writers* (London: printed for J. Johnson, 1798).

14 Schabas, *Natural Origins of Economics*.

15 Malthus, *Essay on the Principle of Population*, C1.

16 S. Hollander, *The Economics of Thomas Robert Malthus* (Toronto: University of Toronto Press, 1997).

17 N. Crafts and T.C. Mills, From Malthus to Solow: How Did the Malthusian Economy Really Evolve? (*Journal of Macroeconomics* 2009, 31: 68–93). N.F. Møller and P.R. Sharp, *Malthus in Cointegration Space: A New Look at Living Standards and Population in Pre-Industrial England*, Discussion Paper No. 08-16 (Copenhagen: University of Copenhagen, Department of Economics, 2008).

18 F. Hirsch, *Social Limits to Growth* (Cambridge, MA: Harvard University Press, 1976).

19 Ibid., p. 19.

20 I. Seidl and C.A. Tisdell, Carrying Capacity Reconsidered: From Malthus' Population Theory to Cultural Carrying Capacity (*Ecological Economics* 1999, 31, 3: 395–408).

21 R.L. Meek, Smith, Turgot and the 'Four Stages' Theory (*History of Political Economy* 1971, 3: 9–27).

22 A. Maddison, *The World Economy: A Millennial Perspective* (Paris: OECD, 2001).

23 N. McKendrick, J. Brewer and J.H. Plumb, *The Birth of a Consumer Society: The Commercialization of Eighteenth-Century England* (Bloomington: Indiana University Press, 1982).

24 Beinhocker, *Origin of Wealth*, p. 316.

25 P. Burkett, *Marx and Nature: A Red and Green Perspective* (London: Palgrave Macmillan, 1999). J.R.T. Hughes, *Ecology and Historical Materialism* (Cambridge: Cambridge University Press, 2000).

26 C. Tilly, *Popular Contention in Great Britain, 1758–1834* (Cambridge, MA: Harvard University Press, 1995).

27 M. Perelman, Marx, Malthus, and the Organic Composition of Capital (*History of Political Economy* 1985, 17, 3: 461–490).

28 A. Maddison, Measuring and Interpreting World Economic Performance 1500–2001 (*Review of Income and Wealth* 2005, 51, 1: 1–35).

29 G.M. Meier and D. Seers (eds), *Pioneers in Development* (Washington, DC: World Bank, 1984), p. 8.

30 W.W. Rostow, *Stages of Economic Growth: A Non-Communist Manifesto* (Cambridge: Cambridge University Press, 1971). W.W. Rostow (ed.), *The Economics of Take-Off into Sustained Growth* (London: Macmillan, 1963).

31 C.P. Kindleberger, *Marshall Plan Days* (London: Allen & Unwin, 1987), p. 27.

32 Dynamics of Socio-Economic Development: An Introduction [program] (Cambridge: Cambridge University Press, 2005).

33 Maddison, *World Economy*.

34 J. Williamson, What Washington Means by Policy Reform, in *Latin American Readjustment: How Much Has Happened?*, ed. J. Williamson (Washington, DC: Institute for International Economics, 1989: 5–20).

35 J. Williamson, *A Short History of the Washington Consensus*, Conference 'From the Washington Consensus towards a New Global Governance' [hosted by Fundación CIDOB] (Barcelona: Institute for International Economics, 2004), p. 2.

36 B. Fine and Jomo K.S. (eds), *The New Development Economics: Post Washington Consensus Neoliberal Thinking* (London: Zed Books, 2006).

37 T.R. Malthus, *Population: The First Essay* (Ann Arbor: University of Michigan Press, 1959), p. x.

38 K.E. Boulding, *The Meaning of the Twentieth Century: The Great Transition* (New York: Harper & Row, 1964); *Ecodynamics: A New Theory of Societal Evolution* (Beverly Hills, CA: Sage, 1978).

39 G. Liagouras, Socio-Economic Evolution and Darwinism in Thorstein Veblen: A Critical Appraisal (*Cambridge Journal of Economics* 2009, 33, 6: 1047–1064). G. Hodgson, Veblen and Darwinism (*International Review of Sociology* 2004, 14, 3: 343–361).

40 Liagouras, Socio-Economic Evolution and Darwinism in Thorstein Veblen.

41 K.E. Boulding, B.F. Skinner: A Dissident View (*Behavioral and Brain Sciences* 1984, 7: 483–484).

42 F.A. Ninkovich, *Modernity and Power: A History of the Domino Theory in the Twentieth Century* (Chicago: University of Chicago Press, 1994).

43 K.E. Boulding, *Ecodynamics: A New Theory of Social Evolution* (Beverly Hills, CA: Sage, 1978).

44 D.H. Meadows, D.L. Meadows, J. Randers and W.W. Behrens, *The Limits to Growth: A Report for the Club of Rome's Project on the Predicament of Mankind* (New York: Universe Books, 1972).

45 M. Singer, Eco-nomics: Are the Planet-Unfriendly Features of Capitalism Barriers to Sustainability? (*Sustainability* 2010, 2, 1: 127–144).

46 D.H. Meadows, D.L. Meadows and J. Randers, *Beyond the Limits: Global Collapse or a Sustainable Future* (London: Earthscan, 1992).

47 D. Kahneman and A. Tversky, *Choices, Values, and Frames* (New York: Cambridge University Press, 2000). C. Camerer, G. Loewenstein and M. Rabin, *Advances in Behavioral Economics* (Princeton, NJ: Princeton University Press, 2004).

48 R.H. Thaler, *Quasi Rational Economics* (New York: Russell Sage Foundation, 1994), p. 137.

49 Smith, *Inquiry into the Nature and Causes of the Wealth of Nations*, p. 84.

50 L. Tiger, *Optimism: The Biology of Hope* (New York: Simon & Schuster, 1979), p. 15.

51 C. Spash, The Development of Environmental Thinking in Economics (*Environmental Values* 1999, 8: 413–435).

52 K. Mayumi, *The Origins of Ecological Economics: The Bioeconomics of Georgescu-Roegen* (London: Routledge, 2001).

53 N. Georgescu-Roegen, Energy and Economic Myths (*Southern Economic Journal* 1975, 41, 3: 347–381).

54 P. Samuelson, *The Collected Scientific Papers* (Cambridge, MA: MIT Press, 1972), p. 450.

55 N. Georgescu-Roegen, *Utility and Value in Economic Thought* (New York: Scribner's, 1973), p. 457.

56 J. Rockstrom, W. Steffen, K. Noone, A. Persson, F.S. Chapin, E.F. Lambin *et al.*, A Safe Operating Space for Humanity (*Nature* 2009, 461, 7263: 472–475).

57 K. Arrow, B. Bolin, R. Costanza, P. Dasgupta, C. Folke, C.S. Holling *et al.*, Economic Growth, Carrying Capacity, and the Environment (*Environment and Development Economics* 1996, 1, 1: 104–110).

58 H.E. Daly, *Beyond Growth: The Economics of Sustainable Development* (Boston, MA: Beacon Press, 1996); *Steady State Economics* (Boston, MA: Island Press, 1991).

59 T. Jackson, *Prosperity without Growth: Economics for a Finite Planet* (London: Earthscan, 2009). J. Martínez-Alier, U. Pascual, F.-D. Vivien and E. Zaccai, Sustainable De-growth: Mapping the Context, Criticisms and Future Prospects of an Emergent Paradigm (*Ecological Economics* 2010, 69, 9: 1741–1747).

60 P. Lawn, Is Steady-State Capitalism Viable? A Review of the Issues and an Answer in the Affirmative (*Annals of the New York Academy of Sciences* 2011, 1219, 1: 1–25).

61 T.W. Schultz, The Economics of Being Poor (Lecture to the memory of Alfred Nobel, 8 December 1979).

62 M.S. Archer and J.Q. Tritter (eds), *Rational Choice Theory: Resisting Colonization* (London: Routledge, 2000).

63 B. Fine, Economics Imperialism and Intellectual Progress: The Present as History of Economic Thought? (*History of Economics Review* 2000, 32: 10–36).

64 G. Tett, *Fool's Gold: How Unrestrained Greed Corrupted a Dream, Shattered Global Markets and Unleashed a Catastrophe* (London: Little, Brown, 2009). S. Johnson and J. Kwak, *13 Bankers: The Wall Street Takeover and the Next Financial Meltdown* (New York: Random House, 2011).

65 F. Fukuyama and S. Colby, What Were They Thinking? The Role of Economists in the Financial Debacle (*American Interest* 2009, September/October).

66 P. Krugman, How Did Economists Get It So Wrong? (*New York Times* 2009, 2 September).

67 P. Söderbaum, A Financial Crisis on Top of the Ecological Crisis: Ending the Monopoly of Neoclassical Economics (*Real-World Economics Review* 2009, 49: 8–19).
68 T. Lawson, The Current Economic Crisis: Its Nature and the Course of Academic Economics (*Cambridge Journal of Economics* 2009, 33, 4: 759–777).
69 Johnson and Kwak, *13 Bankers.*
70 A. Kessler, Cognitive Dissonance, the Global Financial Crisis and the Discipline of Economics (*Real-World Economics Review* 2010, 54: 2–18).
71 G. Epstein and J. Carrick-Hagenbarth, *Financial Economists, Financial Interests and Dark Corners of the Meltdown: It's Time to Set Ethical Standards for the Economics Profession* (Amherst: University of Massachusetts, 2010).
72 S. Sorrell, Energy, Economic Growth and Environmental Sustainability: Five Propositions (*Sustainability* 2010, 2, 6: 1784–1809).
73 C.R. Spash and A. Ryan, *Ecological, Heterodox and Neoclassical Economics: Investigating the Differences* (Munich: Munich Personal RePEc Archive, 2010).
74 N. Stern, *The Stern Review of the Economics of Climate Change: Final Report* (London: HM Treasury, 2006).
75 E. Beinhocker, *The Origin of Wealth: Evolution, Complexity, and the Radical Remaking of Economics* (Boston, MA: Harvard Business School Press, 2006).
76 E.U. von Weizsächer, A.B. Lovins and L.H. Lovins, *Factor Four: Doubling Wealth, Halving Resource Use: The New Report to the Club of Rome* (London: Earthscan, 1996). P. Hawken, *The Ecology of Commerce: A Declaration of Sustainability*, 1st edn (New York: Harper Business, 1993). P. Hawken, A. Lovins and L.H. Lovins, *Natural Capitalism: Creating the Next Industrial Revolution* (London: Earthscan, 1999).
77 M. Ridley, *The Rational Optimist: How Prosperity Evolves* (New York: HarperCollins, 2010).
78 Spash and Ryan, *Ecological, Heterodox and Neoclassical Economics.*
79 Keynes, *General Theory of Employment, Interest, and Money.*
80 W. Kopczuk and E. Saez, Top Wealth Shares in the United States, 1916–2000: Evidence from Estate Tax Returns (*National Tax Journal* 2004, LVII, 2, part 2: 445–487).
81 R. Cockett, *Thinking the Unthinkable: Think-Tanks and the Economic Counter-Revolution, 1931–1983* (London: HarperCollins, 1994).
82 Ridley, *Rational Optimist.*
83 A. Reynolds, Has U.S. Income Inequality Really Increased? (*Policy Analysis* 2007, 586: 1–24).
84 J. Rawls, *A Theory of Justice* (Cambridge, MA: Harvard University Press, 1971). A. Sen, *The Standard of Living* (Cambridge: Cambridge University Press, 1987).
85 F. MacCarthy, *William Morris: A Life for Our Time* (London: Faber and Faber, 1994).
86 D. Card, A. Mas, E. Moretti and E. Saez, *Inequality at Work: The Effect of Peer Salaries on Job Satisfaction*, Working Paper 16396 (Washington, DC: National Bureau of Economic Research, 2010).
87 I. Roberts and P. Edwards, *The Energy Glut: The Politics of Fatness in an Overheating World* (London: Zed Press, 2010). P. Gluckman and M. Hanson, *Mismatch: Why Our World No Longer Fits Our Bodies*, 1st edn (Oxford: Oxford University Press, 2006).
88 J. Burnett, *A History of the Cost of Living* (Harmondsworth: Penguin, 1969). International Labour Office, *The Worker's Standard of Living*, Studies and Reports Series B (Economic Conditions) (Geneva: International Labour Office of the League of Nations, 1938).
89 W.O. Atwater, *Methods and Results of Investigations on the Chemistry and Economy of Food*, US Department of Agriculture Bulletin 21 (Washington, DC: Department of Agriculture, 1895); *Foods, Nutritive Value and Cost*, US Department of Agriculture Bulletin 23 (Washington, DC: US Department of Agriculture, n.d.). W.O. Atwater and C.D. Woods, *Investigations upon the Chemistry and Economy of Foods* (Storrs, CT: Agricultural Experimental Station, 1891).
90 B.S. Rowntree, *Poverty: A Study of Town Life* (London: Macmillan, 1902); *How the Labourer Lives* (London: Thomas Nelson & Sons, 1913); *Poverty and Progress* (London: Longmans, 1941). W.A. Astor and B.S. Rowntree, *British Agriculture: A Report of an*

Inquiry Organised by Viscount Astor and B. Seebohm Rowntree, abridged edn (Harmondsworth: Pelican, 1939).

91 T. Lang, D. Barling and M. Caraher, *Food Policy: Integrating Health, Environment and Society* (Oxford: Oxford University Press, 2009), ch. 8.

92 C. Lindsay, A Century of Labour Market Change: 1900 to 2000 (*Labour Market Trends* 2003 (March): 133–144).

93 J. Kuczynski, *A Short History of Labour Conditions in Great Britain 1750 to the Present Day* (London: Frederick Muller, 1942).

94 H.W. Heinrich, *Industrial Accident Prevention: A Scientific Approach* (New York: McGraw-Hill, 1931).

95 F.A. Manuele, *Heinrich Revisited: Truisms or Myths* (Washington, DC: US National Safety Council, 2002).

96 Health and Safety Executive, *Statistics 2009/10*, http://www.hse.gov.uk/statistics/overall/hssh0910.pdf (London: Health and Safety Executive, 2010).

97 J. Peto, C. Rake, C. Gilham and J. Hatch, *Occupational, Domestic and Environmental Mesothelioma Risks in Britain: A Case-Control Study* (London: Health and Safety Executive, 2008).

98 S. Wong, J. Liu, T. Culpan, M. Lee, Y. Zhao, C. Guglielmo *et al.*, iPhone Workers Say 'Meaningless' Life Sparks Suicides (*Bloomberg News* 2010, 3 June).

99 China Labor Watch, *Annual Report 2010* (New York: China Labor Watch, 2011).

100 House of Commons Transport Committee, *Ending the Scandal of Complacency: Road Safety beyond 2010* (London: Stationery Office, 2008).

101 T. Driscoll, S. Marsh, B. McNoe, J. Langley, N. Stout, A.M. Feyer *et al.*, Comparison of Fatalities from Work Related Motor Vehicle Traffic Incidents in Australia, New Zealand, and the United States (*Injury Prevention* 2005, 11, 5: 294–299).

102 H. Naci, D. Chisholm and T.D. Baker, Distribution of Road Traffic Deaths by Road User Group: A Global Comparison (*Injury Prevention* 2009, 15, 1: 55–59).

103 Y.M. Kishashu, A. Franzblau, T. Robins and G. Smith, Work-Related Road Traffic Injuries in Tanzania: Evidence for Improving Workers Compensation Law in Developing Countries (*Injury Prevention* 2010, 16 (Supplement 1): A101).

104 J. Takala, Global Estimates of Fatal Occupational Accidents (*Epidemiology* 1999, 10, 5: 640–646).

105 W.E. Deming, *The New Economics for Industry, Government, Education*, 2nd edn (Cambridge, MA: MIT Press, 2000), p. xv.

106 International Labour Organization, *Facts on Agriculture*, http://www.ilo.org/public/english/bureau/inf/download/wssd/pdf/agriculture.pdf [accessed 14 August 2011] (Rome: International Labour Organization, n.d. [*c*. 2004]); *Wage Workers in Agriculture: Conditions of Employment and Work* (Geneva: International Labour Organization, 1996).

107 Health and Safety Executive, *Statistics 2009/10*.

108 P. Hurst, P. Termine and M. Karl, *Agricultural Workers and Their Contribution to Sustainable Agriculture and Rural Development* (Rome and Geneva: Food and Agriculture Organization, International Union of Foodworkers, International Labour Organization, 2005).

109 M.G. Marmot, G. Rose, M. Shipley and P.J. Hamilton, Employment Grade and Coronary Heart Disease in British Civil Servants (*Journal of Epidemiology and Community Health* 1978, 32, 4: 244–249).

110 R. Clarke, J. Emberson, A. Fletcher, E. Breeze, M. Marmot and M.J. Shipley, Life Expectancy in Relation to Cardiovascular Risk Factors: 38 Year Follow-Up of 19,000 Men in the Whitehall Study (*BMJ* 2009, 339).

111 A.M. Heraclides, T. Chandola, D.R. Witte and E.J. Brunner, Work Stress, Obesity and the Risk of Type 2 Diabetes: Gender-Specific Bidirectional Effect in the Whitehall II Study (*Obesity (Silver Spring)* 2011, 19 May).

112 J.K. Boehm, C. Peterson, M. Kivimaki and L.D. Kubzansky, Heart Health When Life Is Satisfying: Evidence from the Whitehall II Cohort Study (*European Heart Journal* 2011, 32, 21 (November): 2672–2677).

113 S. Stringhini, A. Dugravot, M. Shipley, M. Goldberg, M. Zins, M. Kivimaki *et al.*, Health Behaviours, Socioeconomic Status, and Mortality: Further Analyses of the British Whitehall II and the French GAZEL prospective cohorts (*PLoS Medicine* 2011, 8, 2: e1000419).

114 J.R. Elliott, The Work of Cities: Underemployment and Urban Change in Late-20th-Century America (*Cityscape: A Journal of Policy Development and Research* 2004, 7, 1: 107–133).

115 B. Mandal, P. Ayyagari and W.T. Gallo, Job Loss and Depression: The Role of Subjective Expectations (*Social Science and Medicine* 2011, 72, 4: 576–583).

116 C.R. Wanberg, The Individual Experience of Unemployment (*Annual Review of Psychology* 2012, 63 (January): 369–396).

117 F. Luo, C. Florence, M. Quispe-Agnoli, L. Ouyang and A. Crosby, Impact of Business Cycles on US Suicide Rates, 1928–2007 (*American Journal of Public Health* 2011, 101, 6: 1139–1146). A. Barth, L. Sögner, T. Gnambs, M. Kundi, A. Reiner and R. Winker, Socioeconomic Factors and Suicide: An Analysis of 18 Industrialized Countries for the Years 1983 through 2007 (*Journal of Occupational and Environmental Medicine* 2011, 53, 3: 313).

118 E. Ford, C. Clark, S. McManus, J. Harris, R. Jenkins, P. Bebbington *et al.*, Common Mental Disorders, Unemployment and Welfare Benefits in England (*Public Health* 2011, 124, 12: 675–681). P. Butterworth, L.S. Leach, J. Pirkis and M. Kelaher, Poor Mental Health Influences Risk and Duration of Unemployment: A Prospective Study (*Social Psychiatry and Psychiatric Epidemiology* 2011 (online 17 June)).

119 K. Eder, *The New Politics of Class: Social Movements and Cultural Dynamics in Advanced Societies* (Beverly Hills, CA: Sage, 1993), p. 91.

120 Z. Bauman, *Work, Consumerism and the New Poor* (Buckingham: Open University Press, 1998).

121 D. Walsh, M. Taulbut and P. Hanlon, The Aftershock of Deindustrialization: Trends in Mortality in Scotland and Other Parts of Post-Industrial Europe (*European Journal of Public Health* 2010, 20, 1: 58–64).

122 T. Lang, E. Dowler and D. Hunter, *Review of the Scottish Diet Action Plan: Progress and Impacts 1996–2005*, Report 2005/2006 RE036 (Edinburgh: NHS Scotland, 2006). Scottish Office, *Scotland's Diet*, Report of the Scottish Health Service Advisory Council Working Group on the Scottish Diet, chaired by Professor Philip James (the James Report) (Edinburgh: Scottish Office, 1993).

9 Nutrition Transition

1 B. Popkin, *The World Is Fat: The Fads, Trends, Policies and Products That Are Fattening the Human Race* (New York: Avery/Penguin, 2009); An Overview on the Nutrition Transition and Its Health Implications: The Bellagio Meeting (*Public Health Nutrition* 2002, 5, 1A: 93–103).

2 B.M. Popkin and P. Gordon-Larsen, The Nutrition Transition: Worldwide Obesity Dynamics and Their Determinants (*International Journal of Obesity and Related Metabolic Disorders* 2004, 28 (Supplement 3): S2–9).

3 Ibid.

4 G. Rayner, C. Hawkes, T. Lang and W. Bello, Trade Liberalisation and the Diet Transition: A Public Health Response (*Health Promotion International* 2006, 21 (Supplement 1): 67–74).

5 B.M. Popkin and J.R. Udry, Adolescent Obesity Increases Significantly for Second and Third Generation U.S. Immigrants: The National Longitudinal Study of Adolescent Health (*Journal of Nutrition* 1998, 128: 701–706). B.M. Popkin and S.J. Nielsen, The Sweetening of the World's Diet (*Obesity Research* 2003, 11, 11: 1–8).

6 G. Rayner and T. Lang, Obesity: Using the Ecologic Public Health Approach to Overcome Policy Cacophony, in *Clinical Obesity in Adults and Children*, 3rd edn, ed.

P.G. Kopelman, I.D. Caterson and W.H. Dietz (Oxford: John Wiley & Sons, 2009: 452–470).

7 J. Jones-Smith, P. Gordon-Larsen, A. Siddiqi and B.M. Popkin, Cross-National Comparisons of Time Trends in Overweight Inequality by Socioeconomic Status among Women Using Repeated Cross-Sectional Surveys from 37 Developing Countries (1989–2007) (*American Journal of Epidemiology* 2011, 173: 667–675).

8 R.W. Fogel and D.L. Costa, A Theory of Technophysio Evolution, with Some Implications for Forecasting Population, Health Care Costs, and Pension Costs (*Demography* 1997, 34, 1: 49–66).

9 R. Floud, R.W. Fogel, B. Harris and S.C. Hong, *The Changing Body: Health, Nutrition, and Human Development in the Western World since 1700* (Cambridge: Cambridge University Press, 2011), p. 6.

10 R.W. Fogel, *Forecasting the Cost of U.S. Health Care in 2040*, NBER Working Paper No. 14361 (Washington, DC: National Bureau of Economic Research, 2008).

11 Floud *et al.*, *Changing Body*, p. 370.

12 E.C. Burnet and W.R. Ackroyd, *Nutrition and Public Health* (London: Allen & Unwin, 1935). League of Nations, *The Problem of Nutrition: Interim Report of the Mixed Committee on the Problem of Nutrition*, vol. 1, A.12.1936.II.B (Geneva: League of Nations, 1936); Final Report of the Mixed Commission of the League of Nations on the Relation of Nutrition to Agriculture, Health and Economic Policy (Geneva and London: League of Nations and Allen & Unwin, 1937).

13 A. Keys, Coronary Heart Disease in Seven Countries (*Circulation* 1970, 41 (Supplement 1): 1–211); *Seven Countries: A Multivariate Analysis of Death and Coronary Heart Disease* (Cambridge, MA: Harvard University Press, 1980).

14 M. Nestle, Paleolithic Diets: A Sceptical View (*Nutrition Bulletin* 2000, 25: 43–47). S.B. Eaton, M. Konner and M. Shostak, Stone Agers in the Fast Lane: Chronic Degenerative Diseases in Evolutionary Perspective (*American Journal of Medicine* 1988, 84, 4: 739–749).

15 H.C. Trowell and D.P. Burkitt (eds), *Western Diseases: Their Emergence and Prevention* (London: Edward Arnold, 1981), p. 428.

16 M. Crawford and S. Crawford, *What We Eat Today* (London: Neville Spearman, 1972). M. Crawford and D. Marsh, *The Driving Force: Food, Evolution and the Future* (London: Heinemann, 1989).

17 M. Gurven and H. Kaplan, Hunter-Gatherers: A Cross-Cultural Examination (*Population and Development Review* 2007, 33, 2: 321–365).

18 Ibid.

19 H.C. Trowell, Hypertension, Obesity, Diabetes Mellitus and Coronary Heart Disease, in *Western Diseases: Their Emergence and Prevention*, ed. D.P. Burkitt and H.C. Trowell (London: Edward Arnold, 1981: 3–32).

20 B. Popkin, *The World Is Fat: The Fads, Trends, Policies and Products that Are Fattening the Human Race* (New York: Avery/Penguin, 2009).

21 B. Caballero and B.M. Popkin (eds), *The Nutrition Transition: Diet-Related Diseases in the Modern World* (New York: Elsevier, 2002).

22 J. Duffy, Yellow Fever in the Continental United States during the Nineteenth Century (*Bulletin of the New York Academy of Medicine* 1968, 44, 6: 687–701).

23 J. Komlos, *On the Biological Standard of Living of Eighteenth-Century Americans: Taller, Richer, Healthier*, Discussion Papers in Economics (Munich: University of Munich, Department of Economics, 2003).

24 Fogel and Costa, Theory of Technophysio Evolution.

25 A. de Tocqueville, *Democracy in America* (London: Penguin Classics, 2003 [1835/1840]).

26 N.S. Scrimshaw, Historical Concepts of Interactions, Synergism and Antagonism between Nutrition and Infection (*Journal of Nutrition* 2003, 133, 1: 316S–321).

27 R.W. Welch and P.C. Mitchell, Food Processing: A Century of Change (*British Medical Bulletin* 2000, 56, 1: 1–17).

28 A.S. Beard and M.J. Blaser, The Ecology of Height: The Effect of Microbial Transmission on Human Height (*Perspectives in Biology and Medicine* 2002, 45, 4: 475–498).

29 E.M. Crimmins and C.E. Finch, Infection, Inflammation, Height, and Longevity (*Proceedings of the National Academy of Sciences of the United States of America* 2006, 103, 2: 498–503).

30 T.J. Hatton, *Infant Mortality and the Health of Survivors: Britain 1910–1950* (Bonn: Institute for the Study of Labor, 2010).

31 J. Komlos, *The Biological Standard of Living in Europe and America 1700–1900*, Studies in Anthropometric History (Aldershot: Variorum Press, 1995).

32 J. Komlos and M. Baur, From the Tallest to (One of) the Fattest: The Enigmatic Fate of the American Population in the 20th Century (*Economics and Human Biology* 2004, 2, 1: 57–74).

33 S.A. Carson, Health during Industrialization: Evidence from the Nineteenth-Century Pennsylvania State Prison System (*Social Science History* 2008, 32, 3: 347–372).

34 J.G. Elmore and A.R. Feinstein, Joseph Goldberger: An Unsung Hero of American Clinical Epidemiology (*Annals of Internal Medicine* 1994, 121, 5: 372–375).

35 CDC, *US Obesity Trends among US Adults 1985–2009*, http://www.cdc.gov/nccdphp/dnpa/obesity/trend/maps/index.htm (Atlanta, GA: Centers for Disease Control and Prevention, 2010).

36 Y. Wang, M.A. Beydoun, L. Liang, B. Caballero and S.K. Kumanyika, Will All Americans Become Overweight or Obese? Estimating the Progression and Cost of the US Obesity Epidemic (*Obesity (Silver Spring)* 2008, 16, 10: 2323–2330).

37 Foresight, *The Future of Food and Farming: Challenges and Choices for Global Sustainability*, Final report (London: Government Office for Science, 2011).

38 FAO, *The State of Food Insecurity in the World* (Rome: Food and Agriculture Organization, 2011).

39 A. Trichopoulou, T. Costacou, C. Bamia and D. Trichopoulos, Adherence to a Mediterranean Diet and Survival in a Greek Population (*New England Journal of Medicine* 2003, 348, 26: 2599–2608). N. Alexandratos, The Mediterranean Diet in a World Context (*Public Health Nutrition* 2006, 9, 1A: 111–117).

40 Ibid.

41 R.H. Hall, *Food for Nought: The Decline in Nutrition* (Cambridge: Polity, 1990). M. Nestle, *Food Politics* (Berkeley: University of California Press, 2002).

42 W.C. Willett, M.J. Stampfer, J.E. Manson, G.A. Colditz, F.E. Speizer, B.A. Rosner *et al.*, Intake of Trans Fatty Acids and Risk of Coronary Heart Disease among Women (*Lancet* 1993, 341, 8845: 581–585). D. Mozaffarian, M.B. Katan, A. Ascherio, M.J. Stampfer and W.C. Willett, Trans Fatty Acids and Cardiovascular Disease (*New England Journal of Medicine* 2006, 354, 15: 1601–1613).

43 A.-M. Mayer, Historical Changes in the Mineral Content of Fruit and Vegetables (*British Food Journal* 1997, 99, 6: 207–211).

44 M. Lawrence, Synthetic Folic Acid vs. Food Folates (*Public Health Nutrition* 2007, 10, 5: 533–534).

45 R.H. Hall, *Food for Nought: The Decline in Nutrition* (Hagerstown, MD: Harper & Row, 1984).

46 R.J. Hammond, *Food: The Growth of Policy* (London: HMSO/Longmans, Green & Co., 1951). L. Allen, B. de Benoist, O. Dary and R. Hurrell (eds), *Guidelines on Food Fortification with Micronutrients* (Rome: World Health Organization/Food and Agriculture Organization, 2004).

47 Ibid., p. xiv.

48 C. Hawkes, *Marketing Food to Children: Changes in the Global Regulatory Environment 2004–2006* (Geneva: World Health Organization, 2007).

49 P.D. Gluckman and M.A. Hanson, Living with the Past: Evolution, Development, and Patterns of Disease (*Science* 2004, 305, 5691: 1733–1736).

50 D. Gibbs, Rickets and the Crippled Child: An Historical Perspective (*Journal of the Royal Society of Medicine* 1994, 87: 729–732).

51 J. Snow, On the Adulteration of Bread as a Cause of Rickets (*Lancet* 1857, ii: 4–5; reprinted in *International Journal of Epidemiology* 2003, 32: 336–337).

52 R.A. Guy, The History of Cod Liver Oil as a Remedy (*American Journal of Disease of Children* 1923, 26, 2: 112–116).

53 A. Hardy, Commentary: Bread and Alum, Syphilis and Sunlight: Rickets in the Nineteenth Century (*International Journal of Epidemiology* 2003, 32, 3: 337–340).

54 G. Wolf, The Discovery of Vitamin D: The Contribution of Adolf Windaus (*Journal of Nutrition* 2004, 134, 6: 1299–1302).

55 B.P. McEvoy and P.M. Visscher, Genetics of Human Height (*Economics and Human Biology* 2009, 7, 3: 294–306).

56 D.J. Gunnell, G.D. Smith, S. Frankel, K. Nanchahal, F.E.M. Braddon, J. Pemberton *et al.*, Childhood Leg Length and Adult Mortality: Follow Up of the Carnegie (Boyd Orr) Survey of Diet and Health in Pre-War Britain (*Journal of Epidemiology and Community Health* 1998, 52, 3: 142–152).

57 J. Garcia and C. Quintana-Domeque, The Evolution of Adult Height in Europe: A Brief Note (*Economics and Human Biology* 2007, 5, 2: 340–349).

58 P. Townsend, *Poverty in the United Kingdom: A Survey of Household Resources and Standards of Living* (Hemel Hempstead: Harvester Wheatsheaf, 1993).

59 A. Sen, *The Standard of Living*, Tanner Lectures on Human Values (Cambridge: Cambridge University Press, 1985).

60 G. Federico, Heights, Calories and Welfare: A New Perspective on Italian Industrialization, 1854–1913 (*Economics and Human Biology* 2003, 1, 3: 289–308).

61 T.J. Hatton and B.E. Bray, Long Run Trends in the Heights of European Men, 19th–20th Centuries (*Economics and Human Biology* 2010, 8, 3: 405–413).

62 M. Hermanussen, J. Burmeister and V. Burkhardt, Stature and Stature Distribution in Recent West German and Historic Samples of Italian and Dutch Conscripts (*American Journal of Human Biology* 1995, 7, 4: 507–515).

63 H. de Beer, Observations on the History of Dutch Physical Stature from the Late-Middle Ages to the Present (*Economics and Human Biology* 2004, 2, 1: 45–55).

64 I. Vaartjes, M. O'Flaherty, D.E. Grobbee, M.L. Bots and S. Capewell, Coronary Heart Disease Mortality Trends in the Netherlands 1972–2007 (*Heart* 2011, 97, 7: 569–573).

65 Komlos and Baur, From the Tallest to (One of) the Fattest.

66 I. Roberts and P. Edwards, *The Energy Glut: The Politics of Fatness in an Overheating World* (London: Zed Press, 2010).

67 L. Akil and H.A. Ahmad, Effects of Socioeconomic Factors on Obesity Rates in Four Southern States and Colorado (*Ethnicity and Disease* 2011, 21, 1: 58–62).

68 Millennium Ecosystem Assessment, *Ecosystems and Human Well-Being: Synthesis* (Washington, DC: Island Press, 2005). UNDP, *Human Development Report 2006: Beyond Scarcity – Power, Poverty and the Global Water Crisis* (Washington, DC: United Nations Development Programme, 2006). UNEP, C. Nellemann, M. MacDevette, T. Manders, B. Eickhout, B. Svihus *et al.*, *The Environmental Food Crisis: The Environment's Role in Averting Future Food Crises – A UNEP Rapid Response Assessment* (Arendal, Norway: United Nations Environment Programme/GRID-Arendal, 2009). Foresight, *The Future of Food and Farming: Challenges and Choices for Global Sustainability – Final Report* (London: Government Office for Science, 2011).

69 T. Lang, D. Barling and M. Caraher, *Food Policy: Integrating Health, Environment and Society* (Oxford: Oxford University Press, 2009), ch. 4.

70 C. Monteiro, The Big Issue Is Ultra-Processing (*World Nutrition* 2010, 1, 6: 237–269).

71 WHO/FAO, *Diet, Nutrition and the Prevention of Chronic Diseases*, Report of the joint WHO/FAO expert consultation, WHO Technical Report Series No. 916 (TRS 916) (Geneva: World Health Organization/Food and Agriculture Organization, 2003).

72 WHO, *Global Strategy on Diet, Physical Activity and Health*, 57th World Health Assembly, WHA 57.17, agenda item 12.6 (Geneva: World Health Assembly, 2004).

73 UN, *UN High Level Meeting on Non Communicable Diseases*, 18 and 19 September 2011,

http://www.un.org/en/ga/president/65/issues/ncdiseases.shtml (New York: United Nations, 2011).

10 Biological and Ecological Transition

1 R. Burian, *The Epistemology of Development, Evolution, and Genetics* (Cambridge: Cambridge University Press, 2004).

2 T.G. Dobzhansky, *Genetics and the Origin of Species* (New York: Columbia University Press, 1937).

3 T.G. Dobzhansky, Nothing in Biology Makes Sense except in the Light of Evolution (*American Biology Teacher* 1973, 35: 125–129).

4 D.W. McShea, The Minor Transitions in Hierarchical Evolution and the Question of a Directional Bias (*Journal of Evolutionary Biology* 2001, 14: 502–518).

5 J. Maynard Smith and E. Szathmáry, *The Major Transitions in Evolution* (Oxford: Oxford University Press, 1997).

6 G.S. Omenn, Evolution and Public Health (*Proceedings of the National Academy of Sciences* 2009, 107 (Supplement 1): 1702–1709).

7 E.R. Choffnes, D.A. Relman and A. Mack, *Antibiotic Resistance: Implications for Global Health and Novel Intervention Strategies: Workshop Summary*, Forum on Microbial Threats, Board on Global Health (Washington, DC: Institute of Medicine (US) Forum on Microbial Threats, 2010).

8 H.F. Dowling, *Fighting Infection: Conquests of the Twentieth Century* (Cambridge, MA: Harvard University Press, 1977).

9 WHO, *Smallpox*, Fact sheets, http://www.who.int/mediacentre/factsheets/smallpox/en/ [accessed 24 June 2011] (Geneva: World Health Organization, 2001).

10 J.P. Mackenbach, The Origins of Human Disease: A Short Story on 'Where Diseases Come From' (*Journal of Epidemiology and Community Health* 2006, 60, 1: 81–86).

11 D.H. Crawford, *Deadly Companions: How Microbes Shaped Our History* (Oxford: Oxford University Press, 2009).

12 B. Spellberg, R. Guidos, D. Gilbert, J. Bradley, H.W. Boucher, W.M. Scheld *et al.*, The Epidemic of Antibiotic-Resistant Infections: A Call to Action for the Medical Community from the Infectious Diseases Society of America (*Clinical Infectious Diseases* 2008, 46, 2: 155–164).

13 P.W. Ewald, Evolution of Virulence (*Infectious Diseases Clinics of North America* 2004, 18: 1–15).

14 W.B. Cannon, *The Wisdom of the Body* (London: Kegan Paul, Trench, Trübner, 1932).

15 J.N. Thompson, Ecology: Mutualistic Webs of Species (*Science* 2006, 312, 5772: 372–373).

16 D.H. Boucher, *The Biology of Mutualism: Ecology and Evolution* (London: Croom Helm, 1985).

17 ICIPE, *Insects and Africa's Health: 40 Years of ICIPE* (Nairobi: International Centre of Insect Physiology and Ecology, 2011), p. 64.

18 R. Hofstadter, *Social Darwinism in American Thought* (New York: George Braziller, 1955).

19 C. Webster (ed.), *Biology, Medicine and Society 1840–1940* (Cambridge: Cambridge University Press, 2003), p. 2.

20 G. Mitman, *The State of Nature: Ecology, Community, and American Social Thought, 1900–1950* (Chicago: University of Chicago Press, 1992).

21 T. Veblen, *The Theory of the Leisure Class* (London: George Allen & Unwin, 1925 [1899]).

22 T.C. Leonard, Mistaking Eugenics for Social Darwinism: Why Eugenics Is Missing from the History of American Economics (*History of Political Economy* 2005, 37 (Supplement): 200–233).

23 A.H. Halsey, Sociology, Biology and Population Control (*Eugenics Review* 1967, 59, 3: 155–164).

24 R.A. Soloway, *Demography and Degeneration: Eugenics and the Declining Birthrate in Twentieth Century Britain* (Chapel Hill and London: University of North Carolina Press, 1995), p. xx.

25 Editors of the *Lancet*, Retraction: Ileal-Lymphoid-Nodular Hyperplasia, Non-Specific Colitis, and Pervasive Developmental Disorder in Children, http://press.thelancet.com/wakefieldretraction.pdf (*Lancet* 2010 (2 February)).

26 C.-E.A. Winslow, Man and the Microbe (*Popular Science Monthly* 1914: 5–20), p. 7.

27 N. Howard-Jones, Robert Koch and the Cholera Vibrio: A Centenary (*British Medical Journal* 1984, 288: 379–381).

28 A. Hardy, Cholera, Quarantine and the English Preventive System, 1815–1895 (*Medical History* 1993, 37: 250–269).

29 Choffnes, Relman and Mack, *Antibiotic Resistance*, p. 4.

30 D. Mazel, Integrons: Agents of Bacterial Evolution (*Nature* 2006, 4: 608–620).

31 L.F. McCaig and J.M. Hughes, Trends in Antimicrobial Drug Prescribing among Office-Based Physicians in the United States (*Journal of the American Medical Association* 1995, 273, 3: 214–219).

32 S. Leekha, C.L. Terrell and R.S. Edson, General Principles of Antimicrobial Therapy (*Mayo Clinic Proceedings* 2011, 86, 2: 156–167).

33 H.C. Wegener, F.M. Aarestrup, P. Gerner-Smidt and F. Bager, Transfer of Antibiotic Resistant Bacteria from Animals to Man (*Acta Veterinaria Scandinavica Supplementum* 1999, 92: 51–57).

34 WHO, *World Health Day 2011: Combat Antimicrobial Resistance* (Geneva: World Health Organization, 2011).

35 Spellberg *et al.*, Epidemic of Antibiotic-Resistant Infections.

36 J. Davies, G. Yim and D. Davies, Look Who's Talking! (*Microbiology Today* 2009 (February): 24–27).

37 Ewald, Evolution of Virulence.

38 UNAIDS, *Joint UN Programme on HIV/Aids*, http://www.unaids.org/en/ (New York: UNAIDS, 2011).

39 UNAIDS, *Countdown to Zero: Global Plan towards the Elimination of New HIV Infections among Children by 2015 and Keeping Their Mothers Alive* (New York: UN Joint Programme on HIV/AIDS, 2011).

40 Crawford, *Deadly Companions*.

41 Ibid., p. 15.

42 S. Williamson, *The Vaccination Controversy: The Rise, Reign and Fall of Compulsory Vaccination for Smallpox* (Liverpool: Liverpool University Press, 2007), p. 13.

43 E.L. Scott, Edward Jenner, FRS, and the Cuckoo (*Notes and Records of the Royal Society of London* 1974, 28, 2: 235–240).

44 Crawford, *Deadly Companions*, p. 175.

45 A.M. Stern and H. Markel, The History of Vaccines and Immunization: Familiar Patterns, New Challenges (*Health Affairs* 2005, 24, 3: 611–621).

46 D.R. Hopkins, *The Greatest Killer: Smallpox in History* (with a new introduction) (Chicago: University of Chicago Press, 1983).

47 W.G. Smillie, *Public Health, Its Promise for the Future* (New York: Macmillan, 1955).

48 Stern and Markel, History of Vaccines and Immunization.

49 Hopkins, *Greatest Killer*, p. 86.

50 N. Durbach, *Bodily Matters: The Anti-Vaccination Movement in England, 1853–1907* (Durham, NC: Duke University Press, 2005).

51 R.M. Wolfe and L.K. Sharp, Anti-Vaccinationists Past and Present (*British Medical Journal* 2002, 325, 7361: 430–432).

52 A.R. Wallace, *The Wonderful Century: Its Successes and Its Failures* (New York: Dodd, Mead & Co., 1898), p. 1.

53 M. Fichman and J.E. Keelan, Resister's Logic: The Anti-Vaccination Arguments of Alfred Russel Wallace and Their Role in the Debates over Compulsory Vaccination in England, 1870–1907 (*Studies in History and Philosophy of Biological and Biomedical Sciences* 2007, 38, 3: 585–607).

54 Centers for Disease Control and Prevention, Ten Great Public Health Achievements: United States, 1900–1999 (*Journal of the American Medical Association* 1999, 281, 16: 1481–1483).

55 S. Funk, M. Salathé and V.A.A. Jansen, Modelling the Influence of Human Behaviour on the Spread of Infectious Diseases: A Review (*Journal of the Royal Society Interface* 2010, 7, 50: 1247–1256).

56 S. Calandrillo, Vanishing Vaccinations: Why Are So Many Americans Opting Out of Vaccinating Their Children? (*University of Michigan Journal of Law Reform* 2004, 37, 1: 353–440).

57 Hopkins, *Greatest Killer*, p. 95.

58 A. Raufu, Polio Cases Rise in Nigeria as Vaccine Is Shunned for Fear of AIDS (*BMJ* 2002, 324, 7351: 1414).

59 Anon., Yes, Vaccinations Are a CIA Plot (*Economist* 2011 (20 July)).

60 J.W. Bennett, *The Ecological Transition: Cultural Anthropology and Human Adaptation* (Edison, NJ: Transaction Publishers, 2005), p. 5.

61 U. Bronfenbrenner, *The Ecology of Human Development* (Cambridge, MA: Harvard University Press, 1979), p. 26.

62 B. Dayrat, The Roots of Phylogeny: How Did Haeckel Build His Trees? (*Systematic Biology* 2003, 52, 4: 515–527).

63 T.H. Huxley, Darwin and Haeckel (*Popular Science Monthly* 1875: 592–598).

64 J. Bascompte, Disentangling the Web of Life (*Science* 2009, 325, 5939: 416–419).

65 A.G. Tansley, The Use and Abuse of Vegetational Concepts and Terms (*Ecology* 1935, 16, 3: 284–307).

66 M. Bampton, Anthropogenic Transformation, in *Encyclopedia of Environmental Science*, ed. D. Alexander, E. Fairbridge and R.W. Fairbridge (New York: Springer, 1999: 22–27).

67 G.P. Marsh, *Man and Nature; or, Physical Geography as Modified by Human Action* (New York: Charles Scribner, 1864).

68 D. Lowenthal, *George Perkins Marsh, Prophet of Conservation* (Seattle: University of Washington Press, 2000).

69 C.L. Redman, *Human Impact on Ancient Environments* (Tucson: University of Arizona Press, 1999).

70 P.M. Vitousek, H.A. Mooney, J. Lubchenco and J.M. Melillo, Human Domination of Earth's Ecosystems (*Science* 1997, 277, 5325: 494–499).

71 C. Tudge, *Neanderthals, Bandits and Farmers: How Agriculture Really Began* (London: Weidenfeld & Nicolson, 1998).

72 J. Doughty, Decreasing Variety of Plant Foods in Developing Countries (*Plant Foods for Human Nutrition*, formerly *Qualitas Plantarum*, 1979, 29, 1–2: 163–177).

73 C. Fowler and C. Mooney, *Shattering: Food, Politics, and the Loss of Genetic Diversity* (Tucson: University of Arizona Press, 1990).

74 FAO, *Dimensions of Need: An Atlas of Food and Agriculture* (Rome: Food and Agriculture Organization, 1995). UNFPA, *Footprints and Milestones: Population and Environmental Change – The State of World Population* (Geneva: United Nations Population Fund, 2001).

75 H.G. Wilkes, Plant Genetic Resources over Ten Thousand Years: From a Handful of Seeds to the Crop-Specific Mega Gene Banks, in *Seeds and Sovereignty: The Use and Control of Plant Genetic Resources*, ed. J.G. Kloppenburg (Durham, NC: Duke University Press, 1988).

76 ETC, *The World's Top 10 Seed Companies – 2006*, http://www.etcgroup.org/en/materials/publications.html?pub_id=656 [accessed 12 July 2007] (Amsterdam: ETC Group, 2007).

77 P.J. Edwards and C. Abivardi, The Value of Biodiversity: Where Ecology and Economy Blend (*Biological Conservation* 1998, 83, 3: 239–246).

78 UNESCO, *World Water Development Report 3: Water in a Changing World* (Paris: World Water Assessment Programme, UNESCO, 2009).

79 Millennium Ecosystem Assessment, *Ecosystems and Human Well-Being: Synthesis* (Washington, DC: Island Press, 2005).

80 UNESCO, *World Water Development Report 3*, p. 101.

81 J. Tibbetts, Water World 2000 (*Environmental Health Perspectives* 2000, 108, 2: A69–73).

82 M. Hvistendahl, China's Three Gorges Dam: An Environmental Catastrophe, http://www.scientificamerican.com/article.cfm?id=chinas-three-gorges-dam-disaster [accessed 2 August 2011] (*Scientific American* 2008 (25 March)).

83 J. Qiu, China Admits Problems with Three Gorges Dam, http://www.nature.com/news/2011/110525/full/news.2011.315.html (*Nature* 2011 (25 May)).

84 D. Worster, Water in the Age of Imperialism and Beyond, in *A History of Water: The World of Water*, ed. T. Tvedt and T. Oestigaard (London: I.B. Taurus, 2006: 5–37).

85 E. Goldsmith and N. Hildyard, *The Social and Environmental Effects of Large Dams* (Wadebridge: Wadebridge Ecological Centre, 1984). J. Watts, China Warns of 'Urgent Problems' Facing Three Gorges Dam: Chinese Villagers Driven Off Land Fear Food May Run Out (*Guardian* 2011 (20 May)).

86 T. Huxley, *Address to the International Fisheries Exhibition: The Fisheries Exhibition Literature* (London: W. Clowes and Sons, 1884).

87 C. Clover, *The End of the Line: How Overfishing Is Changing the World and What We Eat* (London: Ebury, 2004). Pew Oceans Commission, *America's Living Oceans: Charting a Course for Sea Change* (Washington, DC: Pew Charitable Trusts, 2003). Royal Commission on Environmental Pollution, *Turning the Tide: Addressing the Impact of Fishing on the Marine Environment*, 25th report (London: Royal Commission on Environmental Pollution, 2004). FAO, *State of World Fisheries and Aquaculture 2010* (Rome: Food and Agriculture Organization, 2010).

88 Convention on Biological Diversity, *Text of the Convention on Biological Diversity* (Rio de Janeiro: United Nations, 1992).

89 F. Pearce, *Green Warriors: The People and the Politics behind the Environmental Revolution* (London: Bodley Head, 1991).

90 Secretariat of the Convention on Biological Diversity, *Global Biodiversity Outlook 3* (Montreal: United Nations Convention on Biological Diversity, 2010).

91 I.M. Goklany, *The Improving State of the World: Why We're Living Longer, Healthier, More Comfortable Lives on a Cleaner Planet* (Washington, DC: Cato Institute, 2007).

92 F. Pearce, Climate Myths: Global Warming Is Down to the Sun, Not Humans, http://www.newscientist.com/article/dn11650-climate-myths-global-warming-is-down-to-the-sun-not-humans.html (*New Scientist* 2007 (16 May)).

93 N. Lawson, *An Appeal to Reason: A Cool Look at Global Warming* (London: Gerald Duckworth & Co., 2008).

94 WHO, *WHO Framework Convention on Tobacco Control* (Geneva: World Health Organization, 2003).

95 FAO, *Voluntary Guidelines to Support the Progressive Realization of the Right to Adequate Food in the Context of National Food Security*, Adopted by the 127th Session of the FAO Council, November 2004 (Rome: Food and Agriculture Organization, 2004).

96 M. Hulme, Reducing the Future to Climate: A Story of Climate Determinism and Reductionism (*Osiris* 2011 (Summer)).

97 E.A. Frison, J. Cherfas and T. Hodgkin, Agricultural Biodiversity Is Essential for a Sustainable Improvement in Food and Nutrition Security (*Sustainability* 2011, 3, 1: 238–253).

98 H.V. Kuhnlein, B. Erasmus and D. Spigelski (eds), *Indigenous Peoples' Food Systems: The Many Dimensions of Culture, Diversity and Environment for Nutrition and Health* (Rome: Food and Agriculture Organization/Centre for Indigenous Peoples' Nutrition and Environment, 2009).

99 H. Girardet, *Creating Sustainable Cities* (Totnes: Green Books for the Schumacher Society, 1999); *Cities People Planet: Urban Development and Climate Change*, 2nd edn (Chichester: John Wiley & Sons, 2008). J. Seymour and H. Girardet, *Blueprint for a Green Planet* (London: Dorling Kindersley, 1987). J. von Uexküll and H. Girardet, *Shaping Our Future: Creating the World Future Council*, rev. and expanded edn (Totnes: Green Books for the World Future Council Initiative, 2005).

100 C. Steel, *Hungry City: How Food Shapes Our Lives* (London: Chatto & Windus, 2008).

101 TEEB, *The Economics of Ecosystems and Biodiversity: Mainstreaming the Economics of Nature: A Synthesis of the Approach, Conclusions and Recommendations of TEEB* (Nairobi: UN Environment Programme, 2010), p. 27.

102 Ibid.

103 M. Ridley, *The Rational Optimist: How Prosperity Evolves* (New York: HarperCollins, 2010).

104 Voltaire, *Candide, or Optimism* (London: Penguin Classics, 1995 [1759]).

105 R.S. Ostfeld, Biodiversity Loss and the Rise of Zoonotic Pathogens (*Clinical Microbiology and Infection* 2009, 15, s1: 40–43).

106 J. Rockstrom, W. Steffen, K. Noone, A. Persson, F.S. Chapin, E.F. Lambin *et al.*, A Safe Operating Space for Humanity (*Nature* 2009, 461, 7263: 472–475).

11 Cultural Transition

1 G. Hastings, M. Stead, L. Macdermott, A. Forsyth, A.M. Mackintosh, M. Rayner *et al.*, *Review of Research on the Effects of Food Promotion to Children*, Final Report to the Food Standards Agency by the Centre for Social Marketing, University of Strathclyde (London: Food Standards Agency, 2004).

2 C. Lévi-Strauss, *Structural Anthropology* (Chicago: University of Chicago Press, 1983).

3 J. Prochaska and C. DiClemente, Stages and Processes of Self-Change of Smoking: Toward an Integrative Model of Change (*Journal of Consulting and Clinical Psychology* 1983, 51, 3: 390–395).

4 G. Taylor, *Building the Case for the Prevention of Chronic Disease*, http://preventdisease.com/pdf/Chronic_Disease_P.pdf (Ottawa: Health Canada, Disease Intervention Division, Centre for Chronic Disease Prevention and Control, 2002).

5 A. Bandura, Health Promotion from the Perspective of Social Cognitive Theory (*Psychology and Health* 1998, 13: 623–649).

6 National Cancer Institute, *Theory at a Glance: A Guide for Health Promotion Practice*, 2nd edn (Washington, DC: National Institutes of Health, 2005).

7 WHO, *WHO Framework Convention on Tobacco Control* (Geneva: World Health Organization, 2003).

8 BAT, *Modern Tobacco Marketing*, http://www.bat.com/group/sites/uk__3mnfen.nsf/vwPagesWebLive/DO78BDW6?opendocument&SKN=1 [accessed 29 July 2011] (London: British American Tobacco, 2011).

9 K.D. Brownell and K.E. Warner, The Perils of Ignoring History: Big Tobacco Played Dirty and Millions Died. How Similar Is Big Food? (*Milbank Quarterly* 2009, 87, 1: 259–294).

10 G. Hastings, *Social Marketing: Why Should the Devil Have All the Best Tunes?* (London: Butterworth-Heinemann, 2007).

11 J. Dewey, *The Later Works, 1925–1953*, ed. J.A. Boydston and P. Kurtz (Carbondale: Southern Illinois University Press, 1984 [1922]), p. 62.

12 W. Lippmann, *Public Opinion* (New York: Free Press, 1965 [1922]).

13 J.S. Mill, *Autobiography* (Philadelphia: Pennsylvania State University, 2004 [1873]), p. 144.

14 J.W. Bertens, *The Idea of the Postmodern: A History* (London: Routledge, 1995), p. 3.

15 A.L. Kroeber and C. Kluckhohn, *Culture: A Critical Review of Concepts and Definitions*

(Boston, MA: Harvard University, Peabody Museum of American Archaeology and Ethnography, 1952).

16 R. Williams, *Keywords: A Vocabulary of Culture and Society* (London: Fontana, 1976), p. 87.

17 R. Inglehart and C. Welzel, *Modernization, Cultural Change and Democracy* (New York: Cambridge University Press, 2005).

18 R. Inglehart, Globalization and Postmodern Values (*Washington Quarterly* 2000, 23, 1: 215–228).

19 R. Layard, *Happiness: Lessons from a New Science* (London: Allen Lane, 2005). T. Jackson, *Prosperity without Growth: Economics for a Finite Planet* (London: Earthscan, 2009).

20 P. Norris, The Globalization of Comparative Public Opinion Research, in *The Sage Handbook of Comparative Politics*, ed. T. Landman and N. Robinson (London: Sage, 2009: 522–544).

21 K. Marx, *The Communist Manifesto* (London: Penguin, 2002).

22 M. Weber, *The Protestant Ethic and the Spirit of Capitalism* (London: Unwin University Books, 1930).

23 R. Inglehart and W.E. Baker, Looking Forward Looking Back: Continuity and Change at the Turn of the Millennium (*American Sociological Review* 2000, 65, 1: 19–51).

24 S.P. Huntington, The Clash of Civilisations? (*Foreign Affairs* 1993, 72, 3: 22–28), p. 22.

25 D. Senghaas, *The Clash within Civilizations: Coming to Terms with Cultural Conflicts* (London: Routledge, 2002).

26 Inglehart and Baker, Looking Forward Looking Back.

27 R.E. Nisbett, Living Together versus Going It Alone, in *Intercultural Communication: A Reader*, ed. L.A. Samovar, R.E. Porter and E.R. McDaniel (Boston, MA: Cengage Learning, 2008: 134–144), p. 134.

28 H.J. Chang, *Bad Samaritans: The Myth of Free Trade and the Secret History of Capitalism* (London: Bloomsbury Press, 2008).

29 A. de Tocqueville, *Democracy in America* (London: Penguin Classics, 2003 [1835/1840]).

30 R.D. Putnam, Bowling Alone: America's Declining Social Capital (*Journal of Democracy* 1995, 6: 65–78).

31 R.D. Putnam, The Prosperous Community: Social Capital and Public Life (*American Prospect* 1993, 4, 13: 35–42).

32 J. Pretty, Social Capital and the Collective Management of Resources (*Science* 2003, 302, 5652: 1912–1914).

33 J. Dewey, *The School and Society* (Chicago: University of Chicago, 1915), p. 104.

34 J. Beasley-Murray, Value and Capital in Bourdieu and Marx, in *Pierre Bourdieu: Fieldwork in Culture*, ed. N. Brown and I. Szeman (Lanham, MD: Rowman & Littlefield, 2000: 100–119).

35 P. Bourdieu, The Forms of Capital, in *Handbook of Theory and Research for Sociology of Education*, ed. J. Richardson (New York: Greenwood Press, 1986: 241–258).

36 A. Sampson, *Who Runs This Place? The Anatomy of Britain in the 21st Century* (London: John Murray, 2005), p. 199.

37 G.S. Becker, *Human Capital* (Chicago: Chicago University Press, 1975).

38 Putnam, Prosperous Community.

39 R.D. Putnam, The Strange Disappearance of Civic America (*American Prospect* 1996, 24: 34–48).

40 R. Inglehart, *Modernization and Postmodernization: Cultural, Economic, and Political Change in 43 Societies* (Princeton, NJ: Princeton University Press, 1997), p. 189.

41 F. Sarracino, *Social Capital and Subjective Well-Being Trends: Evidence from 11 European Countries* (Siena: University of Siena, 2009).

42 R.D. Putnam (ed.), *Democracies in Flux: The Evolution of Social Capital in Contemporary Society* (New York: Oxford University Press, 2002), p. 12.

43 S. Bowles, Endogenous Preferences: The Cultural Consequences of Markets and Other Economic Institutions (*Journal of Economic Literature* 1998, 36, 1: 75–111).

44 S. Bowles and H. Gintis, Social Capital and Community Governance (*Economic Journal* 2002, 112: F419–F436).

45 G. Simmel, *Conflict* and *The Web of Group-Affiliations* (Glencoe, IL: Free Press, 1950).

46 E. Fehr and U. Fischbacher, Social Norms and Human Cooperation (*Trends in Cognitive Sciences* 2004, 8, 4: 185–190).

47 R. Vine, Totally Wired, www.guardianunlimited.co.uk (*Guardian* 2005 (13 January)).

48 M. Horkheimer and T. Adorno, *The Dialectic of Enlightenment* (New York: Herder and Herder, 1997 [1947]).

49 H. Marcuse, *Eros and Civilization*, 2nd edn (London: Routledge, 1987 [1955]).

50 H. Marcuse, *One-Dimensional Man: Studies in the Ideology of Advanced Industrial Society* (Boston, MA: Beacon Press, 1964).

51 J. Habermas, *The Structural Transformation of the Public Sphere: An Inquiry into a Category of Bourgeois Society* (Cambridge, MA: MIT Press, 1991), p. 36.

52 H.H. Gerth and C.W. Mills (eds), *From Max Weber: Essays in Sociology* (New York: Oxford University Press, 1946), p. 155.

53 J. Habermas, *The Philosophical Discourse of Modernity: Twelve Lectures* (Cambridge, MA: MIT Press, 1990).

54 J. Nubiola, The Reception of William James in Continental Europe (*European Journal of Pragmatism and American Philosophy* 2011, 3, 1: 73–85).

55 G.H. Mead, *On the Influence of Darwin's Origin of Species* (Chicago: Chicago University, 1909), p. 14.

56 A. Honneth, *The Struggle for Recognition: The Moral Grammar of Social Conflicts* (Cambridge, MA: MIT Press, 1996), p. 72.

57 J. Habermas, *Lifeworld and System: A Critique of Functionalist Reason* (Boston, MA: Beacon Press, 2003), p. 188.

58 J. Habermas, *The Future of Human Nature* (Oxford: Blackwell, 2003), p. 10.

59 D. Bell, *The Cultural Contradictions of Capitalism* (New York: Basic Books, 1976), p. 249.

60 F. Nietzsche, *The Will to Power*, trans. Walter Kaufmann (New York: Random House, 1967).

61 M. Foucault and C. Gordon (eds), *Power/Knowledge: Selected Interviews and Other Writings, 1972–1977* (New York: Pantheon Books, 1980).

62 J.L. Cohen and A. Arato, *Civil Society and Political Theory* (Cambridge, MA: MIT Press, 1994), p. 256.

63 L.M.E. Goodlad, *Victorian Literature and the Victorian State: Character and Governance in a Liberal Society* (Baltimore, MD: Johns Hopkins University Press, 2003), p. 4.

64 D. Lupton, Foucault and the Medicalisation Critique, in *Foucault, Health and Medicine*, ed. A. Bunton and R. Petersen (London: Routledge, 1997).

65 S. Orbach, *Fat Is a Feminist Issue* (London: Hamlyn, 1978); *Hunger Strike: The Anorectic's Struggle as a Metaphor for Our Age* (London: Faber and Faber, 1986).

66 J. Mokyr, *The Gifts of Athena: Historical Origins of the Knowledge Economy* (Princeton, NJ: Princeton University Press, 2002).

67 R. Doll and R. Peto, The Causes of Cancer: Quantitative Estimates of Avoidable Risks of Cancer in the United States Today (*Journal of the National Cancer Institute* 1981, 66, 6: 1191–1308).

68 National Cancer Institute (US), *5 a Day for Better Health Program Evaluation Report: Origins*, http://cancercontrol.cancer.gov/5ad_3_origins.html (Rockville, MD: US National Institutes of Health, 2006). WHO, *Promoting Fruit and Vegetable Consumption around the World*, Global Strategy on Diet, Physical Activity and Health (Geneva: World Health Organization, 2004).

69 Centers for Disease Control and Prevention, *5 a Day Works!* (Atlanta, GA: US Department of Health and Human Services, 2005).

70 J.L. Harris, J.L. Pomeranz, T. Lobstein and K.D. Brownell, A Crisis in the Market-place: How Food Marketing Contributes to Childhood Obesity and What Can Be Done (*Annual Review of Public Health* 2009, 30: 211–225).

71 WHO, *Marketing of Food and Non-Alcoholic Beverages to Children*, Report of a WHO Forum and Technical Meeting, Oslo, 2–5 May 2006 (Geneva: World Health Organization, 2006).

72 T. Lobstein, T. Parn and A. Aikenhead, *A Junk-Free Childhood: Responsible Standards for Marketing Foods and Beverages to Children* (London: International Association for the Study of Obesity's StanMark Project, 2011).

73 MarketingCharts, *Global Web Ad Spend to Rise 31% in 2 Yrs*, http://www.marketingcharts.com/television/global-web-ad-spend-to-rise-31-in-2-yrs-18358/ [accessed 27 July 2011] (Thetford Center, VT: Marketing Data Box, 2011).

74 R. Shaw, *Streamlining Advertising Spend to Do More with Less*, https://www.som.cranfield.ac.uk/som/som_applications/somapps/contentpreview.aspx?pageid=13273&apptype=think&article=86 (Cranfield: Cranfield University School of Management, 2009).

75 GroupM, *GroupM Forecasts 2011 Global Ad Spending to Increase 4.8%*, http://www.wpp.com/wpp/press/press/default.htm?guid={b54c1378-c0c0-42e4-b1af-4962ed87df4f} (London: GroupM (WPP), 2011).

76 D. Miller and W. Dinan, *A Century of Spin: How Public Relations Became the Cutting Edge of Corporate Power* (London: Pluto Press, 2008), p. 4.

77 R.W. McChesney and J. Nichols, *The Death and Life of American Journalism: The Media Revolution that Will Begin the World Again* (Washington, DC: Nation Books, 2010).

78 Marcuse, *One-Dimensional Man*.

79 T. Bradshaw, Facebook Strikes Diageo Advertising Deal (*Financial Times* 2011 (18 September)).

80 E.W. Said, The Clash of Ignorance (*Nation* 2001 (22 October): 1–4).

81 M. McLuhan, *Understanding Media: The Extensions of Man*, 1st edn (New York: McGraw-Hill, 1964). M. McLuhan and Q. Fiore, *The Medium Is the Massage: An Inventory of Effects* (Harmondsworth: Penguin, 1967).

82 J. Mill, *James Mill on Education*, ed. W.H.E. Burston (Cambridge: Cambridge University Press, 2010).

83 J.S. Mill, *Utilitarianism* (London: Parker, Son, and Bourn, 1863), ch. 2.

84 Goodlad, *Victorian Literature and the Victorian State*.

85 C. Barnett, *The Lost Victory: British Dreams and British Realities, 1945–50* (Basingstoke: Macmillan, 1995); *The Verdict of Peace: Britain between Her Yesterday and the Future* (Basingstoke: Macmillan, 2001).

86 Manchester Medical Collection, *Manchester and Salford Sanitary Association*, http://archiveshub.ac.uk/permeadhtml/gb133mmc3-mmc-13-p1.shtml (Manchester: Manchester City Archives, 1852).

87 N. Capaldi, The Libertarian Philosophy of John Stuart Mill (*Reason Papers* 1983, 9: 3–19).

88 R. Nozick, *Anarchy, State, and Utopia* (New York: Basic Books, 1974).

89 D. Harsanyi, *Nanny State: How Food Fascists, Teetotaling Do-Gooders, Priggish Moralists, and Other Boneheaded Bureaucrats Are Turning America into a Nation of Children* (New York: Broadway Books, 2007).

90 D. Dyzenhaus, John Stuart Mill and the Harm of Pornography, in *Mill's On Liberty: Critical Essays*, ed. G. Dworkin (Lanham, MD: Rowman & Littlefield, 1997: 31–54).

91 L.M.E. Goodlad, 'Character Worth Speaking Of': Individuality, John Stuart Mill and the Critique of Liberalism (*Victorians Institute Journal* 2008, 36: 7–45).

92 A. Grunseit, *Impact of HIV and Sexual Health Education on the Sexual Behaviour of Young People: A Review Update* (Geneva: UN Programme on HIV/AIDS, 1997).

93 B.F. Skinner, *Beyond Freedom and Dignity* (New York: Vintage Books, 1972).

94 B.F. Skinner, *Walden Two* (New York: Macmillan, 1976 [1948]).

95 A. Bandura, *Social Learning through Imitation* (Lincoln: University of Nebraska Press, 1962); *Principles of Behavior Modification* (New York: Holt, Rinehart and Winston, 1969).

96 Bandura, Health Promotion from the Perspective of Social Cognitive Theory, p. 623.

97 A.R. Andreasen and P. Kotler, *Strategic Marketing for Nonprofit Organizations*, 6th edn (Upper Saddle River, NJ: Pearson Prentice Hall, 2003).

98 A.R. Andreasen, *Social Marketing in the 21st Century* (Thousand Oaks, CA: Sage, 2006), p. 181.

99 Hastings, *Social Marketing*. G.B. Hastings, E. Devlin and L. McFadyen, Social Marketing, in *The ABC of Behavior Change: A Guide to Successful Disease Prevention and Health Promotion*, ed. J. Kerr, R. Weitkunat and M. Moretti (Edinburgh: Churchill Livingstone, 2005).

100 K.D. Brownell and K.B. Horgen, *Food Fight: The Inside Story of the Food Industry, America's Obesity Crisis, and What We Can Do about It* (Chicago: Contemporary Books, 2004).

101 N. Cavill and E.W. Maibach, VERB: Demonstrating a Viable National Option for Promoting Physical Activity among Our Children (*American Journal of Preventive Medicine* 2008, 34, 6: S173–S174). J.L. Collins and H. Wechsler, The VERB Campaign (*American Journal of Preventive Medicine* 2008, 34, 6: S171–S172).

102 CDC, *VERB*, http://www.cdc.gov/youthcampaign/ [accessed 29 July 2011] (Atlanta, GA: Centers for Disease Control and Prevention, 2006).

103 M.E. Huhman, L.D. Potter, J.C. Duke, D.R. Judkins, C.D. Heitzler and F.L. Wong, Evaluation of a National Physical Activity Intervention for Children: VERB Campaign, 2002–2004 (*American Journal of Preventive Medicine* 2007, 32, 1: 38–43).

104 K. Krisberg, Successful CDC Verb Campaign in Danger of Losing Funding: Budget Cuts Likely (*Nation's Health* 2005, 35, 8).

105 Department of Health, *Change4Life*, http://www.dh.gov.uk/en/News/Currentcampaigns/ Change4Life/index.htm (London: Department of Health, 2008).

106 Department of Health, *Change4Life One Year On* (London: Department of Health, 2010).

107 EPODE European Network, *Changing Behaviour in the Context of EPODE-Like Programmes*, http://www.epode-european-network.com/es/noticias-een/158-een-key-activities-january-2011.html [accessed 30 July 2011] (Paris: EPODE European Network, 2011).

108 M. Romon, A. Lommez, M. Tafflet, A. Basdevant, J.M. Oppert, J.L. Bresson *et al.*, Downward Trends in the Prevalence of Childhood Overweight in the Setting of 12-Year School- and Community-Based Programmes (*Public Health Nutrition* 2009, 12, 10: 1735–1742).

109 M. Romon, A. Duhamel, J. Salleron, A. Lommez, J. Meyer and J.-M. Borys, Évolution de la prevalence du surpoids et de l'obésité chez les enfants de 4 à 11 ans entre 2005 et 2010 dans les villes EPODE (*Nutrition clinique et métabolisme* 2010, 24, S1 (December)).

110 T. Alam, Quand l'expert montre la lune, le sociologue regarde le doigt. L'expertise d'un 'think tank' européen destiné à la promotion d'un PPP en santé (*Lien Social et Politiques* 2011, 66).

111 World Health Day 2010: 1000 cities – 1000 lives, http://www.creatingsharedvalue. org/post/2010/04/07/World-Health-Day-2010-1000-cities-1000-lives.aspx.

112 J.-M. Borys, Y. Le Bodo, S. De Henauw, L. Moreno, M. Romon, J. Seidell *et al.* (eds), *Preventing Childhood Obesity: EPODE European Network Recommendations* (Cachan: Lavoisier Publishing, 2011).

113 House of Lords Science and Technology Select Committee, *Behaviour Change*, Report of the House of Lords Science and Technology Select Committee, 2nd Report of Session 2010–12 (London: Stationery Office, 2011), p. 7.

114 M. Huisman, F.J. Van Lenthe, K. Giskes, C.B.M. Kamphuis, J. Brug and J.P. Mackenbach, Explaining Socio-Economic Inequalities in Daily Smoking: A Social-Ecological Approach (*European Journal of Public Health* 2011 (online 7 April)).

115 WHO, *WHO Framework Convention on Tobacco Control*.

116 C.J.L. Murray and A.D. Lopez, Alternative Projections of Mortality and Disability by Cause 1990–2020: Global Burden of Disease Study (*Lancet* 1997, 349: 1498–1504).

117 M. Favin and M. Griffiths, *Communication for Behavior Change in Nutrition Projects: A Guide for World Bank Task Managers* (Washington, DC: Human Development Network, World Bank, 1999).

118 R.D. Galloway, Health Promotion: Causes, Beliefs and Measurements (*Clinical Medicine and Research* 2003, 1, 3: 249–258).

119 A.R. Andreasen, The Marketing of Social Marketing in the Social Change Marketplace (*Journal of Public Policy and Marketing* 2002, 21, 1: 3–13).

120 D. Wikler, Who Should Be Blamed for Being Sick? (*Health Education and Behavior* 1987, 14, 1: 11–25).

121 S. Grier and C.A. Bryant, Social Marketing in Public Health (*Annual Review of Public Health* 2005, 26, 1: 319–339).

122 C. Airhihenbuwa and R. Obregon, A Critical Assessment of Theories/Models Used in Health Communication for HIV/AIDS (*Journal of Health Communication* 2000, 5 (Supplement): 5–15).

123 B. Wammes, A. Oenema and J. Brug, The Evaluation of a Mass Media Campaign Aimed at Weight Gain Prevention among Young Dutch Adults (*Obesity (Silver Spring)* 2007, 15, 11: 2780–2789).

124 L.B. Snyder, Health Communication Campaigns and Their Impact on Behavior (*Journal of Nutrition Education and Behavior* 2007, 39, 2S: S32–S40).

125 R. Thaler and C. Sunstein, *Nudge: Improving Decisions about Health, Wealth, and Happiness* (New Haven, CT: Yale University Press, 2008).

126 Ibid., p. 8.

127 House of Lords Science and Technology Select Committee, *Behaviour Change*, p. 12.

128 G. Rayner and T. Lang, Is Nudge an Effective Public Health Strategy to Tackle Obesity? No (*BMJ* 2011 (14 April): 342).

129 N. Elias, *The Civilizing Process* (Oxford: Blackwell, 1978).

130 V. Packard, *The Hidden Persuaders*, 2nd edn (Harmondsworth: Penguin, 1981 [1957]).

131 D. Halpern, C. Bates, G. Mulgan, S. Aldridge, G. Beales and A. Heathfield, *Personal Responsibility and Changing Behaviour: The State of Knowledge and Its Implications for Public Policy* (London: Cabinet Office, Prime Minister's Strategy Unit, 2004). P. Dolan, M. Hallsworth, D. Halpern, D. King and I. Vlaev, *Mindspace* (London: Cabinet Office/ Institute for Government, 2008).

132 Foresight, *Tackling Obesities: Future Choices* (London: Government Office of Science, 2007).

133 R. Thaler, *Rethinking Regulation after the Financial Crisis and Oil Spill: A Behavioral Approach*, Graduate Council Lecture, 20 October 2010, www.youtube.com/ watch?v=zLMephdISTw (Berkeley: University of California at Berkeley, 2010).

134 V. Maher, *The Anthropology of Breast-Feeding: Natural Law or Social Construct* (Oxford: Berg, 1992).

135 L. Dyson, F. McCormick and M. Renfrew, Interventions for Promoting the Initiation of Breastfeeding (*Cochrane Database of Systematic Reviews* 2005, 2).

136 Ibid.

137 IBFAN, *Breaking the Rules, Stretching the Rules 2010* (Penang: International Baby Food Action Network, 2011).

12 Democratic Transition

1 M. McFaul, A. Magen and K. Stoner-Weiss, *Evaluating International Influences on Democratic Transitions: Concept Paper* (Stanford, CA: Center on Democracy, Development and the Rule of Law, Freeman Spogli Institute for International Studies, Stanford University, 2007).

2 J. Bentham, A Comment on the Commentaries and A Fragment on Government, in

The Collected Works of Jeremy Bentham, ed. J.H. Burns and H.L.A. Hart (Oxford: Clarendon Press, 1977), p. 393.

3 D. Acemoglu, S. Johnson and J. Robinson, Disease and Development in Historical Perspective (*Journal of the European Economic Association* 2003, 1, 2–3: 397–405).

4 D. Held, *Models of Democracy*, 3rd edn (Cambridge: Polity, 2006).

5 J. Locke, *John Locke: Political Writings*, ed. David Wootton (London: Penguin Classics, 1993).

6 C.B. Macpherson, *The Political Theory of Possessive Individualism: Hobbes to Locke* (Oxford: Clarendon Press, 1962).

7 J. Locke, *Two Treatises of Government* (London: Whitmore and Fenn and C. Brown, 1821 [1690]), p. 191.

8 D.C. North and B.R. Weingast, Constitutions and Commitment: The Evolution of Institutions Governing Public Choice in Seventeenth-Century England (*Journal of Economic History* 1989, 49, 4: 803–832).

9 J.S. Mill, *Considerations on Representative Government* (London: Longmans, 1919), p. 11.

10 M. Olson, *The Logic of Collective Action: Public Goods and the Theory of Groups* (Cambridge, MA: Harvard University Press, 1971), p. 15.

11 B. Crick, *Democracy: A Very Short Introduction* (Oxford: Oxford University Press, 2002), p. 5.

12 Á. Franco, C. Álvarez-Dardet and M.T. Ruiz, Effect of Democracy on Health: Ecological Study (*British Medical Journal* 2004, 329, 7480: 1421–1423).

13 M. McKee and E. Nolte, Lessons from Health during the Transition from Communism (*BMJ* 2004, 329, 7480: 1428–1429).

14 J.P. Ruger, Democracy and Health (*QJM* 2005, 98, 4: 299–304).

15 L.E. Sieswerda and C.L. Soskolne, Franco *et al.*'s Results Need to Be Re-visited Because Their Analysis Did Not Correctly Model the Relationship between Wealth and Health (*British Medical Journal* 2005 (28 January)).

16 Freedom House, *Freedom in the World 2011: The Authoritarian Challenge to Democracy* (Washington, DC: Freedom House, 2011), p. 3.

17 Economist Intelligence Unit, *Democracy Index 2010: Democracy in Retreat* (London: The Economist, 2010).

18 Ibid.

19 H.G. Wells, *The Rights of Man: or, What Are We Fighting For?* (Harmondsworth: Penguin, 1940).

20 UN, *Universal Declaration of Human Rights*, Adopted and proclaimed by General Assembly Resolution 217 A (III), 10 December 1948 (Geneva: United Nations, 1948).

21 D. Lowe, *Idea to Reality: NED at 25* (Washington, DC: National Endowment for Democracy, 2009).

22 McFaul, Magen and Stoner-Weiss, *Evaluating International Influences on Democratic Transitions.*

23 CDC, *CDC Health Disparities and Inequalities Report: United States, 2011* (Atlanta, GA: US Department of Health and Human Services, Centers for Disease Control and Prevention, 2011: 116).

24 A. Puddington and T.O. Melia, *Today's American: How Free?* (Washington, DC: Freedom House, 2008).

25 Anon., *The Global State of Workers' Rights: Free Labor in a Hostile World* (Washington, DC: Freedom House, 2010).

26 C. Breay, *Magna Carta: Manuscripts and Myths* (London: British Library, 2002).

27 M. Weber, *The Protestant Ethic and the Spirit of Capitalism* (London: Unwin University Books, 1930). R.H. Tawney, *Religion and the Rise of Capitalism* (Harmondsworth: Penguin, 1969 [1922]).

28 C. Hill, *The World Turned Upside Down: Radical Ideas during the English Revolution* (London: Temple Smith, 1972).

29 A.L. Morton, *A People's History of England* (London: Lawrence & Wishart, 1976 [1938]).

30 North and Weingast, Constitutions and Commitment.

31 J. Garrard, *Democratisation in Britain: Elites, Civil Society and Reform since 1800* (London: Palgrave, 2002).

32 D. Acemoglu and J.A. Robinson, *Economic Origins of Dictatorship and Democracy* (New York: Cambridge University Press, 2006).

33 K. Polanyi, *The Great Transformation* (Boston, MA: Beacon Press, 1957).

34 Garrard, *Democratisation in Britain*.

35 Acemoglu and Robinson, *Economic Origins of Dictatorship and Democracy*.

36 A. Lizzeri and N. Persico, Why Did the Elites Extend the Suffrage? Democracy and the Scope of Government, with an Application to Britain's 'Age of Reform' (*Quarterly Journal of Economics* 2004, 119, 2: 707–765).

37 Ibid.

38 Ibid.

39 E.P. Thompson, *The Making of the English Working Class*, new edn (Harmondsworth: Penguin, 1968).

40 A.K. Sen, *Development as Freedom* (Oxford: Oxford University Press, 1999), p. 157.

41 J. Rawls and E. Kelly (eds), *Justice as Fairness: A Restatement* (Cambridge, MA: Harvard University Press, 2001), p. 42.

42 R. Nozick, *Anarchy, State, and Utopia* (New York: Basic Books, 1974).

43 UN, *Universal Declaration of Human Rights*.

44 L. Diamond, *The Spirit of Democracy: The Struggle to Build Free Societies throughout the World* (New York: Times Books, 2008).

45 Garrard, *Democratisation in Britain*, p. 3.

46 J.-J. Rousseau, *Of the Social Contract*, trans. Maurice Cranston (London: Penguin Classics, 1974 [1762]).

47 J. Lind, *A Treatise of the Scurvy, Containing an Inquiry into the Nature, Causes and Cure, of That Disease, together with a Critical and Chronological View of What Has Been Published on the Subject* (3 volumes) (Edinburgh: printed by Sands, Murray and Cochran for A. Kincaid and A. Donaldson, 1753).

48 P. Baldwin, *Contagion and the State in Europe 1830–1930* (Cambridge: Cambridge University Press, 1999).

49 Ibid.

50 E. Blackwell, *Why Hygienic Congresses Fail: Lessons Taught by the International Congress of 1891* (London and New York: G. Bell, 1892), p. 15.

51 S. Declich and A.O. Carter, Public Health Surveillance: Historical Origins, Methods and Evaluation (*Bulletin of the World Health Organization* 1994, 72, 2: 285–304).

52 M. Jelsma, *The Development of International Drug Control: Lessons Learned and Strategic Challenges for the Future* (Geneva: Global Commission on Drug Policies, 2011).

53 J.F. Spillane, *Cocaine: From Medical Marvel to Modern Menace in the United States, 1884–1920* (Baltimore, MD: Johns Hopkins University Press, 2000).

54 M. Kohn, Sex, Drugs and Modernity in London during and after the First World War, in *Cocaine: Global Histories*, ed. P. Gootenberg (London: Routledge, 2002: 105–116).

55 Africa Partnership Forum, *Peace and Security: Drug Trafficking, Piracy and Money Laundering – The International Dimension of Organised Crime* (Paris: OECD, 2009).

56 League of Nations, *Health Organization* (Geneva: League of Nations Information Section, 1931: 32).

57 Anon., An International Health Organization and the League of Nations (*Canadian Medical Association Journal* 1924, 14, 6: 532–533).

58 League of Nations, *Health Organization*, p. 14.

59 J.S. Huxley, *Evolution: The Modern Synthesis* (London: George Allen & Unwin, 1942).

60 J.S. Huxley, *UNESCO: Its Purpose and Its Philosophy* (London: Preparatory Commission of the United Nations Educational, Scientific and Cultural Organization, 1946).

61 A. Huxley, *The Politics of Ecology: A Question of Survival* (Santa Barbara, CA: Center for the Study of Democratic Institutions, 1963).

62 T. Kuokkanen, *International Law and the Environment: Variations on a Theme* (Alphen aan den Rijn: Kluwer Law International, 2002).

63 F.P. Bosselman and A.D. Tarlock, The Influence of Ecological Science on American Law: An Introduction in Symposium, Ecology and the Law (*Chicago-Kent College of Law Review* 1994, 69: 848–873).

64 New York City Public Health Department, *1886–1914: Immigration, the Bacteriological Revolution, and Hermann Biggs* (New York: City of New York, 2005).

65 P. Weindling, Public Health in Germany, in *The History of Public Health and the Modern State*, ed. D. Porter (Amsterdam and Atlanta, GA: Editions Rodopi, 1994: 119–131).

66 J. Cassel, Public Health in Canada, in *The History of Public Health and the Modern State*, ed. D. Porter (Amsterdam and Atlanta, GA: Editions Rodopi, 1994: 276–312).

67 L. Bryder, A New World: Two Hundred Years of Public Health in Australia and New Zealand, in *The History of Public Health and the Modern State*, ed. D. Porter (Amsterdam and Atlanta, GA: Rodopi Editions, 1994: 313–333).

68 V.A. Smith, *The Oxford History of India*, 3rd edn (Oxford: Oxford University Press, 1958). P.J. Marshall, Warren Hastings (1732–1818), in *Oxford Dictionary of National Biography*, ed. H.C.G. Matthew and B. Harrison (Oxford: Oxford University Press, 2004).

69 N. Robins, *The Corporation that Changed the World: How the East India Company Shaped the Modern Multinational* (London: Pluto, 2006).

70 S. Anderson and J. Cavanagh, *Top 200: The Rise of Corporate Global Power* (Washington, DC: Institute of Policy Studies, 2000).

71 UN Centre on Transnational Corporations, The UNCTC: A Historical Collection and Re-collection by Former UNCTC Staff, http://benchpost.com/unctc/ [accessed 11 November 2007], 2003. L. Emmerij and R. Jolly, *The UN and Transnational Corporations*, Briefing Note 17, United Nations Intellectual History Project, http://www.unhistory.org/briefing/17TNCs.pdf (New York: Ralph Bunche Institute for International Studies/CUNY Graduate Center, 2009).

72 T. Sagafi-nejad and J.H. Dunning, *The UN and Transnational Corporations: From Code of Conduct to Global Compact* (Bloomington: Indiana University Press, 2008).

73 A.L. Taylor, *Governing the Globalization of Public Health*, University of Maryland Legal Studies Paper No. 2004-23, 2004.

74 G. Nicholson, An Evil Answer to Human Ills (*British Medical Journal* 1979 (9 June): 1553–1554).

75 P. Knightley, H. Evans, E. Potter and M. Wallace, *Suffer the Children: The Story of Thalidomide* (London: André Deutsch, 1979).

76 M.H. Bernstein, *Regulating Business by Independent Commission* (Princeton, NJ: Princeton University Press, 1955).

77 E. Dal Bó, Regulatory Capture: A Review (*Oxford Review of Economic Policy* 2006, 22, 2: 203–225).

78 E.P. Millstone and T. Lang, Risking Regulatory Capture at the UK's Food Standards Agency? (*Lancet* 2008, 372, 9633: 94–95).

79 P. van Zwanenberg and E. Millstone, *BSE: Risk, Science, and Governance* (Oxford and New York: Oxford University Press, 2005). A. Watterson, Chemical Hazards and Public Confidence (*Lancet* 1993, 342, 8864: 131–132).

80 GlobalGAP, *What Is GlobalGAP?*, http://www.globalgap.org/ [accessed 15 June 2008] (Cologne: GlobalGAP, 2008).

81 GlobalGAP, *EurepGAP Becomes GlobalGAP on Sept 7 2007 at Bangkok Conference*, http://www.globalgap.org/cms/front_content.php?idcat=9&idart=182 [accessed 23 September 2007] (Cologne: GlobalGAP, 2007).

82 S.E. Finer, *The Life and Times of Sir Edwin Chadwick* (London: Taylor & Francis, 1952).

83 R. Cockett, *Thinking the Unthinkable: Think-Tanks and the Economic Counter-Revolution, 1931–1983* (London: HarperCollins, 1994).

84 M. Friedman, *Capitalism and Freedom* (Chicago: University of Chicago Press, 1962).

85 R. Dickinson and S.C. Hollander, Consumer Votes (*Journal of Business Research* 1991, 22: 335–342).

86 D. Shaw, T. Newholm and R. Dickinson, Consumption as Voting: An Exploration of Consumer Empowerment (*European Journal of Marketing* 2006, 40, 9/10: 1049–1067).

87 A.O. Hirschman, *Exit, Voice, and Loyalty: Responses to Decline in Firms, Organizations, and States* (Cambridge, MA: Harvard University Press, 1970), p. 16.

88 J.F. Kennedy, Special Message on Protecting the Consumer Interest, Statement read to Congress by President John F. Kennedy, Washington, DC, 15 March 1962.

89 Consumers International, *Consumer Rights* (London: Consumers International, 2006).

90 A.E. Black and M. Rayner, Coronary Prevention Group, *Just Read the Label: Understanding Nutrition Information in Numeric, Verbal and Graphic Formats* (London: HMSO, 1992).

91 K.D. Brownell and J.P. Koplan, Front-of-Package Nutrition Labeling: An Abuse of Trust by the Food Industry? (*New England Journal of Medicine* 2011, 364, 25: 2373–2375). F. Lawrence, *Not on the Label* (London: Penguin, 2004). J. Wiggins, Retailers Clash with Food Companies over Nutritional Labelling Scheme (*Financial Times* 2006 (11 February): 2); Food Companies Go Their Own Way on Labelling (*Financial Times* 2006 (9 February): 17).

92 C. Gribben and M. Gitsham, Food Labelling: Understanding Consumer Attitudes and Behaviour (Berkhamsted: Ashridge Business School, 2007).

93 Carbon Trust, *Carbon Trust Launches Carbon Reduction Label*, Press launch, London, 15 March 2007, http://www.carbontrust.co.uk/about/presscentre/160307_carbon_label. htm [accessed 18 March 2007] (London: Carbon Trust, 2007).

94 Mars, *Participation in the 'Platform for Good Nutrition Physical Exercise'*, http://www.mars. com/germany/en/commitments/health-and-nutrition/participation-in-the-peb.aspx (Viersen, Germany: Mars, 2011).

95 European Commission, *European Platform for Action on Diet, Physical Activity and Health*, http://ec.europa.eu/health/ph_determinants/life_style/nutrition/platform/platform_ en.htm (Brussels: European Commission, Directorate General for Health and Consumers, Public Health, 2005).

96 WHO European Region, *European Charter on Counteracting Obesity*, Istanbul, 16 November 2006 (Copenhagen: WHO European Region, 2006).

97 R.A. Dahl, *Who Governs?* (New Haven, CT: Yale University Press, 1961); *On Democracy* (New Haven, CT: Yale University Press, 1998).

98 C.W. Mills, *The Power Elite* (New York: Oxford University Press, 1956). P.A. Baran and P.M. Sweezy, *Monopoly Capital: An Essay on the American Economic and Social Order* (New York: Monthly Review Press, 1966).

99 G. Esping-Andersen, *The Three Worlds of Welfare Capitalism* (Princeton, NJ: Princeton University Press, 1990).

100 Dahl, *On Democracy*, p. 86.

101 R.G. Wilkinson and K. Pickett, *The Spirit Level: Why More Equal Societies Almost Always Do Better* (London: Allen Lane, 2009).

102 C. Muntaner, J. Lynch and G. Davey-Smith, Social Capital, Disorganized Communities, and the Third Way: Understanding the Retreat from Structural Inequalities in Epidemiology and Public Health (*International Journal of Health Services* 2001, 31, 2: 213–237).

103 M. Foucault, Governmentality, in *The Foucault Effect: Studies in Governmentality*, ed. G. Burchell, C. Gordon and P. Miller (Chicago: University of Chicago Press, 1991: 87–104).

104 M. Hillman, *How We Can Save the Planet* (London: Penguin, 2004).

13 The implications of Ecological Public Health

1 M. Wolf, The Grasshoppers and the Ants: A Modern Fable, www.FT.com (*Financial Times* 2010 (22 May)).

2 G. Eliot, *The Mill on the Floss* (Edinburgh and London: William Blackwood and Sons, 1860), book 6, ch. 44.

3 J.B.S. Haldane, *Daedalus; or, Science and the Future: A Paper Read to the Heretics, Cambridge on February 4th, 1923* (New York: E.P. Dutton & Co., 1923).

4 G.H. Brundtland, *Our Common Future*, Report of the World Commission on Environment and Development (WCED) chaired by Gro Harlem Brundtland (Oxford: Oxford University Press, 1987).

5 T. Jackson, *Prosperity without Growth: Economics for a Finite Planet* (London: Earthscan, 2009).

6 J.P. Vandenbroucke, H.M. Eelkman Rooda and H. Beukers, Who Made John Snow a Hero? (*American Journal of Epidemiology* 1991, 133, 10: 967–973).

7 WHO, *Obesity: Preventing and Managing the Global Epidemic*, Report of a WHO Consultation, WHO Technical Series 894 (Geneva: World Health Organization, 2000); *Global Strategy on Diet, Physical Activity and Health*, 57th World Health Assembly, WHA 57.17, agenda item 12.6 (Geneva: World Health Assembly, 2004).

8 R.J. Dubos, *Man Adapting* (New Haven, CT: Yale University Press, 1980 [1965]); *Mirage of Health: Utopias, Progress and Biological Change* (New York: Rutgers University Press, 1987 [1959]).

9 G. Gardner and B. Halweil, *Underfed and Overfed: The Global Epidemic of Malnutrition*, Worldwatch Paper 15 (Washington, DC: Worldwatch Institute, 2000).

10 FAO, *State of World Food Insecurity 2010* (Rome: Food and Agriculture Organization, 2010).

11 WHO, *Obesity and Overweight*, Fact Sheet 311 (Geneva: World Health Organization, 2011).

12 National Audit Office, *Tackling Obesity in England* (London: Stationery Office, 2001).

13 L. Donaldson, *Annual Report of the Chief Medical Officer for England 2002* (London: Department of Health, 2003).

14 Health Committee of the House of Commons, *Obesity*, Third Report of Session 2003–04, HC 23-1,vol. 1 (London: Stationery Office, 2004).

15 Foresight, *Tackling Obesities: Future Choices* (London: Government Office of Science, 2007).

16 Obesity 'as Bad as Climate Risk', *BBC News*, http://news.bbc.co.uk/1/hi/health/7043639.stm (London: BBC, 2007 (14 October)).

17 Department of Health, *Healthy Weight, Healthy Lives: A Cross-Government Strategy for England* (London: Department of Health, 2008).

18 Department of Health, *Healthy Lives, Healthy People: A Call to Action on Obesity in England*, http://www.dh.gov.uk/health/2011/10/call-to-action/ (London: Department of Health, 2011).

19 R. Lang, *An Economic Analysis of Obesity on Wages*, Working Paper Series 1 (Rochester, NY: Social Science Research Network, 2002). T. Lang and G. Rayner, Obesity: A Growing Issue for European Policy? (*Journal of European Social Policy* 2005, 15, 4: 301–327); Overcoming Policy Cacophony on Obesity: An Ecological Public Health Framework for Policymakers (*Obesity Reviews* 2007, 8 (Supplement): 165–181). G. Rayner and T. Lang, Obesity: Using the Ecologic Public Health Approach to Overcome Policy Cacophony, in *Clinical Obesity in Adults and Children*, 3rd edn, ed. P.G. Kopelman, I.D. Caterson and W.H. Dietz (Oxford: John Wiley & Sons, 2009: 452–470).

20 UN Habitat, *Global Report on Human Settlement 2011: Cities and Climate Change* (Nairobi: UN Habitat, 2011). E.G. Krug, L.L. Dahlberg, J.A. Mercy, A.B. Zwi and R. Lozan (eds), *World Report on Violence and Health* (Geneva: World Health Organization, 2002).

21 UNEP, C. Nellemann, M. MacDevette, T. Manders, B. Eickhout, B. Svihus *et al.*, *The Environmental Food Crisis: The Environment's Role in Averting Future Food Crises – A UNEP Rapid Response Assessment* (Arendal, Norway: United Nations Environment Programme/GRID-Arendal, 2009).

22 E. de Bakker and H. Dagevos, Reducing Meat Consumption in Today's Consumer Society: Questioning the Citizen–Consumer Gap, www.springerlink.com/content/b1347017pu125304/ (*Journal of Agricultural and Environmental Ethics* 2011 (online 24 September)).

23 D. Fennell, *Investigation into the King's Cross Underground Fire*, Report to the Department of Transport (London: Her Majesty's Stationery Office, 1988).

24 G. Rose, *The Strategy of Preventive Medicine* (Oxford: Oxford University Press, 1992).

25 P. Farmer, *Pathologies of Power: Health, Human Rights, and the New War on the Poor* (Berkeley: University of California Press, 2004).

26 T. Farley and D. Cohen, *Prescription for a Healthy Nation: A New Approach to Improving Our Lives by Fixing Our Everyday World* (Boston, MA: Beacon Press, 2005). D.A. Cohen and T.A. Farley, Eating as an Automatic Behavior (*Preventing Chronic Disease* 2008, 5, 1: 1–7).

27 W. Winkelstein, Jr, The Development of American Public Health, a Commentary: Three Documents that Made an Impact (*Journal of Public Health Policy* 2009, 30, 1: 40–48).

28 A.L. Fairchild, D. Rosner, J. Colgrove, R. Bayer and L.P. Fried, The Exodus of Public Health: What History Can Tell Us about the Future (*American Journal of Public Health* 2010, 100, 1: 54–63).

29 A.R. Wallace, *The Wonderful Century: Its Successes and Its Failures* (New York: Dodd, Mead & Co., 1898), p. iv.

30 A. Bevan, *In Place of Fear* (London: William Heinemann, 1952).

31 Ibid., pp. 167–168.

32 O. James, *Affluenza: How to Be Successful and Stay Sane* (London: Vermilion, 2007). R. Layard, *Happiness: Lessons from a New Science* (London: Allen Lane, 2005).

33 WHO, *The World Health Report 2001 – Mental Health: New Understanding, New Hope* (Geneva: World Health Organization, 2001).

34 Jackson, *Prosperity without Growth*.

35 J. Pretty, M. Griffin, M. Sellens and C. Pretty, *Green Exercise: Complementary Roles of Nature, Exercise and Diet in Physical and Emotional Well-Being and Implications for Public Health Policy*, CES Occasional Paper 2003-1 (Colchester: University of Essex Centre for Environment and Society, 2003).

36 W. Bird, *Natural Thinking: Investigating the Links between the Natural Environment, Biodiversity and Mental Health*, 1st edn (Sandy: Royal Society for the Protection of Birds, 2007); *Natural Fit* (London: Natural England, 2007).

37 R.C. Brownson, E. Baker, K.N. Gillespie and W.R. True, *Evidence-Based Public Health* (Oxford: Oxford University Press, 2011).

38 J. Green, The Role of Theory in Evidence-Based Health Promotion Practice (*Health Education Research* 2000, 15, 2: 125–129). M.P. Kelly, V. Speller and J. Meyrick, *Getting Evidence into Practice in Public Health* (London: Health Development Agency, 2004), p. 12.

39 P. Wells, *New Labour and Evidence Based Policy Making* (Sheffield: University of Sheffield Political Economy Research Centre, 2004).

40 C.S. Peirce, *Philosophical Writings of Peirce* (Mineola, NY: Dover Publications, 1955).

41 T. Huxley, The Valuation of Evidence (*The Times* 1853).

42 C.-E.A. Winslow, *The Conquest of Epidemic Disease: A Chapter in the History of Ideas* (Princeton, NJ: Princeton University Press, 1943), p. 249.

43 Kelly, Speller and Meyrick, *Getting Evidence into Practice in Public Health*.

44 M. Sweet and R. Moynihan, *Improving Population Health: The Uses of Systematic Reviews* (New York: Millbank Memorial Fund, 2007).

45 D.L. Sackett, W.M.C. Rosenberg, J.A.M. Gray, R.B. Haynes and W.S. Richardson, Evidence Based Medicine: What It Is and What It Isn't (*BMJ* 1996, 312, 7023: 71–72). R. Manser and E.H. Walters, What Is Evidence-Based Medicine and the Role of the Systematic Review: The Revolution Coming Your Way (*Monaldi Archives for Chest Disease* 2001, 56, 1: 33–38).

46 B. Djulbegovic, G.H. Guyatt and R.E. Ashcroft, Epistemologic Inquiries in Evidence-Based Medicine (*Cancer Control* 2009, 16, 2: 158–168).

47 C.M. Martin and C. Peterson, The Social Construction of Chronicity: A Key to Understanding Chronic Care Transformations (*Journal of Evaluation in Clinical Practice* 2009, 15, 3: 578–585).

48 S. Mickenautsch, Systematic Reviews, Systematic Error and the Acquisition of Clinical Knowledge (*BMC Medical Research Methodology* 2010, 10: 53).

49 A. Bhidé, The Judgment Deficit (*Harvard Business Review* 2010 (September): 44–53).

50 A.L. Malabre, *Lost Prophets: An Insider's History of the Modern Economists* (Boston, MA: Harvard Business Press, 1995), p. 220.

51 A.N. Whitehead, *An Introduction to Mathematics* (London: Williams and Northgate, 1911), p. 61.

52 Winkelstein, Development of American Public Health.

53 J.L. Mackay, Lessons from the Private Statements of the Tobacco Industry (*Bulletin of the World Health Organization* 2000, 78, 7: 902–910).

54 UNESCO, *The Precautionary Principle*, Report of the World Commission on the Ethics of Scientific Knowledge and Technology (COMEST) (Paris: UN Educational, Scientific and Cultural Organization, 2005).

55 P. Bennett and K. Calman (eds), *Risk Communication and Public Health* (Oxford: Oxford University Press, 1999).

56 R.E. Ulanowicz, S.J. Goerner, B. Lietaer and R. Gomez, Quantifying Sustainability: Resilience, Efficiency and the Return of Information Theory (*Ecological Complexity* 2009, 6, 1: 27–36).

57 G. Bateson, *Steps to an Ecology of Mind* (London: Intertext Books, 1972). S.S. Tognetti, Science in a Double-Bind: Gregory Bateson and the Origins of Post-Normal Science (*Futures* 1999, 31, 7: 689–703).

58 N. Krieger, *Epidemiology and the People's Health: Theory and Context* (New York: Oxford University Press, 2011).

59 J.M. Eyler, *Sir Arthur Newsholme and State Medicine, 1885–1935* (Cambridge: Cambridge University Press, 1997).

60 A. Newsholme, *Public Health and Insurance: American Addresses* (Baltimore, MD: Johns Hopkins University Press, 1920), p. 3.

61 B. Russell, *Icarus, or The Future of Science* (London: Spokesman Books, 1973 [1923]).

62 WHO, *Global Strategy on Diet, Physical Activity and Health*.

63 WHO, *Obesity*; *Diet, Nutrition and the Prevention of Chronic Diseases* (Geneva: World Health Organization, 1990); *World Health Report 2003: Shaping the Future* (Geneva: World Health Organization, 2003).

64 T. Lang, G. Rayner and E. Kaelin, *The Food Industry, Diet, Physical Activity and Health: A Review of Reported Commitments and Practice of 25 of the World's Largest Food Companies* (London: City University Centre for Food Policy, 2006).

65 UNEP, *Financing of UNEP*, http://www.unep.org/rms/en/Financing_of_UNEP/Environment_Fund/index.asp [accessed 19 August 2011] (Nairobi: UN Environment Fund, 2011).

66 A. Blundell-Wignall, An Overview of Hedge Funds and Structured Products: Issues in Leverage and Risk (*Financial Market Trends* 2007, 92, 1: 37–57).

67 Ibid., p. 41.

68 G. Tett, *Fool's Gold: How Unrestrained Greed Corrupted a Dream, Shattered Global Markets and Unleashed a Catastrophe* (London: Little, Brown, 2009).

69 I. Graham, *Automotive Industry: Trends and Reflections*, Global Economic Crisis: Sectoral Coverage (Geneva: International Labour Organization, 2010).

70 I. Roberts and P. Edwards, *The Energy Glut: The Politics of Fatness in an Overheating World* (London: Zed Press, 2010).

71 H.E. Sigerist, *Preface to Landmarks in the History of Hygiene* (Oxford: Oxford University Press, 1956).

72 Fairchild *et al.*, Exodus of Public Health.

73 J.J. Hanlon, An Ecologic View of Public Health (*American Journal of Public Health* 1969, 59, 1: 4–11).

74 K. Calman, The 1848 Public Health Act and Its Relevance to Improving Public Health in England Now (*British Medical Journal* 1998, 317, 7158: 596–598).

75 National Library of Medicine, *Profiles in Science: The Reports of the Surgeon General: Changing Conceptions of Public Health*, http://profiles.nlm.nih.gov/NN/Views/Exhibit/narrative/conceptn.html [accessed 12 March 2010] (Bethesda, MD: United States National Library of Medicine, 2010).

76 Faculty of Public Health, *What Is Public Health*, http://www.fph.org.uk/what_is_public_health [accessed 19 August 2011] (London: Faculty of Public Health, 2010).

77 R. Stanwell-Smith and D. Hine, Public Health Medicine in Transition (*Journal of the Royal Society of Medicine* 2001, 94, 7: 319–321).

78 G. Rayner, Multidisciplinary Public Health: Leading from the Front? (*Public Health* 2007, 121, 6: 449–454).

79 R.A.W. Rhodes, The Hollowing Out of the State (*Political Quarterly* 1994, 65, 2: 138–151). C. Skelcher, Changing Images of the State: Overloaded, Hollowed-Out, Congested (*Public Policy and Administration* 2000, 15, 3: 3–19).

80 K. Jones, *The Making of Social Policy in Britain: From the Poor Law to New Labour* (London: Continuum, 2006), p. 22.

81 Dubos, *Mirage of Health*, p. 148.

82 S.E. Finer, *The Life and Times of Sir Edwin Chadwick* (London: Taylor & Francis, 1952), p. 236.

83 W. James, *Great Men and Their Environment* (Kila, MT: Kessinger Publishing, 2005 [1880]), p. 174.

84 C.-E.A. Winslow, The Untilled Fields of Public Health (*Science* 1920, 51, 1306: 23–33).

85 D.E. Taylor, *The Environment and the People in American Cities, 1600s–1900s: Disorder, Inequality, and Social Change* (Durham, NC: Duke University Press, 2009).

86 I.L.E. Paulus, *The Search for Pure Food: A Sociology of Legislation in Britain* (Oxford: Martin Robertson, 1974).

87 P. Redfern, *The Story of the C.W.S.: The Jubilee History of the Co-operative Wholesale Society, Limited, 1863–1913* (Manchester: Co-operative Wholesale Society, 1913). J. Birchall, *Co-op: The People's Business* (Manchester: Manchester University Press, 1994).

88 G. Jones, *Social Hygiene in Twentieth Century Britain* (London: Croom Helm, 1986), p. 6.

89 DHMD, *Deutsches Hygiene-Museum Dresden*, http://www.dhmd.de/?id=211 (Dresden: Deutsches Hygiene-Museum, 2011).

90 R. Proctor, *Racial Hygiene: Medicine under the Nazis* (Cambridge, MA: Harvard University Press, 1988).

91 G. Burchell, C. Gordon and P. Miller (eds), *The Foucault Effect: Studies in Governmentality* (Chicago: University of Chicago Press, 1991).

92 M. Foucault, *Discipline and Punish: The Birth of the Prison* (New York: Vintage Books, 1995).

93 C. Taylor, *Sources of the Self: The Making of Modern Identity* (Cambridge, MA: Harvard University Press, 1989), p. 396.

94 M. Kaye, *1807–2007: Over 200 Years of Campaigning against Slavery* (London: Anti-Slavery International, 2005).

95 J. Habermas, *The Structural Transformation of the Public Sphere: An Inquiry into a Category of Bourgeois Society* (Cambridge, MA: MIT Press, 1991).

96 R.R. Colwell, Biocomplexity and a New Public Health Domain (*EcoHealth* 2004, 1, 1: 6–7).

97 E. Stokstad, Will Malthus Continue to Be Wrong? (*Science* 2005, 309, 5731: 102).

98 T.C. Okeahialam, Children with Protein-Calorie Malnutrition Evacuated to Gabon during the Nigerian Civil War (*Journal of Tropical Pediatrics* 1972, 18, 2: 169–184).

INDEX